"Americans are totally confused by what to eat because most of current dietary recommendations are rarely supported by the real facts. Randy Karp has performed an extremely valuable service, by debunking much of the mythology that surrounds our food supply. If you are truly interested in nutrition, then you should definitely read this book."

—Dr. Barry Sears, Author, *The Zone*

"If you were to read only one book on food and supplements this is it! Author Karp connects all the dots, revealing the powerful information we need to know and the misinformation you may wish you didn't."

—Bill Kurtis, TV Journalist

"Startling, shocking, and enlightening are the words that best describe this book, which challenges much of the conventional wisdom in the field of nutrition today. You will not be able to put this book down! Even with advanced degrees in Public Health and Nutrition and 30 years in the field, I learned a lot from *Misinformed About Food*. A fascinating and compelling must-read, that's well-written, despite containing technical, scientific information that really hits home. At the conclusion, Randy lays out a practical, step-by-step plan to increase your intake of the best nutrients for health and longevity."

—Dr. Roy Vartabedian, Author, *New York Times* bestseller *Nutripoints: Healthy Eating Made Simple*
www.Nutripoints.com

"Food is essential to life and health, and yet, until we're sick, we spend almost no time learning about it and debunking the myths that surround it. Randy Karp provides startling information about foods we thought we knew and the program we need to restore our health now. Randy shows us how to bulletproof our bodies, from the inside out, and stay healthy."

—**Glen Tullman**, Chief Executive Officer, Allscripts

"This book is awesome! Don't wanna put it down. It asks (and answers) so many of my questions: Soy—friend or foe? GMOs, carbs vs. proteins, supplements... Definitely one of the most helpful, insightful books I've read in ages."

—**Mary Louise English**, www.BoomerHealthTips.com

~~MIS~~INFORMED
ABOUT
FOOD

MISINFORMED ABOUT FOOD®

THE SHOCKING TRUTH

ABOUT THE FOOD WE EAT

AND THE POWER OF

SUPER-NUTRIENTS

Debunks the Myths!
Supercharge Immunity,
Reverse Signs of Aging,
Harness the Power of Purposeful Eating!

RANDY KARP

GLOBAL
SOLUTIONS
PRESS

PRESCOTT, AZ

Misinformed About Food
© 2010 Randy Karp

Global Solutions Press LLC
303 E. Gurley Street #261
Prescott, AZ 86301-3804

First Edition

Karp, Randy.
  Misinformed about food : the shocking truth about the food we eat
and the power of super-nutrients / Randy Karp. -- 1st paperback ed.
  -- Prescott, AZ : Global Solutions Press, c2010.
    p. ; cm.
    ISBN: 978-0-9819219-3-8
    "Debunks the myths, supercharge immunity, reverse signs of aging,
       harness the power of purposeful eating."
    Includes bibliographical references and index.
    1. Nutrition. 2. Functional foods. 3. Diet. 4. Dietary supplements.
  5. Self-care, Health. I. Title.
RA784 .K37 2009   2009921375
613.2--dc22   2009

Printed in the United States of America

Cover and Book Design: Patricia Bacall
Author Photo: Mark Halpern

TO THE READER

While this book was based on extensive research, neither the author nor the publisher is qualified to give medical advice or to provide any type of professional or personal service. It is sold with the understanding that the reader will consult a medical and or a health care professional before putting into practice any of the suggestions or opinions in this book. Even doing so does not insure that you will experience the same results as indicated. The importance of taking tests suggested in this book and or those suggested by a health care professional before initiating the changes detailed in this book can't be underscored.

The publisher and author disclaim all responsibility for any problems that may be associated with the application of any recommendations and suggestions, or any use of the information found herein; and further disclaim any liability for any consequence that may be incurred by putting any information found in this book to work, either indirectly or directly; or by the reader or anyone else who may learn or apply or make inferences based on the information or principles found in this book.

This book is dedicated to the memory of my father, Dr. Edward Karp, DN, the man who inspired it, and to my mother, the late Bonnie Karp, who put up with us.

CONTENTS

Chapter 1

Is soy your friend or foe? Is soy milk the miracle we're told it is? What science really says about eating fish. The world's healthiest protein foods. And the worst... Does calcium cause osteoporosis and make you arthritic? Is too much cholesterol robbing you of life? Or too little? Do eggs raise your cholesterol level or lower it? Are bodybuilders right about protein overload? Or does it cause bone loss?

Chapter 2

Can saturated fat be healthful? Are low-fat foods zapping your youth? Cooking with olive oil—or is Canola oil the best choice? Learn the one common denominator of good health. The truth about statin drugs. The truth about olives and the real scoop on olive oil. The most radioactive food in the world. Recapture your youth—the startling facts. Revitalize your skin and hair —recapture the glow.

Chapter 3

Carbohydrates—building blocks or wrecker's ball? • Can love build "love handles"? The truth about "the Weirdberries," from Gogi to Acai. The facts, science, health value and history of our foods. The truth about organics—are they *really* better than conventionally grown foods? The truth about juice machines. Can cooking cause wrinkles? How to bring our agricultural system back to its roots. • Is celery aging you?

Chapter 4

The startling truth about genetically modified foods. The danger of "drift." The death of the "Flavr-Savr" tomato. Are living things the technology of the future? Can trees clear our waterways? How do bacteria unlock the door to the future? The brave new world of biotechnology—examine ethical issues on both sides of the equation and decide for yourself. Can we really end cancer in our lifetime? Explore the exciting potential of super foods!

PREFACE

By the time you've completed reading this book you'll know more about the power of food and supplements than most of the experts. And you'll need to. At the time of this writing, Fidelity Investments estimates that the average couple will need $215,000 when they retire just to cover their health care costs. That's up 7.5 percent from the year before. And the company expects those costs to continue to rise 7 percent a year for the foreseeable future. That's if our current Medicare program remains intact. It may not. Add another $17,000–$56,000 a year for long-term health care, a cost that varies considerably by state according to the Metlife Institute in an interview with CNN Money's senior writer Jeanne Sahadi.

Today, our average life expectancy is just under 78 years of age according to the National Center for Health Statistics (2005, Final Data). While the gap in lifespan between men and women and between blacks and whites continues to narrow (approximately five years apart for each set of groups), the estimated years of life of a newborn child continue to grow longer.

But there's good news. You can avoid danger—and you'll find the tools to do so here, without the use of medicine or fad diets. If drugs and diets worked, there would be no need for new ones each year. *Misinformed About Food* is based on hard facts—not hype, news headlines, or marketing testimonials from multi-level sales organizations. It's about setting the record straight through intensive investigation using published research performed by some of the world's greatest minds in the field of health care. Not studies using three mice or five human subjects.

The steady stream of contradictory information we're bombarded with each day, often misinformation, leaves us confused. Perplexed, we buy books only to discover they have little value we can apply. Others promise miracles that don't occur. We try, we fail, and we try again. We become frustrated. Worse, we give up. When we follow a system that fails to deliver, some of us mistakenly blame ourselves.

The tremendous amount of misinformation we've all been forced to swallow, and the consequences that befall those who do so, prompted the writing of this book. Unlocking the real power of food and supplements and knowing how to harness them gives you the power to age gracefully and avert disaster. *Misinformed About Food* is about taking control of your life rather than accepting things as they are. Because the way things are isn't working. It's about you and your loved ones and a system that's failed to protect us. And about a new form of health care, where *you* care for you.

Our dependence on conventional medicine is unhealthy. It's permitted us to hand off the responsibility of health care to others. Many of us have walked away from the task of caring for the most important thing in our lives: our lives. So confident are we that the present system will *fail* us that we bet on it—paying outrageous premiums to insurance companies to insure our death, while neglecting to eat the right foods to insure our life. Though medicine plays an important role, it's often a detour, patching us up so we can overcome another hurdle that might have been easily avoided. Instead, we remain misinformed.

Oncologists, cardiologists, and other life-saving professionals work wonders when we need them to and we should be grateful for their help. But they do little to help us prevent the root of the problem. After all, it's not their job. But if it's not their job, then whose job is it? Our present approach, fixing the symptoms rather than precluding them, is like an old shoe that no longer fits. It's been an expensive approach that's cost us and our loved ones dearly. And it makes prevention the bargain of a lifetime.

Fortunately, a new brand of health care professional is emerging. It includes many of those above with an enlightened and integrated approach to their healing; as well as homeopaths, naprapaths, anti-aging physicians, acupuncturists, naturopaths, modern day internists and more. But their numbers and voice will only grow as we demand they do.

Yet sadly, most of us will take time for everything in our lives—*except* our lives. Few of us appear to be willing to commit even an hour a day for a longer one. My father keenly understood this. A pioneer in health and nutrition, he remained troubled by our lack of regard for ourselves. He felt that the average parent spent more time preventing their cars from malfunctioning than they do their children. Our current system of treatment counts on that. Rather than paying our doctor each month for keeping us well (as was done centuries ago in parts of China), we seek them out when we're broken. Then we go and get fixed. But we don't really get fixed. Few health care practitioners are paid to determine how it began—and to prevent it from beginning again.

Most of us know someone who found religion, embracing a rigid program of exercise and an unwavering commitment to diet after suffering a heart attack or stroke. Must we face death before taking our health to heart? A patient of my father's once told him that his dad smoked and drank and lived to be 93. To that Dad replied, "If he hadn't, he'd have lived to be 104!"

He made sure that my mother Bonnie read food labels to avoid purchasing products with preservatives and red dye #2. I was only five years old. Anyone who knew him knew he "walked the talk." He was proud of his involvement with Chicago's School of Naprapathy. He and his colleagues subscribed to the old adage that an ounce of prevention is worth a pound of cure. A forefather of what was to become a revolution of sorts, he died before he could see trans fats banned in New York, and before the FDA said it was okay to clone our food.

We're a culture based on doing what we want when we want to. And we want it now. But the harder we push ourselves, the more difficult it is to live thoughtfully. While my father knew that, he felt powerless to change it. But this book, the one that he inspired, can. When we truly understand the power of food, the process of eating becomes more deliberate and purposeful.

The universe hands us rocket fuel. We can spray it, process it, transport it, chop it to death, shoot it with antibiotics, overcook it, denature it, add additives and preservatives to it—or not. The choice is ours. Today, that choice is harder to make, but it's more important to do so now than at any other time in our history.

Recently, a best-selling book written by a well-known expert in the medical field was under fire. The substance of the allegations appeared credible. But the author's response was less than constructive. Instead he attacked the credentials of those that dared to challenge his work. After all, who were they to find fault in his assertions? He's a doctor! They were not. Fortunately, most doctors are bright, caring professionals, who are open-minded, and welcome debate.

So permit me to address my credentials. I'm a person, like many of you, who wanted answers. I was no longer willing to sacrifice my life out of some sort of blind respect for what I came to regard as misinformation, ambiguity, and the absence of a definitive health plan. What was needed was a solid plan based on qualified research enabling us to live truly longer and healthier lives.

We have a distinct advantage in our mission to find self-care—we have no cross to burn—and no tunnel vision based on a particular school of training. Training that today may fall short in its ability to keep us well.

We seek answers, not testimonials. Our lack of affiliation with institutions and convention permits us to approach our quest as open-minded students, unencumbered by grants and special interest groups.

We need a coherent system, capable of extending our lives based on real data from solid research, discovered in cutting edge laboratories throughout the world.

The information you need to know is about to unfold, along with a simple yet incredibly powerful program to help you get there. Walking this talk will immediately begin to reverse the signs of aging and fatigue and build an immune system beyond what you may have imagined possible.

So join me now as we unlock the real power of food.

TIPS ON READING THIS BOOK:

Get your highlighter out (you'll be glad you did). This book is loaded with information that you might find helpful to capture, based on your needs or the needs of others. The first portion lays the groundwork. You may find parts to be technical in some areas. While each chapter lays a certain amount of ground-work for those that follow it, don't hesitate to skip over such discussions if you wish. The book unfolds into a fascinating read, and a powerful program that will change your life.

The information contained herein, is based on the author's opinion, after reviewing the information he chose to include and should not be relied upon. All opinions stated in this book were based on information the author considers correct, but neither the author nor the publisher can warrant its accuracy, nor should it, again, be relied upon. The reader acknowledges their understanding that any study the author has used to support a position, may be partially or fully refuted or proven otherwise by other studies the author was not aware, did not accept, or failed to consider. Any references to products and the manner in which they are produced, grown, processed, developed or tested is not intended to refer to all items in the same category, produced by all persons or all makers, who may use other means than those the author reviewed or considered to produce, create, preserve, transport, test, or market, that product or similar products.

ACKNOWLEDGMENTS

First, my thanks goes to my wife Kelly, for her encouragement, love, and support that permitted me to complete this extensive work. An impossible task, if not for her willingness to sacrifice a more normal life. Most nights and weekends these past few years were either interrupted or abandoned to give me the time required to complete it. Kelly, thank you. I love you more than you know.

To my daughter Lauren, a very special thank you. I'm so proud of you. Your unselfish willingness to help your father in the final edit process with a second set of well-educated eyes is gratefully acknowledged. A fine journalist and reporter for a Houston newspaper, her assistance was invaluable. Working nights and weekends to avoid interference with her other important duties, my daughter's assistance was unflinchingly there when her dad needed it most, despite her already over-burdened schedule.

Sincere appreciation to my dear friend Marc Fine. Without his insight and willingness to share his true thoughts as each chapter unfolded, this book would not been possible. His painstaking effort editing this book's important bibliography is deeply appreciated.

And to my friend, Paul Dixon, whose encouragement and focus on the marketing aspects of the brand are gratefully acknowledged.

The valuable contribution of many leaders in their fields throughout the world is equally acknowledged. Special thanks to Dr. Udo Erasmus for taking time out of his busy schedule to help me better understand important technical information on the subject of fats. And to Dr. Tony O'Donnell, CNC Naturopath, for his friendship, mentoring, and valuable information that helped this first-time author gain a better understanding of the process.

A special thanks as well to Chicago's National College of Naprapathic Medicine for the support, passion, and inspiration you gave to my father, the late Edward Raymond Karp (DN). And to his wife, the late Bonnie Karp, who taught me to never quit.

And I'd like to extend a special thanks to the captain of our very small team, Patricia Bacall, who gave this rookie the time and attention normally reserved for best-selling authors. In creating the great cover graphics and layout, Patricia went beyond the call of duty.

CHAPTER 1

PROTEIN

"The human mind treats a new idea
the way the body treats a strange protein; it rejects it."
—Peter B. Medawar,
Brazilian-born British Zoologist, 1915–1987

At some point in time we become aware that the machinery we know as *us*, no longer works like it used to. Suddenly, a condition becomes acute enough for us to discover it. But whatever *it* is didn't occur overnight. Like baldness or weight gain, disease is a gradual process that unfolds over time. Infections are medicated, blockages are surgically removed, and back pain manipulated away. While each approach may provide relief, at least temporarily, the source of the problem (or how it occurred and what will prevent it from returning) is rarely the focus. To do so requires an understanding of the shocking misinformation that's gotten us there. The answers are here. Once you know the facts, you've begun the journey on the incredible road to self care. So start your engines; and prepare yourself for an eye-opening roadmap to wellness.

Humans can't exist without protein … no protein, no life. When life's requirements are the greatest, so is our corresponding need for protein. When we're distressed or diseased, protein comes to the rescue to aid us in repairing ourselves. A high fever, a deep depression, a severe infection, surgery, and other stressful events impinge on the body and result in a more rapid consumption of protein. An even greater ratio of protein to body weight is required in the early stages of our life when our children are growing and building tissue. As we grow older our tissues break down and protein is needed to properly repair and restore them. Our protein requirements are affected by the impact of ongoing change.

Optimum digestion requires enzymatic action, and all enzymes are made of protein. Hence, all life requires enzymatic action to sustain itself. The Law of Adaptive Secretion of Digestive Enzymes, developed by the physiological laboratory at Northwestern University in 1941, and confirmed by researchers throughout the world, holds that our body produces just enough of the enzymes necessary to accomplish a particular task. The more digestive enzymes we get from raw foods, the more effectively those produced by our body are in carrying out important metabolic functions, according to Dr. Edward Howell (1985, Avery Nutrition, *Enzyme Nutrition*). Howell suggests that a good deal of what we call disease can be prevented by the proper utilization and distribution of enzymes produced by our body. The more we are able to get from our food, the less our body must work to produce them. Continually forcing our organs to produce a greater amount than they normally would diminishes their ability to do so over time, and requires more effort to accomplish less. At the same time, it distracts them from focusing on other important duties. According to Howell, good health largely depends on our ability to ensure that nothing interferes with the ability of our enzymes to do their job. We can assist them by eating the right foods, or hinder them by eating the wrong ones.

Processed or pasteurized foods are stripped of nutrients and void of enzymes. They've been exposed to heat and devitalized. The lower the amount of digestive enzymes we receive from our diet, the harder the pancreas must work to produce them.

Researchers at the University of Minnesota's Department of Anatomy have shown that rats fed for 135 days on a diet of 80 percent cooked food had an increase in pancreatic weight of 20 to 30 percent. The pancreas overworked to produce enzymes, which could have been used to optimize our metabolic processes. Instead they were used to digest cooked food that was void of them. Nutritional studies by Dr. Francis Pottenger from 1932 to 1942 (1997, Keats Publishing, *Nutrition and Physical Degeneration*, Weston A. Price) suggest that the regular consumption of processed, cooked, or canned food causes the development of degenerative disease and premature death.

The pancreas is not the only organ that gets overtaxed by poor food choices devoid of enzymes and other important nutrients. The stomach compensates by producing a large amount of hydrochloric acid. In the short term, undigested or poorly digested food may create bloating, abdominal fullness or pain, heartburn, gas, and even belching, known as indigestion or dyspepsia. In the long run, using too much of the stomach's hydrochloric acid for digestion reduces the amount available to produce its own digestive enzyme, known as pepsin. The latter requires a large amount of hydrochloric acid to create a low pH so it can properly function. An absence of pepsin can lead to a number of problems ranging from digestive tract issues to allergies. A vicious cycle ensues.

In the end, poor digestion affects every organ in our body. We're all captains of our very own ship. Our organs are our foot soldiers. Each decision you make directly affects their ability to do their jobs.

While raw foods can pose problems of their own, such as possible contamination, washing them thoroughly is easy enough. Some foods also provide less vitamins and phytonutrients than their slightly cooked counterparts. Heat breaks down the cell walls in certain foods that release chemicals that are not as available in those same foods when they're eaten raw, such as the lycopene found in tomatoes. A balanced diet with a high percentage of raw foods is the first step toward the effective utilization of protein. Lightly cooking other foods as an equal or lower percentage of our total intake of carbohydrates is optimal.

Many hormones and all the antibodies that help fight disease are made of protein as are our fingernails, skin, muscles, cartilage, and even hemoglobin, the iron-carrying portion of our blood. Our blood can't clot or rid itself of impurities without it. Protein is that important. The word *protein* itself originates from the Greek words that mean "of first importance." It's second only to water as a percentage of our body, occupying about one sixth of the total weight of an average adult.

IF OUR BODIES DON'T GET THE PROTEIN THEY REQUIRE, THEY STEAL IT FROM MUSCLE TISSUE.

Protein, and what we need to do to consciously get what we need out of it, is often misunderstood. Protein molecules consist of twenty-two amino acids. A protein molecule doesn't become a protein molecule until each one of these comes together to form one. When this occurs, it's a blessed event. Twenty-one won't do; you need to have twenty-two.

Some bacteria and all plants have twenty-two; but humans don't. Our body is only capable of producing thirteen. The other nine are available, but they must come from our food, which is why they're referred to as "essential." It's *essential* we obtain them elsewhere. The thirteen that are produced by our body are known as "non-essential."

Unlike fats and carbohydrates, you *can't store* protein. You can eat it until the cows come home, but the process of loading up on protein isn't like a camel storing water. It won't ensure that a particular amino acid, needed at a given point in time, will be present at the precise moment your body requires it. So what's a body to do?

Our amino acid "pool" is in a constant state of flux, continually changing and regularly depleting itself on demand. It's made up of any or all of the potentially available thirteen non-essential amino acids our body is capable of producing, as well as what's left of the nine "essential" ones *after* our digestive system has broken them down from our food.

If our bodies don't get the protein they require, they *steal* it from muscle tissue. You can see the ravaging affects of this protein *pull* in the gaunt and hopeless faces of the hungry. Photos depicting poor children from third-world countries capture the emaciated look that so often characterizes its victims. Malnourishment is the severe consequence of a diet woefully lacking in protein, and the leading cause of death in third-world countries.

According to the United Nations Children's Fund (UNICEF), one in ten children will die of hunger before their fifth birthday. About 24,000 people will die from hunger or hunger related illnesses each day, or one death every 3.6 seconds. In a world where one out of four people (1.6 billion at the time of this writing) survives on less than $1 a day, we must find ways to educate them. They need to be able to afford a staple diet. Sadly, this condition isn't limited to unfortunate people living in under-developed countries. In the United States, 12 million children suffer from hunger. One child out of every 165 will die before the age of five. In this land of plenty, many of our children are quite literally starving to death.

While malnutrition and death are extreme examples of deficiency, they aren't the only way a poor intake of protein affects our life. Some of us experience fatigue, impaired immunity, or puffiness (known as edema), due to a lack of an adequate intake. Dry hair, cracked fingernails, and skin problems may also indicate an inadequate consumption or utilization of protein.

Although it's unlikely you suffer from such symptoms, it's quite possible that you're malnourished. Malnutrition is defined by *Webster's Dictionary* (11th edition) as "faulty nutrition due to inadequate or unbalanced intake of nutrients or their impaired assimilation or utilization."

When viewed as defined, malnutrition affects many of us. Understanding this and changing our diets as required, permits us to live longer and healthier lives. People afflicted with bulimia or anorexia nervosa are also malnourished. In a broader

...THE VAST MAJORITY OF AMERICANS ARE MALNOURISHED.

sense, an inadequate diet that hinders our ability to properly absorb our food often leads to deficiency and impairment in other important areas.

According to the 14th Annual State of the World Hunger Report (2004, Bread for the World Institute), "Hunger manifests itself in many ways other than starvation and famine. Most poor people who battle hunger deal with chronic undernourishment and vitamin or mineral deficiencies, which result in stunted growth, weakness and heightened susceptibility to illness." This point is further illustrated by Mark Hyman, MD, and Mark Liponis, MD, co-authors of the book *Ultra Prevention: The 6-Week Plan That Will Make You Healthy for Life* (2005, Atria Books). In industrialized nations where food is plentiful, eating a large volume of food doesn't ensure us of a "balanced" diet. Conversely, eating the right quality of food doesn't necessarily mean we're getting *enough* nutrients. Neither process ensures that our bodies are in the right condition to effectively metabolize, digest, and absorb our food. In summary, *the vast majority of Americans are malnourished.*

Too little protein manifests itself in other ways that may be more difficult to discern. The lack of adequate nutrition is responsible for many of what we commonly refer to as "mental illnesses." But the term "mental health" is an invention of man. While no one has ever seen, touched, smelled, or measured a "mind," an entire field has developed in an effort to study and profit from yours. While cognitive disease and behavioral disorders are very real, many can be prevented or corrected with the proper selection of healthy fats, protein, and other nutrients. The power of our food to affect this area of our life can't be underscored.

To illustrate this point, a recent study led by Dr. Pnina Green of Tel Aviv University and published in the *Journal of Lipid Research* (June, 2005) found that the primary difference in the brain between lab rats that were deliberately bred to be genetically depressed, and those that were not, was the imbalanced ratio of Omega-6 to Omega-3. The study suggests that altering this imbalance would modify or even prevent the onset of this depression. Further research is required. But sufficient data from a host of other studies demonstrates the ability of the right foods to affect desirable change.

Selecting the finest protein foods is just as important as selecting the healthiest fats. An insufficient supply of amino acids in the *pool* that are absent when our body demands them results in some degree of impaired cognition. The absence of three of these (tyrosine, phenylalanine, and tryptophan) is closely related to what we refer to as depression. Tryptophan is converted to serotonin, while tyrosine produces the neurotransmitter known as nor-epinephrine. Proper metabolism of protein directly affects our behavior.

The best way to insure that the right balance of amino acids are present when they're required is to select the highest quality foods, chew them well, and eat them often. Eating them in their raw state allows their digestive enzymes to assist us in the process of digestion. To some extent it reduces the burden placed on our glands to produce them. That enables them to conserve the energy that would otherwise be required to produce them. Energy that can now be applied to other important tasks.

On the other hand, cooked, processed and otherwise denatured food requires our body to produce more enzymes to to permit us to digest them. This requires our body to produce more energy to do so. According to research by Dr. Paul Kouchakoff, cooking food diminishes its enzymes, and forces our bodies to produce white blood cells as part of an actual immune response.

Another way to pre-digest our food is by smelling it! Some of the twenty-two enzymes produced by our body to help us digest our food are found in our saliva. Smelling food stimulates the production of pre-digestive enzymes.

So it's true. Those that savor their food, chew it well, and enjoy its aroma, will likely digest more, require less to become satisfied, and have more energy than those that don't.

Food has the power to heal and energize you, and reduce or even reverse the scourge of premature aging—a condition that often begins by making poor choices of protein foods. Conversely, the proper selection of the highest quality proteins is an important step in building the best machine we can to stand the test of time.

Beyond aging, the greatest danger for most of us is the slow, invisible disease that quietly takes its toll long before it's visible. The pace of our lives and our other priorities distract us from seeing the accident looming around the corner. This gradual creeping of disease eventually produces symptoms conspicuous enough for physicians to diagnose. To us, this means our condition has arrived. But fixing the *appearance* of disease is not the same as *determining* what caused it, and taking the appropriate action required to prevent it from returning. This slowly forming deficiency leads to internal inflammation, which creates the foundation for illness. But disease can often be prevented and reversed without surgery, HMOs, PPOs, and intervening health care.

ASK NOT WHAT YOUR PROTEIN MOLECULES CAN DO FOR YOU BUT WHAT YOU CAN DO FOR YOUR PROTEIN MOLECULES.

While the traditional American diet has more than twice the amount of protein we require daily, that doesn't mean we can properly utilize it. We eat protein, digest it, break it down, metabolize it, absorb it, and create new proteins. But again, eating protein doesn't mean we're building protein. Some protein foods have more essential amino acids than others and are therefore more complete. Failure to eat enough of these leaves us in a deficient state, creating an imbalance easily corrected by eating properly.

But there are other important considerations. We discussed how your mouth lends a helping hand to your stomach and how the stomach's ability to digest your food depends on what it's given to work with. Not just the type of food but also its condition. Like a hand-off in a relay, the ability of your food to perform, and the way it crosses the finish line, is only as good as the collective effort made by each member of the team.

Your stomach is required to produce more enzymes to attack a greater surface area, because the food you chose was only partially predigested. Now it's your small intestine's turn to emulsify the fats it received from the bile acids produced in your liver. If your liver was unable to produce enough of these, and your pancreas didn't produce a sufficient amount of the right enzymes required to break them down, the protein that began the journey won't achieve its performance potential by the time it crosses the finish line. It's a group effort; a tag team of organs properly handing off to each other.

Ask not what your protein molecules can do for you, but what you can do for your protein molecules.

While opinions vary on the average amount of protein required, a good rule of thumb for a healthy adult is 0.8 grams of protein for each kilogram of body weight.[1] A person weighing 150 pounds requires around 55 grams of protein each day. A 175-pound adult requires approximately 64 grams of protein a day (175 lbs. ÷ 2.2 lbs. × 0.8 grams).

It appears the 55 grams required daily by the average adult is just that ... enough for the average adult. More protein is required as body mass increases. Body builders will need to increase the amount of protein they require for each pound they gain. But the amount required to do so is moderate. The rest of us needn't do so. The key is to effectively utilize this material. Doing so requires that the highest quality protein be available. The capacity to properly utilize it depends on the individual's health, and their ability to digest, metabolize, and absorb it.

To put 55 grams of protein in perspective, First Databank (1996, Protein Content of Common Foods) publishes a food chart that lists the amount of protein in many foods, based on a 3-ounce serving size (roughly the size of a standard deck of playing cards). A 3-ounce serving of sirloin steak, for example, contains 26 grams. Unfortunately, the average size we're served in most restaurants is 9 ounces, or 78 grams; more than the stomach can hold at any given time. It's also more protein than we need in an entire day. The remainder sits in your intestines and putrefies.

FOR THOSE WHO OVERLOAD ON PROTEIN, IT'S IMPORTANT TO UNDERSTAND THAT THE BODY TURNS EXCESS AMINO ACIDS INTO FAT AND SUGAR.

Sharing an entrée of animal protein is a sensible approach to good eating. In this example, that shared 9 ounce portion of steak found in most restaurants would provide 39 grams of protein, leaving a balance of 16 grams for the remainder of the day. That would allow you to eat a couple of eggs for breakfast (12 grams), plenty of vegetables, and approximately one ounce of nuts (5 grams). A 3-ounce portion of turkey breast, chicken, and venison contribute an identical amount of protein as steak. But there's no need to share as much seafood—a 3-ounce serving of salmon has only 18 grams of protein (the same portion of crab has 13 grams and scallops have 14 grams). Make sure to hang onto your ham—a 3-ounce portion has a measly 2 grams of protein. Nuts average between 4 to 7 grams for just 1 ounce and are a terrific choice as you'll see shortly.[2]

For those who overload on protein, it's important to understand that the body turns excess amino acids into fat and sugar. As you've learned, amino acids don't hang around; if they could, we wouldn't need to continually eat protein to get more of them. Our kidneys break them down into organic molecules that acidify your bloodstream. Because our bloodstream maintains a balanced pH, it's the kidney's job to neutralize the acidity that results from this process. When the kidney is on a mission, there's no reasoning with it. It needs calcium to neutralize all this acid in the urine so it gets it where it can. It *steals* it from our skeleton. Bone loss is the natural by-product of the over-consumption of highly acidic *animal* protein.

The average adult is not fully absorbing the protein they eat and not eating often enough to have the right supply of amino acids on hand to build muscle. Most body builders process the amount of protein they require more efficiently. But again, *only* the amount they require. The remainder is converted to fat.

According to Dr. Carmen Castanada Sceppa, MD PhD (2007, *International Journal of Medical Science 2.1*: 19–27) of the Jean Mayer USDA/Human Nutrition Research Center on Aging at Tufts School of Medicine, not all exercise is created equal. "In resistance training, you are building up muscle and protein is used more efficiently." In other words, the standard amounts of protein we require are more than most of us utilize. Resistance training helps maximize the potential value of protein more effectively.

In summary, the need for additional protein, beyond that required by the previous formula, is of questionable value. Since it's not stored, the remainder (which is not fully utilized) is converted by your body to fat and sugar. But is there really any danger from eating too much protein? Few issues in this book are as complex and eagerly debated. Many theories claim that excess protein leaches calcium from your bones and reduces skeletal density. But tell that to the Masai warriors, a handsome people with lean and unblemished skeletal structure. How do we reconcile this? We're told that too much protein creates a corresponding loss of calcium that's excreted through the urine. In fact, some experts are very clear and specific about this: "The body loses approximately 1.75 milligrams of calcium in the urine for every 1 gram increase in animal protein," according to Connie Weaver, PhD, head of foods and nutrition at Purdue University. (*American Journal of Clinical Nutrition 61* (4): (1995), "Dietary protein increases production of acid in the blood which can be neutralized by calcium mobilized from the skeleton.")

Researchers discovered that women who ate more than 95 grams of protein a day were 20 percent more likely to break a wrist over a twelve-year period

THE BODY LOSES APPROXIMATELY 1.75 MILLIGRAMS OF CALCIUM IN THE URINE FOR EVERY 1 GRAM INCREASE IN ANIMAL PROTEIN.

of time than those who ate an average amount of daily protein (less than 68 grams a day). Dr. David A. Bushinsky, professor of pharmacology and physiology from Rochester University (*Journal of Physiology*, November 1999), found that protein generates more acid than other nutrients in the bloodstream. As Bushinsky explains, when this occurs, calcium and other minerals are taken from bone to allow the blood to return to its normal pH level. He notes that bone loss can occur within minutes of consuming a protein-rich meal. If you're a body builder, this might cause concern. According to these experts, the massive structure you've worked so hard to achieve is crumbling. So, does protein leach calcium? Or does it not? And if so, why doesn't it appear to affect the Masai?

The facts are clear.

Different proteins have different consequences when they're synthesized. Some are highly acidic, while others are alkaline. When acidic proteins are metabolized, they're known as *acidic ash*. Such foods contain large concentrations of sulphur, chloride, or phosphorous, which are used by your body to produce acids.

Ash has the potential to create chronic acidic stress, inducing the kidneys to excrete their own acid as well as ammonium and titratable acid, according to researchers Uriel S. Barzel and Linda K. Massey and colleagues (*Journal of Nutrition*, June 1998).

BONE LOSS CAN OCCUR WITHIN MINUTES OF CONSUMING A PROTEIN RICH MEAL.

In their landmark study, the researchers state that "alkali buffers, whether chemical salts or dietary fruits and vegetables high in potassium, reverse acid-induced obligatory urinary calcium loss. We conclude that excessive dietary protein from foods with high potential renal acid load adversely affects bone, unless buffered by the consumption of alkali-rich foods or supplements."

So body builders and others on protein-overload will only leach calcium from bone to buffer cells if their overload comes from an excess intake of high acidic ash foods. This means it's best to avoid too much protein from eggs, meat, fish, and other sources, including whole wheat bread, lentils, cranberries, crackers, maize, plums, prunes, rice, peanuts, pasta, cheese and walnuts. Note that *the single most acidic food of all common foods is Parmesan cheese.*

More importantly, the danger from high-acidic ash foods can be *countered* (assuming no other toxins are present) by eating them in conjunction with high-alkaline foods. These include most fruits and vegetables (except asparagus, barley, and most beans). This also includes foods prepared with baking powder or bicarbonate of soda. Strong evidence exists that the effects of high-protein diets are mediated through changes in acid-based balance.

This also unravels the Masai paradox. Despite a diet high in acidic ash protein, they indulge in a special after dinner drink; a soup they produce by boiling the skin of a shrub or tree known as acacia (also known as wattle or thorn tree). Acacia gum arabic is a leading alkaline ingredient found in many antacid preparations. In effect, the Masai are *buffering* the high acidic ash of their protein.

Ngela Cheung, MD, PhD, director of the osteoporosis program and associate director of the women's health program at the University Health Network agrees: "An acid environment in the body contributes to inflammation. It exacerbates conditions such as rheumatoid arthritis. Steak, pork, and chicken have acidic ash. An acid environment is also associated with kidney stones. The acid leaches minerals from the bones, and then the blood levels of the minerals supersaturate and coalesce in the kidneys."

Fortunately, this acidic condition can be mediated by certain supplements as well. Researchers Thomas Remer and Freiderich Manz ("High Meat Diet, Acid-Base Status and Calcium Retention," *Journal of Nutrition*, October 2003) discuss the effects of highly acidic ash foods. The scientists note that "this is the case if the acidifying potential of elevated protein is not counterbalanced by an adequate intake of base-forming minerals like potassium or magnesium."

While intake of high alkaline foods helps offset the ravages of metabolic acidosis, researchers Rylander et al. (*Journal of Nutrition*, September 2006) have shown a corresponding *loss* of magnesium and potassium, too. The Masai get both nutrients from drinking the blood of their cattle (fortunately, there are easier ways to do so!). Many potassium-rich foods are generally magnesium-rich. These include avocados, brussels sprouts, kiwi, bananas, tomatoes, cantaloupe, lima beans, plain yogurt, and more. And supplements containing both are available.

But aside from skeletal density, does too much protein compromise the ability of our body to carry out other important functions? High-intake users are often warned that protein overload can impair their liver and kidneys. A study conducted by Brigham and Women's Hospital (BWH) showed that kidney decline in women with *previously* impaired kidney function was worsened. No decline in kidney function resulted from the consumption of excessive amounts of non-animal protein. "The potential impact of protein consumption on renal function has important public health implications given the prevalence of high-protein diets and use of protein supplements," said Eric C. Knight, BWH researcher. "We found that among women with mildly reduced kidney function—about 25 percent of individuals in our study—a higher-protein diet may lead to accelerated decline in kidney function compared with a lower-protein diet."

... MANY FORMS OF KIDNEY AND LIVER DISEASE ARE EXACERBATED BY INCREASED PRESSURE TO THE ORGAN, AND THAT PRESSURE IN THE BLOOD COMES FROM ANIMAL PROTEIN.

A large body of evidence suggests that many forms of kidney and liver disease are further impaired by increased pressure to the organ, and that pressure in the blood comes from animal protein. Most diets designed to slow the progression of kidney disease call for an extremely low consumption of protein.

Dr. Barry Brenner, MD Emeritus Chief of Nephrology at Brigham and Women's Hospital's Department of Medicine discussed this connection in an interview: "Dr. Henry Christian, PBBH's first Chief of Medicine, and his colleague Dr. James White, had the answer back in 1913 when they prescribed low-protein diets, but they didn't know why they worked. In their diet clinic for those with kidney disease, they saw that lowering dietary protein enabled those with illness to live longer. Eventually they discovered why: "Protein increases glomerular pressure, and the glomerulus normally works best under low pressure."

We're told that diets high in animal protein exacerbate kidney and liver disease. Sulphur-rich animal proteins have also been linked to cancer and other ailments, while plant proteins have not. But are acidic ash animal proteins the real culprit? Or, is disease due to the imbalance caused by a corresponding deficiency in countering alkaline based plant proteins?[3] I believe it's the latter. It's not that the glass is half full with animal protein but half empty, with an insufficient amount of offsetting potassium-rich, plant-based alkaline protein. A failure to *balance* that ratio in our diet, leads to an imbalance. *Overloading* on acidic ash protein *isn't* healthy. Balancing the right proteins is. It's an important distinction worth noting. Eating an *excessive amount* of acidic protein also affects our bodies' ability to absorb other nutrients.

According to the *American Journal of Kidney Diseases* (August 2002), the body's ability to absorb calcium is reduced after only 6 weeks of excessive protein intake. This suggests that overloaders may need more protein just to absorb normal amounts of calcium, leading to a vicious cycle requiring more of the bad stuff to get the good stuff. An important distinction between animal protein and plant protein is that the former contains large amounts of sulphur. Sulphur is found in two of the primary amino acids: methionine and cysteine. Excess sulfur in the diet has been linked to inflammation and may play a role in disease, particularly cancer. But a reasonable amount of sulfur is healthful.[4]

Osteoporosis is a progressive deterioration of bone matrix, eventually resulting in thin and brittle bone that's easily broken, effecting approximately 10 million Americans (80 percent are women). But it's *not* a normal part of growing old as we've been told. An excessive amount of acidic ash protein causes our body to leach calcium from bone to alkalize our blood. Research shows that eating an unbalanced ratio of animal to plant protein appears to be one of three factors primarily responsible for diminished bone density.[5,6] The next is the absence of a sufficient amount of estrogen. Estrogen regulates the excessive uptake of calcium in our bone. Remember, good health is all about balance. Finally, the more calcium taken in, particularly in the absence of a sufficient amount of estrogen, the more we must export. As long as this 'tug of war" remains balanced, we enjoy healthy bone. But the majority of the cells responsible for absorbing calcium, **the osteoblasts, die in the process of being challenged to absorb more calcium than they were genetically intended to**; while their counterparts, the *osteoclasts*, continue to export calcium and other minerals out. The longer you have this imbalance, the faster your bones age prematurely. This also explains why women have an increased risk for bone fracture after menopause, when their estrogen level plummets; and how too much calcium can actually cause osteoporosis.

CAN EATING EXCESSIVE AMOUNTS OF PROTEIN AFFECT OUR BODY'S ABILITY TO ABSORB IMPORTANT NUTRIENTS? THE ANSWER IS YES.

Not surprisingly, societies with the highest rates of osteoporosis eat the largest amount of animal protein. They also drink the largest amount of milk .[7, 8, 9, 10, 11]

While a poor diet, high in acidity and low in alkalinity, and the lack of exercise may reduce bone mass, there are other culprits. Chief among them is a reduced level of protective estrogen, remedied by replacing what you've lost with bio-identical hormones. Other causes include calcium overload from supplements, particularly after our formative years, which destroys osteoblasts. These are the cells that deposit calcium from your diet into bone building matrix. Can too much calcium also cripple your heart? Research sheds new light on why so many of those suffering with osteoporosis, (thinning of bone from calcium loss), are also afflicted by "atherosclerosis" (thickening of arterial walls from calcium deposits)[25]. The missing link…vitamin D and K2. Without each, dietary calcium can end up precisely where you wish it wouldn't—in your arteries, veins, and heart. Adding the right amount of these nutrients, along with an adequate intake of calcium, has been shown to reduce rates of hip fracture, rekindle bone mineralization and increase bone density.

The best course of action is to eat the proper type and optimum amount of protein, based on your needs and weight. While our requirement for protein is clear, we eat far more than we need. Today, the average American eats more than 195 grams a day. Too much protein can also overpower your liver's ability to metabolize it, ultimately producing potentially toxic ammonia. Science shows that most of us need less than 60 grams a day from the highest quality sources. That's 25-30 percent of what you're likely eating now. While these foods will cost more, you'll be eating far less and will actually save money. In the longer term, the savings are even greater. You'll increase your life span, earn more years of income, and reduce the amount of money your insurance company won't cover for needless hospital stays. Spending more per gram and reducing the amount of protein in your diet, will permit you to spend less. Research suggests that a diet largely consisting of processed foods lays the groundwork for internal inflammation and, in the end, sows the seeds of our destruction.

The movie Soylent Green (1973) takes us to a time when the only food source that remained in the world was human. This fictional apple hasn't fallen too far from today's fake food tree. In fact, scientists have found several toxins, from the food we eat today, in our bodies' tissue from fake foods, literally making "you are what you eat," a grim reality. With this understanding, let's turn our attention to one of the most important aspects of this discussion. *What* protein *should* we eat? First, it's important to understand the interplay of the food chain. We truly are what we eat. But for the purpose of this discussion, it's equally important to understand another important fact—we are, actually, what we eat *ate*.

Not long ago, the U.S. government issued a statement designed to calm a beleaguered public about the threat of mad cow disease (bovine spongiform encephalopathy). We were told that our food supply is safe. But it's not true. Again, we were *Misinformed About Food*. While mad cow disease may not become widespread anytime soon, our food supply is anything but safe. You and your loved ones are threatened. The government won't protect you. Tobacco remains legal—and so does the industrialized processing and sale of red meat.

BEEF—IT'S WHAT'S FOR DINNER®!

Beef is a complete protein. It contains *all* of the essential amino acids we require. But what else does it contain? Eating beef seems as American as apple pie—but so are heart disease and cancer. Just ask the Chinese who have become "Westernized" in recent years.

According to a study by researchers Jiang He, MD, et al. (*The New England Journal of Medicine*; Major Causes of Death among Men and Women in China Volume 353:1124-1134; Number 11; September 15, 2005) "Adverse changes in lifestyle (such as a high intake of dietary fat and increased physical inactivity) that tend to accompany industrialization and urbanization have become increasingly prevalent in these countries, and such changes may have increased the risk of chronic disease, including vascular disease and cancer." They conclude: "Our study indicates that diseases of the heart, malignant neoplasms, and cerebrovascular disease are the leading causes of death in the Chinese population of adults 40 years of age and older. Together, they account for approximately two thirds of the total mortality in the study population."

McDonald's is expanding so rapidly in China that the demand for the metal nickel used to make stainless steel for food counters and kitchens has gone through the roof. According to the Nickel Institute ("Fast Food in China," March 2005), the average McDonald's uses two tons of stainless steel.

The United States Department of Agriculture ("FAS Worldwide," July 2006), Yum! Brands, owners of fast food restaurants such as KFC (over 1,000 locations), Pizza Hut, Taco Bell, and others, have nearly tripled the number of outlets over the past four years from 650 to well over 2,000. Yum! China, which includes locations in Thailand and Taiwan, currently boasts over 2,700 locations. According to the company, China is their number one market targeted for new restaurant growth worldwide. The explosive incidence of heart disease has risen in direct proportion to the increased consumption of fast food. India is right behind them. According to Sandeep Kohli, managing director for Yum! Restaurants International India, "Pizza Hut is an international brand that is part of India's local fabric and our customers' lives." On the surface, this almost sounds like a new brand of religion. But, if I were betting man, I'd say the company will achieve its objective of 1,000 locations by 2014.

Closer to home, we eat steak from feedlot cattle because it tastes good, and find comfort in the fact that everyone else does. But if we lived in parts of India, we might not—yet. In an interview entitled "Taking the Pulse of the Planet" by Bill McKibben (*Audubon* 1999), Lester R. Brown, the founder of the Worldwatch Institute, Washington, DC, shared some profound thoughts on this subject. According to McKibben, "Brown's life is devoted to tracking what he calls the vital signs: the stock price of the earth, the sales per square foot of the planet." Brown continues: "If everyone in the world consumed meat, eggs, and cheese the way we do in this country, it would take about three planets the size of this one to satisfy our needs. It takes a lot of grain to grow all that meat. But that's the direction the world is going in. When income goes up one of the first things that happens in every society is that the consumption of livestock products goes up. Last year the world ate 26 percent more meat than it did just eight years ago."

Marketing is a powerful tool of persuasion. Lung cancer seems to be popping up all over the place. But before the advent of the cigarette, it was virtually unheard of (according to a study by LeAnn D. Anderson et al. in "Assessing a Decade of Progress in Cancer Control," *Oncologist*, June 2002): "If the trends of the past decade continue, more women will die of lung cancer than men do by the end of the next decade."

Bad habits die hard—and so do we. The way we eat tops the list of one of the worst habits known to mankind. It's my belief that the regular consumption of certain fatty, processed, saturated fats (like those found in some highly processed, fatty industrialized meats, suet, and vegetable oil) contributes to internal inflammation. This wrong fat interferes with the body's ability to protect itself. The right fat (including certain healthy saturated fat as you'll soon discover) protects us. You've heard about the correlation between high levels of cholesterol serum in our blood and heart disease. There's also a similar correlation between *high levels* of certain saturated fat and LDL (bad cholesterol). Red meat from grain-fed beef is one of the largest sources of fat in the human diet.

According to the USDA Economic Research Service, the average American consumes 200 pounds of meat annually (of which, almost 67 pounds is beef). A 6-ounce broiled Porterhouse steak is a great source of complete protein—38 grams. That's a good thing. Beef contains all the amino acids your body needs to form a complete molecule of protein. But it also delivers 44 grams of fat; 16 grams from the wrong kind of saturated fat. That's almost three quarters of the recommended daily intake for saturated fat (*American Journal of Public Health 87*(6): 992–997, 1997). So, why do Americans consume so much beef? Well, in large part, because it's a tasty and readily available source of dense protein. Red meat is also a leading source of Omega-6 fatty acids. An excessive amount of Omega-6s interferes with your body's ability to produce Omega-3 fatty acids. The right balance of these fats is required to achieve optimal health. Cancer needs Omega-6 fatty acids to flourish.

IF EVERYONE IN THE WORLD CONSUMED MEAT, EGGS, AND CHEESE THE WAY WE DO IN THIS COUNTRY, IT WOULD TAKE ABOUT THREE PLANETS THE SIZE OF THIS ONE TO SATISFY OUR NEEDS.

To put our dietary evolution in perspective, a million years ago prehistoric man enjoyed a ratio of 1 Omega-6 fatty acid to every 1 Omega-3 fatty acid. Today, this ratio is estimated to be, on average, as much as 25 Omega-6s to each Omega-3. This is an imbalance as out of hand as our health. We need to take control *now*. But there's no need to give up red meat. The right red meat eaten in moderation, provides healthier Omega-3 fatty acids and other important nutrients than fish; but industrialized red meat does not.

What's industrialized meat? An article written by Michael Pollan for the *New York Times* tells it all. Many years ago, cattle roamed the plains and ate what nature intended. These animals were well equipped by nature. Because they are *ruminants* (grazing animals that eat what their stomachs already digested, later regurgitate it, and eat it again), grasses from the plains are an ideal food source. Their digestive system (stomach) contains "healthy" bacteria, which breaks down grasses and turns them into useful acids and protein. But in our modern world, farm lot "cities" have made grazing in the grass a fond memory.

The 1950s saw the advent of huge commercial feedlots. The owners bought calves from farmers who raised yearlings from birth.

But somewhere around this time, the cow's worst nightmare began. Big business got involved—and time became money. A century ago, most cattle were 4 to 5 years old by the time they were slaughtered. But today a calf goes from 80 pounds to 1400 pounds in as little as 14 months. Nearly 80 percent of the cattle born in the United States are ultimately slaughtered by four huge meatpacking houses: IBP (a subsidiary of Tyson), National, Excel, or Monfort. After the free-range stage of infancy is over, the cattle are weaned from a natural diet of grass they can ruminate to a mix of alfalfa, corn, and hay with a tad of ruminant on sprawling feedlots. Pollan explains that "a cattle feedlot is a kind of city, populated by as many as 100,000 animals. It is very much a pre-modern city, however—crowded, filthy and stinking, with open sewers, unpaved roads and choking air."

Because corn and grain are not made for ruminants, the cattle often suffer from acute gastritis. They're forced to eat stuff they weren't made to digest. According to researchers at Cornell University, acidosis can occur, which results in the accumulation of as much as 300 times the amount of *Escherichia coli* (E. Coli) bacteria found in grass-fed cattle. Is this reason enough to switch to grass-fed beef?

A farmer in Iowa once explained to me how he needed to occasionally cut open one of the four stomach compartments of his livestock to eliminate a potentially deadly explosion of gas. Many things can go wrong when an animal is forced to eat food they can't digest, including dangerous, life-threatening, bloat. As John B. Hall and Susan Silver, Virginia Tech University, point out (Virginia Cooperative Extension, June 2001): "Changing rapidly from a forage-based diet to a grain-based diet causes millions of fiber-digesting microbes to die-off as they cannot digest the starch, and there are too few starch-digesting microbes to use the grain so the grain sours in the rumen. As a result, rumen pH decreases, the rumen stops working, and the animal becomes ill. In severe cases, cattle can develop acidosis and founder or die."

Commonly referred to as "twisted stomach," this condition occurs in the animal's abomasum, also known as their "true stomach." Cattle that develop acidosis often find that their abomasum actually "floats out of place." Researchers describe the process as "[they become] torsioned, stopping the flow of digesta." This condition can only be repaired surgically. But this living hell of industrialized cattle involves much more than surviving acidosis and mad cow disease.

According to Pollan: "Growing the vast quantities of corn used to feed livestock in this country takes vast quantities of chemical fertilizer, which in turn takes vast quantities of oil—1.2 gallons for every bushel. So, the modern feedlot is really a city floating on a sea of oil."

Remember—you are what you eat—ate. This is just the tip of the iceberg. *Antibiotics* (estimated to be upward of 5,000 tons a year), as well as *hormones* such as diethylstilbestrol (DES), a sex hormone, legal until the FDA banned its use in 1979, and *cattle parts* were introduced to the feed. Hormones such as testosterone, oestradiol 17-a, progesterone, zeranol, melengesterone, and trenbalone acetate are perfectly legal today. Although cattle parts are no longer allowed (prohibited to reduce the spread of mad cow disease), other animal proteins such as chicken manure, pig, and chicken parts are still permitted by law. While we can't legally use steroids, the cattle you eat can. How many estrogen pellets have been injected in how many cattle? The FDA still permits feedlots to use hormones to induce growth in cattle but does not permit its use for raising turkey, chicken, pigs, and other wildlife. Should we be surprised when we hear that human cancers have been linked to an imbalance of our hormones?

Unfortunately, a similar fate awaits most commercially raised animal sources of protein. Seeing other farm animals such as sheep, pigs, and veal calves raised this way is horrifying, particularly for the animals themselves. If you'd like to get involved, there are a number of national organizations fighting for the rights of farm animals, such as The Humane Farming Association (www.hfa.org).

I'll spare you the details of the nightmare they call the "kill floor"—and the castration stun guns, manure laden carcasses, and more. It is, quite literally, a living hell. So what's a red meat lover to do?

Retooling the phrase to "You are what you eat has eaten" can be a good thing. Some happy cattle fit for consumption are still grazing the plains as their ancestors did before them, but there aren't many. Grass-fed cattle raised naturally have even more Omega-3 fatty acids than fish, according to a review conducted by University of California Cooperative Extension and California State University, Chico. While industrialized beef has a ratio of 1:25, grass-fed beef still boasts an Omega profile similar to their ancestors' ratio of 1:1. Omega-3 fatty acids reduce inflammation and help prevent heart disease, cancers, arthritis, and other inflammatory conditions. Omega-6 fatty acids promote inflammation, blood clotting (which can be a good thing), and tumor growth. Just like other substances in your body, you need the right balance of both to achieve optimal health.

I'LL SPARE YOU THE DETAILS OF THE NIGHTMARE THEY CALL THE "KILL FLOOR"—AND THE CASTRATION STUN GUNS, MANURE LADEN CARCASSES, AND MORE. IT IS, QUITE LITERALLY, A LIVING HELL.

Grass-fed beef is also an incredible source of usable iron, known as absorbable "heme" iron. Forty percent of Americans are iron deficient in this form of iron. An iron deficiency leaves us weak and tired. If a food is high in iron, but not the absorbable form, it won't help you satisfy this requirement. We should also be aware that regular exercise depletes our zinc reserves. Non-heme iron—from vegetables, fruits, grains, and supplements is far more difficult for the body to absorb. Only 3 ounces of beef provides a greater amount of heme iron than approximately ½ cup of spinach. But absorption from non-heme sources can be improved by adding foods with vitamin C to your meal.

Grass-fed beef is also one of the highest sources of usable zinc. A 4-ounce serving is equivalent to three 4-ounce cans of tuna.

It's also an excellent source of beta-carotene. Beta-carotene is converted to vitamin A when it's available and when our body requires it. A study by two California State University, Chico, students with the UC Cooperative Extension (funded by the W. K. Kellogg Foundation of California Food and Fiber Future) concluded that there's almost *twice* as much beta-carotene in grass-fed beef than its industrialized counterpart. A good source of vitamin E, grass-fed beef contains more than three times the vitamin E (9.3 micrograms) per gram than its cow-city cousins. This powerful antioxidant offers proven protection against cancer-causing nitrosamines that form from the grilling or frying of meat and other foods.

Much of the beef sold in health food stores has been raised *naturally*, on a diet of organic grains. Don't be misled by health food stores touting organic grain-fed beef. They can try to convince you, but you'll never convince a cow. There's nothing *natural* about grain to a cow. We know ruminants such as cattle were not meant to eat grain. What good is organic grain if it can't be properly digested? Nearly void of Omega-3s, grain-fed beef has few of the vitamins and minerals found in the grass-fed alternative.

So what's the healthiest source of beef? You won't find it on industrialized feedlots that clock production from birth to your freezer section in 14 months or less; nor in feedlot cities serving up *natural* organic grain. Only farmed-raised grass-fed beef without hormones, antibiotics, and additives allowed to freely graze will do. Because grass-fed beef is far lower in fat, it's also lower in calories. It trumps the feedlot gang with 60 percent to 85 percent more of these important fatty acids. According to a 2001 study by Iowa State University, grass-fed beef contains almost *3 times less* Omega-6 fatty acids. Today's modern Omega imbalance ("Omega-3 Information Service," Larson, 2002) is a major cause of most disease. Grass-fed cattle also retain important nutrients from the prairie grasses they eat. These vitamins and minerals allow them to create conjugated linoleic acids (CLA), a fat that helps reduce the risk of obesity, diabetes, heart disease, and cancer in animals while super charging their immunity. To achieve this same benefit, the average person would need to eat approximately 5 grams of CLA per day (the daily requirement). A 3.5-ounce serving of grass-fed beef provides 1.23 grams of CLA, or 25 percent of the daily requirement. The same amount of conventionally raised beef provides less than 10 percent of the daily requirement. While the importance of the correct fats is getting a lot of attention, Omega-3s have certainly grabbed the spotlight. But the importance of *CLA* needs to be emphasized as well.

Animal studies demonstrate the power of "synthetic" CLA to prevent a number of cancers, including prostrate, colorectal, breast cancer, and more. Naturally occurring CLA has been found to lower low-density lipoprotein (LDL) and triglyceride levels while boosting immunity and increasing the density of healthy bone formation in cattle. CLA has also been shown to reverse the symptoms of diabetes in laboratory animals who were genetically predisposed to heart disease by improving glucose utilization. In many animals, tumor growth is inhibited by even small amounts of CLA. Tumors were suppressed as much as 50 percent when only half of one percent was in their diet. But a scant amount of published data exists to support these same claims in humans.

In a Finnish study, women reduced their risk of breast cancer by 60 percent when levels of CLA were high, in contrast to those women with low levels of this amino acid. In the absence of additional research, eating grass-fed beef for its Omega balance and its ability to reduce or eliminate most major diseases in livestock might be reason enough to make the switch. CLA is an essential amino acid, so our body must break it down from the food we eat. Grass-fed beef packs a powerful punch of this potential cancer fighter. Larry Satter, an agricultural research scientist at the Dairy Forage Research Institute in Madison, Wisconsin, found that grazing dairy cattle had an incredible 500 percent more CLA than those that ate a diet of grain, hay, and silage. In her book, *Why Grass-fed Is Best,* famed author and grass-fed beef proponent Jo Robinson states: "Is there enough CLA in grass-fed products to reduce your risk of cancer? Probably so. It has been estimated that people eating ordinary grain-fed meat and dairy products consume about 1 gram of CLA a day. Judging by animal studies, this is one third of the amount required to reduce the risk of cancer. Switching to grass-fed animal products would increase your CLA intake three to five times, which could make the all-important difference."

In addition to grass-fed beef, lamb and certain dairy products are excellent sources of CLA. But dairy cattle and other livestock require the same free-range grass-fed diet as beef cattle. Cheese made from grazing grass-fed dairy cattle is an excellent choice for additional CLA. The compound was first isolated in 1983 (from ground beef) by a research team led by Michael W. Pariza, PhD, of the University of Wisconsin. Researchers have not only confirmed CLA's anticarcinogenicity in experimental animals—it's the only fatty acid consistently shown to inhibit cancer growth in such animals—but have also explored ways to increase the amount of CLA in your diet. If you replace industrialized protein with naturally grass-fed sources now, you'll put the brakes on the damaging effects of internal inflammation. In the short term, it will cost you more money. But it's well worth the cost and easier to find than you think. The finest product of its kind, Tallgrass Beef® (served at one of President Obama's inaugural dinners) can be delivered to your front door (www.RKInformedLiving.com). The best choice is to purchase from a local ranch near you, or you may wish to consider working with a local farming family. For some, a weekend trip down a rural road might be the start of ushering in a lifestyle with a new sense of priority—you.

WILD GAME

Animals that are typical grass grazers, such as elk, mule deer, and antelope, have considerably more Omega-6s as grain-fed beef do per serving. Bison have half the amount of saturated fat as grass-fed beef and slightly more Omega-6s but only half the amount of beneficial Omega-3s. While bison are typically leaner, they have a ratio of approximately 6 to 1 of Omega-6s to Omega-3s. Grass-fed beef remains the most balanced choice of a healthy protein in a diet that includes meat.

Item, per 100 grams	Pronghorn Antelope	Mule Deer	Elk	Bison	Range-Grazed beef	Grain fed beef
Saturated	875	972	664	421	933	2028
Stearic	441	401	172	197	327	651
Myristic/Palmitic	434	571	492	224	606	1377
Monounsaturated	582	732	508	444	754	2114
Polyunsaturated	530	463	399	182	19	291
Omega-6	442	359	343	156	139	275
Omega-3	88	104	56	26	52	16
Cholesterol	52	54	48	45	49	48
Calories	117	119	112	104	112	136
Protein, g	22.4	22.6	22.4	21.9	21.8	21.7
Fat, g	2.5	2.7	2.0	1.4	2.4	5.0

From Medeiro, L.C. (2002). "Nutritional content of game meat." B-920R. College of Agriculture, University of Wyoming.

POULTRY

The process used to mass produce industrialized poultry is just as tragic as cattle. Fortunately, you'll find no sacrifice in taste or texture in turkey and other poultry raised the old-fashion way. They're among the most flavorful sources of protein available. The process of getting today's mass-market version of turkey from the feedlot to your dinner table is still another race against the clock. Broiler chickens are loaded with bacteria and fattened up with antibiotics. According to LCA Justice for Animals, turkeys are often so fat that their legs can't withstand the weight. Over time, it's too difficult for them to walk around and their legs just break. Their legs aren't much use to them anyway because they're often confined in such small cribs. Most receive little fresh air and are forced to breath in ammonia day after day. They're often put into sheds with no windows and little ventilation from the day they're born; a practice that makes them more than a little aggressive. Some are literally de-beaked and eventually starve to death. Droppings are accumulated on a floor of wood shavings or similar material, provide a breeding ground for bacteria. The life of an industrialized turkey is brutal.

It's hard to imagine a life that could be any worse than this, unless you're an industrialized *layer* chicken (the kind that lays eggs). Approximately 250 million chickens are born to do so each year. Most live on feedlots. After birth, they're often snatched[12] from their moms and thrown on conveyor belts. The females that lay eggs are sorted by workers from the males that don't. Because the males don't plump up and can't lay eggs, many are thrown in a bag and suffocated, ground in a macerator and fed to their sisters, gassed, or drowned. Millions are thrown in the garbage each year. Male chicks are dumped by the hundreds of thousands into trash bins where they slowly suffocate.

Life for a female layer chick is somewhat longer but equally tortured. After the separation, they're often de-beaked without anesthetic with a hot soldering iron, which slices through bone and a thin layer of sensitive skin between the horn and the beak. This is done to eliminate aggressive pecking that occurs when chickens are crammed into confining wire cages; some as small as 14 inches long that they may share with six to eight other hens. There's no room for them to stretch a wing. In a typical shed on an egg factory farm, battery cages are stacked one on top of the other. Excrement from birds in cages above can fall onto those below.

The practice of forced molting is a modern technique (though it was first introduced several decades ago), used by an industry that deprives chicks of food from 5 to 21 days at a time, or until they lose 25 percent to 35 percent of their body weight (Webster, 2000, p. 192). This practice of shocking a chick to molt is done to increase the quantity and quality of the eggs they'll continue to produce in a subsequent season. A formal request to stop this inhumane starving of chicks was the subject of a petition to the United States Department of Agriculture (USDA) and FDA by two animal welfare organizations, the United Poultry Concerns and the Association of Veterinarians for Animal Rights. The two groups have evidence showing that "chickens have a complex nervous system and cognitive capacity, and that their ability to suffer from acute and chronic stress, pain, and fear entitles them to relief from the inhumane practice of being deliberately starved."

Researchers at the Biophysics Group at Silsoe Research Institute in England agree. Behavioral studies done by the group showed that chickens are truly intelligent creatures that "can anticipate the future and demonstrate self-control." And according to Dr. Joy Mench, professor and director of the Center for Animal Welfare at the University of California at Davis: "Chickens show sophisticated social behavior ... That's what a pecking order is all about. They can recognize more than a hundred other chickens and remember them. They have more than thirty types of vocalizations."

But the carnage continues—ammonia-filled hen houses compete with the stench of urine and feces for space in their lungs. After egg laying slows down, generally in as little as two years, they're considered useless, though their "natural" life span is between 10 to 15 years. They dehydrate when deprived of water, before being jammed into crates or garbage bags and trucked to the slaughterhouse. Almost suffocating from the weight of other strange birds during transport, their bones are so brittle that even more may break. According to People for the Ethical Treatment of Animals

AFTER EGG LAYING SLOWS DOWN, GENERALLY IN AS LITTLE AS TWO YEARS, THEY'RE CONSIDERED USELESS, THOUGH THEIR "NATURAL" LIFE SPAN IS BETWEEN 10 TO 15 YEARS.

(PETA) in their fact sheet "Factory Farming: Mechanized Madness," when they arrive at the slaughterhouse "their throats are slit by machines, and they are immersed in scalding-hot water for feather removal. They are often conscious throughout the entire process. Often, because their bones are so brittle from egg production that the electric current would cause them to shatter, hens are not even stunned before their throats are slit." According to Barbara Olenjnik ("Dwindling Spent Hen Disposal Outlets Causes Concern," *Poultry Times*, September 2003), about 100 million are slaughtered annually. Their natural pecking order is now an industrialized wrecking order. In 1958, Congress passed the Humane Slaughter Act, which required that "food animals" be stunned or have a metal bolt drilled through their head, so that death came swiftly. But oddly enough, neither poultry, fish nor rabbits were included in this act.

The fate of the almost 9 billion broiler chickens produced each year is no better. According to a report written by David Wallinga, MD, for the Institute of Agriculture and Trade Policy ("Playing Chicken: Avoiding Arsenic in Your Meat," April 2006): "Estimates are that at least 70 percent have been fed arsenic. Some of that arsenic stays in chicken meat."

Wallinga later adds: "We estimate from 1.7 to 2.2 million pounds of roxarsone, a single arsenic feed additive, are given each year to chickens. Arsenic is an element—it doesn't degrade or disappear. Arsenic subsequently contaminates much of the 26 to 55 billion pounds of litter or waste generated each year by the U.S. broiler chicken industry, likely also contaminating the communities where that waste is generated or dispersed. In the chicken-producing town of Prairie Grove, MO, house dust in every one of 31 homes examined was found to contain at least two kinds of arsenic also found in chicken litter."

There are far more humane techniques and healthier alternatives. Although chickens don't graze, some are put in a crib and rotated around a pasture. The practice of doing so the old-fashion way is growing, and this fledgling industry deserves our thanks and support. Turkeys are somewhat better at grazing than chickens and can be put in pens and allowed to really roam. While chickens raised as nature intended are a fine source of protein, farm raised turkey is the number one recommended super-poultry food of choice. Turkey offers us another complete protein that's lower in calories than either beef or chicken. It's also one of the few non-ruminating animals whose meat contains a significantly higher content of CLA than found in chicken, pork, or fish. Unlike cattle, they're not completely grass-fed nor should they be. Fortunately, they can obtain 40 percent of their dietary needs from grass. Chickens can only receive 20 percent to 30 percent from grazing. Because they are not ruminants, their diet should be supplemented with organic grain. Unlike cattle, their systems happily tolerate it.

Pasture-raised, antibiotic-free, and hormone-free turkey is a great source of high-quality protein and is the best of all animal sources that provide calcium. **In fact, there's actually more protein in one gram of turkey than there is in one gram of beef.** Turkeys also graze better than chickens. While emu, ostrich, and bison meat are lower in saturated fat, pasteurized turkeys are, today, generally more accessible. Natural farm-raised turkey is also low in sodium and a good source of niacin and phosphorous.

However, there's often an alarming amount of bacteria found in poultry, regardless of whether they are pasture raised or industrially produced. The best way to guard against this is to cook your turkey thoroughly.

Eating farm-raised turkey raised the old-fashioned way is one of the healthiest sources of animal protein available. According to John D McArthur (*The Eagle, Ben Franklin, and the Turkey*), Ben Franklin regarded the turkey as the most noble bird of them all, and had preferred it to the bald eagle as the new symbol for the United States of America. So eat noble and eat healthy. Eat free-range turkey.

SEAFOOD

In general, *fish stink*! Those advocating that you eat "three servings of fish a week" (the amount found to lower coronary disease in a recent study) are telling you the good but not the bad and the ugly. Decades ago, scientists conducted a 25-year study of 1,800 members of the Inuit Eskimos of Greenland. The results of this research were dramatic, showing a surprisingly low rate of heart disease, multiple sclerosis, bronchial asthma and other chronic disease. Their diet was loaded with fat, primarily from the consumption of fish and other marine animals. This was good fat (you'll learn more in greater detail in Chapter 2), supplying more than 7 grams of Omega-3 fatty acids daily. Sadly, it's estimated that the average American is getting a mere 200 *milligrams* per day in our diet.

The miracle of Omega-3 fatty acids has been heralded by many bestselling authors. But today's recommendations are based on research dating back to 1950. The man that deserves the credit for pulling it all together is Dr. Barry Sears PhD, when he introduced his outstanding book, *The Omega Rx Zone: The Miracle of the New High Dose Fish Oil* (HarperCollins, 2003). You'll learn more about this shortly.

You've also been told that eating fish is good for your health. Yet, what held true in Greenland in 1980 may not hold true in the United States today. Eating fish may lower your risk of coronary heart disease, but what else is it doing to you? Should you eat three servings a week of fish because the Inuit Eskimos of Greenland did so in 1950?

What's so beneficial about eating fish? Simply put, fish are one of the finest sources of Omega-3 fatty acids available. An ever-expanding body of solid research illustrates how a deficiency of this important fat in our diet is one of the leading causes of chronic disease and premature death. Conversely, adding a meaningful amount of this important fat to our daily consumption decreases the incidence of myocardial infarction, depression, and cancer. In addition to diminishing the incidence of this disease, and lengthening our lives, complete reversals of chronic illnesses are well documented. Dr. Barry Sears, Dr. Artemis Simopoulis, and other respected researchers called its discovery one of the most significant events in the twenty-first century. The issue is the balance or ratio of these fatty acids. Recall, our ancestors achieved an almost 1:1 ratio of Omega-6 fatty acids to Omega-3s. Think of Omega-6s as *constrictors*. While needed to carry out important bodily functions (such as clotting), an imbalance creates internal inflammation (more on this in Chapter 2). This inflammation is one of the leading causes of premature death, and most chronic disease. It may also explain why so many of those around us are victims of cancer, heart disease, and other pathological illness. While some restriction from Omega-6 is essential, too much fans the flames of internal inflammation.

THINK OF FISH AS SPONGES, ABSORBING NUTRIENTS (AS WELL AS CONTAMINANTS) IN THEIR FLESH. THE FATTIER THE FLESH, THE MORE NUTRIENTS (AND TOXINS) THEY ABSORB.

But how did our Paleolithic ancestry achieve this balanced ratio of important Omega fatty acids? Much like the Inuit Eskimos did, they ate a great deal of fish. Remember, you are what you eat *-ate*. The fish weren't born with Omega-6s. They *ate* them, and then processed and contained them. Fish eat algae, an organism so powerful it could literally synthesize this fat by itself. While algae are the simplest of organisms, only the size of a single cell, they're also the most powerful food ever introduced on our planet. And the oldest food as well —almost 3 billion years old. Yet only recently have we discovered its intrinsic value.

Since the time fish first swam on this planet, algae became their mainstay. And conversely, fish became the most efficient source of Omega-3 fatty acids. Today, modern man has *discovered* that a diet consisting of three or more servings of fish a week can significantly decrease the onset of heart disease. It's no small wonder that the Inuit Eskimos had a conspicuous absence of heart disease. But here's the good news—you can achieve the same benefits the Inuit Eskimos did simply and safely. Think of fish as sponges, absorbing nutrients (as well as contaminants) in their flesh. The fattier the flesh, the more nutrients (and toxins) they absorb. But what was good news for our ancestors 150,000 years ago (and the Inuit Eskimos of Greenland today) has become a double-edge sword for the average American today. These spongy aquatic harbingers of Omega-3s are soaking up contaminants at an alarming rate. The older the fish, the longer they've soaked them up. Predatory fish have not only retained their own fair share of toxins, but they've also absorbed them from the fish *they* ate. Making the larger, higher order of fish most hazardous to our health.

So, while certain fish are still a rich source of Omega-3 fatty acids, they also provide modern man with a scary proposition. Many of the fish we're told to eat are chocked full of methyl mercury and polychlorinated biphenyls (PCBs) contaminates. The *safer fish*, according to FDA guidelines, are those containing the lowest levels of mercury contamination, such as sole, haddock, and flounder (bottom feeders), but they also provide a far smaller amount of Omega-3 fatty acids.

Where do these contaminants come from and how harmful can they be? Mercury is a powerful neurotoxin. Depending on the form and degree of exposure, mercury can cause profound neurological damage ranging from autism to dementia. If inhaled, as much as 80 percent of it can enter the bloodstream. Research shows that even in small amounts, it suppresses our immune system causing damage to our blood cells, glands, organs, and enzymes. Discarded fever thermometers are one of the largest sources of mercury deposited in our municipal waste system. Some 17 tons are deposited each year. But today, there's no need to continue this practice. There are digital electronic and gas alternatives. Duluth, Minnesota, and San Francisco, California, have banned the use of mercury thermometers. Hopefully, more communities will pass similar resolutions. But mercury exposure comes to us from less visible sources as well.

Some have suggested that an alarming increase in diagnosable autism in the United States may be attributable to the routine use of Thimerosal, a mercury-containing preservative used in several and frequently recommended vaccines for children. On July 7, 1999, a joint statement was issued to the medical community by the U.S. Public Health Service and The American Academy of Pediatrics expressing concern over this issue. Autism was formerly diagnosed in one to three children for every 10,000 births. Today, the frequency of diagnosed autism has risen to between 20 to 40 per 10,000 births, and reports of 1 per 150 births have been reported in several states including New Jersey and California.

No discussion regarding mercury poisoning can be complete without considering toxic poisoning from amalgam, or what we commonly refer to it as the metal fillings in our teeth. While we refer to this material as "silver," a far greater percentage of *mercury* is mixed together to form this compound. Autopsy studies have shown a direct correlation between the amount of mercury found in the brain and the amount of mercury amalgam found in teeth. In November 2001, Congresswoman Diane Watson of Los Angeles introduced legislation that would require labeling and disclosure of these obvious dangers by the dental community, laying the groundwork for a complete phase-out of its usage over a five-year period. The following facts, disclosed in the bill she submitted for approval, cite an alarming misuse of the single most toxic non-radioactive element of our time, and its continued effect on our population: *A teenager with six fillings has six mercury thermometers worth of mercury in his or*

A TEENAGER WITH SIX FILLINGS HAS SIX MERCURY THERMOMETERS WORTH OF MERCURY IN HIS OR HER MOUTH.

her mouth. Mercury is the major ingredient in each filling, about one half gram per cavity. According to Professor Boyd Hayley, University of Kentucky, that is a "colossal" amount of mercury in scientific terms—as much, in fact, as is in a thermometer. A major health risk exists—The Agency for Toxic Substances and Disease Registry of the United States Public Health Service reports that those poisonous vapors go first to the brain and kidneys.

Mercury is volatile, vaporous, and passes from the placenta to mother's milk.

In 1996 the Canadian government recommended that dentists not place fillings in the mouths of children or pregnant women. The 1999 report on mercury by the Agency for Toxic Substances and Disease Registry also says that mercury passes through the placenta into the developing child's brain. In 1997, a major manufacturer of dental amalgam, Dentsply, said that amalgam is *contraindicated* for children and pregnant women, as well as for those with braces, mercury hypersensitivities, or kidney problems. Another manufacturer, Vivadent, added a contraindication for nursing mothers. The American Dental Association, which endorses manufacturers' products they support, for money, does everything possible to keep its members quiet on this issue. As Congresswoman Watson points out: "The ADA has a rule that gags dentists from talking about the risks of mercury amalgam, a rule that some dental boards enforce against dentists who call for the elimination of mercury in dental fillings. I understand that rule is being challenged by dentists in Federal court in Maryland based on the First Amendment."

As you've seen, mercury contamination may be found in our land, air, sea, mouth, brain, and fetuses from many sources, including our food. So, when the FDA sets *allowable* limits far below those set by other responsible governments and organizations, we must wonder—why? If we're not supposed to consume an "undesirable amount of a toxin," then is consuming less than that therefore *acceptable*? Don't many of these sources combine to far exceed the allowable limit of each?

Finally, why wouldn't the government set limits on our consumption of seafood? Thousands of tons of mercury are carried off to our waterways through the air, as a by-product of coal-burning power plants and battery manufacturers. When it reaches our lakes and sea, it's broken down by bacteria and changed to a poisonous organic compound know as methyl mercury. The National Academy of Sciences (*NeuroToxicology*, 2001), estimates that methyl mercury puts 60,000 newborns at risk each year for neurological damage based on their exposure to this toxin in the womb. Overexposure also results in baldness, paraesthesia (a pricking, tingling, or creeping sensation on the skin), depression, and blurred vision. If *we* are permitting thousands of tons of mercury to reach our waterways from power plants in this country, how much more is hitch hiking on air currents from foreign countries? The danger of wind drift is real.

Near the Tapajos River tributary that empties into the Amazon River, ninety-one villagers were tested for exposure to methyl mercury poisoning. Researchers from the University of Montreal discovered neurological damage evident in their mercury levels, which were above 50 micrograms (previously thought to be the clinical threshold). Even these Amazonian villagers, who eat fish as a mainstay, could not escape the danger of the air we breathe from the coal we burn.

Closer to home, Dr. Jane Hightower studied 116 middle to high-income men and woman in her San Francisco medical practice (*Environmental Health Perspectives*, 2003). She found that 90 percent of them had mercury levels in their blood that exceeded the Environmental Protection Agency's (EPA) standards for safety. Patients were chosen for the study based on the amount of fish in their diet, or symptoms that appeared to be consistent with mercury poisoning, including hair loss, depression, memory loss, confusion, and tremors. Most had levels that were more than double the levels the EPA regards as safe, while approximately 15 percent of those studied exceeded it by 400 percent. Of seven children tested, six had blood or hair levels exceeding the EPA's allowable limit.

While both the EPA and the National Academy of Sciences have lead the charge, alerting an already confused public to the growing danger of methyl mercury contamination, the FDA has once again under-reacted. The allowable levels of one part-per-billion (ppb) of mercury contaminant lag far behind the maximum levels considered safe by the EPA and World Health Organization

(WHO). According to the U.S. Department of Health and Human Services, statistics from the National Vaccine Injury Compensation Program show that the federal courts have received 5,263 claims relating to autism from 1988 to January 2008. Only *one* claim resulted in compensation; 4,913 claims were still pending and 350 were dismissed.

In an attempt to protect their citizens, forty-two states have decided it was in the public's best interest to enact their own legislation. Until recently, the FDA didn't even warn pregnant woman and young children (who are at the greatest risk) about the dangers of tuna. When they finally did, they completely omitted tuna *steak* from their warning, which contains an even greater level of methyl mercury contaminant than canned tuna.

The tuna industry is a powerful lobby—and the FDA is clearly dancing to their beat. According to the EPA's standard, a 45-pound child eating just one six-ounce can of white chunk albacore tuna weekly receives *almost four times more mercury* than is considered safe. New test results from the FDA itself on white canned tuna (albacore) show it contains three times more mercury than less expensive tuna products. But canned tuna is the third most popular item on grocery shelves. The FDA claims they're reluctant to deprive Americans of a relatively cheap source of protein. Based on these findings, Jane Houlihan, vice president of Research of the Washington, DC, Environmental Working Group states that "a pregnant woman who eats one 6-ounce can of albacore tuna each week could be exceeding a safe dose of mercury by 30 percent on average." The FDA has been accused of testing as little as twelve pieces of tuna fish. But, Houlihan tells us, they've been aware of the higher mercury content in albacore canned tuna since they first conducted this research in 1993.

In 2001, the FDA issued a mercury advisory for pregnant women and young children to avoid eating shark, swordfish, king mackerel, and tilefish. According to the survey, eating 12 ounces of any other fish (two 6-ounce servings) weekly was within safety limits. They warned pregnant moms to limit their consumption of certain predator fish, but not canned albacore tuna. So let's put this in perspective: People eat tuna for different reasons, of course. Some, at least in part, for the benefit they hope to gain from its valuable fatty acids. So, why is the majority of canned tuna today *low fat*? Now, we can get all the toxins that may be present and only one tenth of the amount of Omega-3s. We continue to be *Misinformed About Food.*

As you've seen, mercury can damage the brain tissue of a developing fetus. But the FDA doesn't want to scare us away from purchasing an inexpensive, healthy source of protein?

Our discussion has focused on mercury levels of ocean fish. But what about contamination of fresh water fish found in our lakes and rivers? Here, in what we still call "fresh water," the contamination can be even greater. According to the EPA, in 2002, 2,800 advisories were issued representing approximately 33 percent of the nation's total lake acreage and over 15 percent of the nation's total river miles. More than 40 states have issued alarming advisories, including Ohio, Illinois, Florida, and Rhode Island, who issued their own warnings in 2003, along with the Micmac Native American Indian tribe of Maine.

The following is an excerpt from a news release issued on April 23, 2003, by the Minnesota Department of Health (MDH): "All fish tested in Minnesota have mercury," said MDH Environmental Scientist Patricia McCann. "In fact, all fish, whether store bought or sport caught have some mercury. The amount depends on what the fish feed on, how old the fish are and to some degree the water they live in," she said. The state advisory applies to both commercially available fish as well as those caught by anglers in local waters.

The following is an example of a responsible local government's desire to protect its own people: "The Ohio Department of Health has issued fish consumption advisories for some area waters due to trace elements of mercury found in some fish. The Chagrin, Cuyahoga, and Ashtabula Rivers, Conneaut Creek, and Mogadore Reservoir south of Kent, are all included in the advisory. This advisory is specifically designed for women of child-bearing age, and children under the age of 6."

Meal Advice for Eating Ohio Sportfish				
Body of Water	Area Under Advisory	Species	Meal Frequency	Contaminant
Mogadore Reservoir	All Waters	Largemouth Bass	One meal a month	Mercury
Conneaut Creek	All Waters	Smallmouth Bass	One meal a month	Mercury

Body of Water	Area Under Advisory	Species	Meal Frequency	Contaminant
Ashtabula River	24th St Bridge to Lake Erie	Smallmouth Largemouth Walleye Channel Catfish Common Carp	One meal/week One meal/month One meal/month Six meals/year Six meals/year	PCBs Mercury, PCBs Mercury, PCBs PCBs PCBs
Mahoning River	Berlin Dam to Pa. border	White Crappie Smallmouth Walleye Spotted Bass	One meal/mo.	
Chagrin River	All Waters	Rock Bass Smallmouth	One meal/month	Mercury Lead
Cuyahoga River	Ohio Edison Dam Pool to Lake Erie	Common Carp, White Sucker 11"+ Largemouth Brown/Yellow Bullheads	One meal/month One meal/month 6 meals/year	PCBs Mercury PCBs

Source: http://geaugalink.com/recreatn/fishing.html

This warning was updated as of March 1998 and was copied in February 2005.

However, contamination from methyl mercury in our air and water, amalgam mercury in our mouth, and the mercury found in thermometers are only a few of the many sources of this toxin. Some fluorescent lamps, athletic shoes, mercury switches, medical and municipal waste facilities, and even old "junk" cars are all sources of this hazardous material. On February 6, 2004, the EPA issued a report stating that approximately 630,000 babies born each year (of nearly 4 million born annually) may be exposed to dangerous levels of mercury in the womb. This is nearly *double* the number the agency previously estimated. While mercury grabs a good deal of attention, there are a number of other metals and toxins in fish that are equally troublesome. They include chemicals such as PCBs, polycyclic aromatic hydrocarbons, pesticides (from run-off), arsenic, furans, and other organic compounds.

If you think farm-raised fish is a safer alternative, think again. Business is booming for fish farmers; so now let's expose still another myth. Today, more fish are produced by fish farms in the Pacific than are found in wild caught fisheries. Growth of farm fishing in countries such as Chile has become explosive. Not surprisingly, industrial production of seafood is often approached in much the same way as other industrialized production of meat and poultry. It's a cheaper, harmful, inhumane process that we support each time we purchase any of these products. It's also anything but *natural*. Farmed salmon often feed on their own waste. And remember, *you* are what you eat—*ate*. According to Greenpeace (Farm Fishing: www.Greenpeace.org): "A typical salmon farm of 200,000 fish produces roughly the same amount of fecal matter as a town of 62,000 people." And like cattle, farmed fish are often fed man-made pellets or meal containing ground fish parts from cheaper fish. That's why most farmed fish contain little in the way of Omega-3 fatty acids. In fact, most are completely void of this important nutrient.

Efforts *are* underway in this country to improve the farm diet of certain fish as they have done in other countries. Trout farmers in North Carolina, Idaho, and elsewhere, are attempting to reduce the amount of fish meal in their farmed diets for example.

Beyond the feed issue, farm-raised fish are often treated with vaccines or antibiotics to stop the spread of bacteria associated with large populations living in cramped caged quarters. According to a report by Michael C. Weber for the Sea Web Aquaculture Clearinghouse, sea lice are almost an epidemic on many salmon farms. Eleven different compounds from five different pesticides are often used to beat them into submission.

All but one of these compounds is toxic. A number of studies have shown that levels of antibiotics in farmed fish exceed allowable safety standards. In addition to antibiotics, metals are used to wash the cages or other structures housing the fish. This is done to stop the build-up of other organisms. Many of these washes or paints contain chemicals from copper derivatives, which are toxic to fish. A recent two-year study using the EPA standards for safety, led by David Carpenter of the University of Albany (*Science*, July 2004), found that farm-raised salmon had **ten times more contamination** than found in wild-caught salmon. You've seen how hazardous this was to a tribe in the Amazon when exposed to even minute concentrations of mercury. Carpenter's team discovered that farm-raised salmon in the United States contain five times the amount of other contaminants based on EPA guidelines.

Not surprisingly, the FDA took issue: "We've looked at the levels found ... and they do not represent a health concern," said Terry Troxell, director of the

FDA's Office of Plant and Dairy Food and Beverages. "In the end, our advice is not to alter consumption of farmed or wild salmon."

According to the study, farm-raised fish that were tested contained far greater levels of the cancer causing contaminant dioxin, as well as PCBs and should be eaten infrequently. The EPA's guidelines for PCBs state that a person who eats fish twice a week should consume no more than 4 to 6 parts per billion of PCBs. But this study found that PCB levels in farmed salmon sold in the United States and Canada averaged about 30 ppb (which, again, is five times the EPA guidelines.)

The researchers also discovered that farm-raised salmon contained ten times more contaminates than wild-caught. No wonder we consumers have become so distrusting. The responsibility of protecting our health can't be passed off to others. A USA Today investigation (December, 2009) revealed that the USDA provides thousands of pounds of "spent hen" (old meat, rejected by chains, such as KFC, over quality concerns) to school lunch programs across the country. Hormones, chemicals, and antibiotics are used to plump up cattle. New ingredients like "natural flavoring" (if it's natural, it needs no flavoring) are introduced on packages that aren't what you thought. Coal-burning power plants continue to belch potentially toxic metals capable of destroying our food, air and well-being.[13]

So do perfluorocarbons (PFCs), an entire class of toxins the government has taken little action on despite overwhelming evidence that they continue to poison us. The next time you hear a claim that Stainmaster,® Teflon,® or Gore-Tex® products are built to last, take it to heart. According to a report by the EWG, they never degrade. If so, your children and your grandchildren will continue to be exposed to these potentially deadly contaminants through our food, air, and water—forever.[14]

The EPA finally took action against a maker who used one such chemical, known as PFO (as the active ingredient), in their Scotch-gard™ fabric repellent. Three makers now use another chemical called PFBS. It also lasts *forever*; and *never* breaks down, though studies indicate they're not toxic.

But big business needn't worry. There's no shortage of other toxic, slippery, indestructible perfluorochemicals. When they say Teflon never sticks, they aren't kidding. While Teflon itself is not pentadecafluorooctanoic acid (PFOA), PFOA is used to produce it. It's released in the air along with other chemicals when you heat it to broiling temperatures. Today it's estimated to be in the blood of 90 percent of all Americans. It also never breaks down. But its makers can also rest easy—it would appear that it was completely legal for them to fill our air and waterways with all the PFCs and other indestructible materials they wish, because it's *unregulated*.

But there's some good news on the horizon. Studies have shown that the benefits of Omega-3 fatty acids in fish can be *safely* taken in *far* greater concentration, virtually free of the toxins found in fish. This supplement gets there through a process of mild distillation. Makers refer to this product as *pharmaceutical* grade fish oil, but there's no regulation that enforces this distinction. There are pure, concentrated products from reputable companies that can indeed help us heal. Of course, Omega-3s are available from other animal foods such as grass-fed beef and free-range turkey. They're also found in walnuts and flaxseed, although in lesser concentrations. So, the question remains, why eat fish? If you love fish as much as I do, then keep eating it—but not the farmed or man-handled versions. There are other healthier, powerful, natural alternatives.

ALASKAN WILD RED SOCKEYE SALMON

Fish without hazardous levels of mercury and PCB's? Yes, there is such a thing. You can still eat fish and enjoy their great health building attributes. However, it generally costs more to eat *real* fish and other high-quality proteins today. But in the end, it will cost you far more if you don't.

Wild fish are uniquely colorful, brimming with robust natural flavor. You'll see and taste the difference. If you've never eaten real Alaskan red, wild, sockeye salmon from an unpolluted river you're in for a real treat. Containing an average of 1.2 to 1.3 grams of eicosapentaenoic acid (EPA) and docosahexaenoic acid (DHA) (totaling a whopping 2.5 grams of Omega-3 fatty acids in one 3.5 ounce serving), these fish have important bragging rights.

Some companies that ship wild red Alaskan salmon packed in ice and delivered to your door step from Alaska's Copper River are Vital Choice® (www.RKInformedLiving.com) and Northwest Seafood (www.northwest-seafood.com). Costco® now offers Alaskan Wild Salmon at a reasonable price. Vital Choice also offers wild halibut and tuna, but they contain a smaller amount of important Omega-3s. Their lab analysis shows that both are also relatively toxin free. Northwest Seafood also features Alaskan king crab legs.

Pharmaceutical grade fish oil, which you'll learn more about in Chapter 3, can provide many times the Omega-3 fatty acids than you can obtain from eating three meals a week of fish, with virtually no toxicity. But I eat both the wild-caught salmon as well as pharmaceutical grade fish oil. While more research is required, there appears to be other yet-to-be-determined mechanisms in fish that work to heal us.

An analysis of the current research indicates that the protection provided by Omega-3 fats comes from the DHA and/or the EPA found in fish oil. In several leading studies showing the merit of this fat, fish oil supplements were the only source. In other research, such as the landmark DART heart study, participants were able to select between fish oil supplements or fish itself. The American Heart Association's latest recommendations suggest we eat two servings of fatty fish a week. This alone is roughly twice the small amount eaten by the average American. Research by Dr. Barry Sears and others show that even greater benefit can accrue to those who supplement with far greater amounts of Omega-3 fish oil to combat certain conditions.

Personally, I supplement with more than 7 grams a day of pharmaceutical grade fish oil. This is in addition to my regular consumption of Alaskan wild red salmon and other foods rich in Omega-3 fats, such as grass-fed beef and walnuts. While this is greater than the amount required to *maintain* good health, the benefits appear to be well worth it. According to Dr. Sears, 5 to 10 grams are recommended based on his own research to optimize *normal* health and reduce chronic inflammation, the cause of most chronic disease. The Harvard Medical school study for bipolar depression observed amazing results when their volunteers had an average of 10 grams of Omega-3s a day.

There are several well-educated people with strong voices that *do* speak out on our behalf and they deserve our thanks, including California's State Attorney General Bill Lockyer. He sued California grocers under the state's anti-toxin laws. Lockyer charged them with violating California's Proposition 65 for their failure to properly label the mercury content in certain types of fish. As a result of his actions, several grocers have each agreed to post warnings at their fish counters.

Isn't it time for each of us to take responsibility for our own health? Are we willing to pay a higher price for eating healthier now, or face a far greater cost for not doing so later?

INDUSTRIALIZED PROTEIN AND ANTIBIOTIC RESISTANCE

By now you know there's a common ground among all industrialized animal sources of protein. Confining creatures such as chickens and other sources of protein in overcrowded environments is brutal stuff. But the big guys have figured out how to deal with poultry when their practice, by its nature, provokes them to.

When fighting breaks out, some ranchers cut their toes and beaks off without analgesics. Their chickens also never, or rarely, breathe fresh air. They spend their days inhaling ammonia and airborne infectious bacteria while feeding, at least in part, on antibiotics and petroleum distillates. Our government appears to allow large feedlot owners to do whatever it takes, which is nothing short of shameful. Research has shown that our overuse of antibiotics is creating a subculture of resistant bacteria, which threatens our ability to fight a number of menacing infections. Bacteria who, like people, do what they can to survive a good fight. Research shows a direct correlation between the antibiotics used to protect our poultry and livestock from infection, and increased antibiotic resistance in humans. Again, *you* are what you eat *ate*.

When feedlot chickens grow ill, potentially infecting tens of thousands of other imprisoned hens in *battle cages,* gallons of antibiotics such as enrofloxacin are often poured into their water supply—presenting a clear and present danger to not only the chickens. Christine Gorman's (Time V.159, N.3 21jan02) excellent article, "Playing Chicken with our Antibiotics Over Treatment," discusses the potential health hazards this creates in your life. When the chickens stop coughing, a different strain of bacteria quietly breeds in their intestines. While causing no *visible* problem in the chickens, this strain of bacteria, known as *Campylobacter,* multiplies like wildfire. When we eat industrialized chicken, it may contaminate the genetic material in our tissue; these bacteria enable themselves to resist enrofloxacin (the animal version of Cipro). You may recall a good deal of press about Cipro. Not long ago, it received much attention as the oral antibiotic of choice for the treatment of Anthrax. Both the animal version and the human version are produced by Bayer AG of Wisconsin. The former is so similar to the human version that bacteria resistance to one frequently spells resistance to the *other.* The implications for human beings are staggering. As resistant bacteria are produced at record rates, our options for fighting off infectious disease have become increasingly limited. At this rate, it's likely that a day will soon come when Cipro will be a worthless ally in our fight against Anthrax.

According to the Union of Concerned Scientists ("Hogging It: Estimates of Antimicrobial Abuse in Livestock"), 70 percent of all antibiotics used in this country are fed to formerly healthy animals on feedlots. That's eight times more than are given to humans (25 million pounds versus 3 million pounds). According to a report by the Environmental Defense Organization ("Resistant Bugs and Antibiotic Drugs, State and County estimated use of Antibiotics in

Agricultural Feed and Animal Waste"), two states, North Carolina and Iowa, are each estimated to use 3 million pounds of antibiotics as feed additives annually. That's more than the amount used for the medical treatment of human beings nationally—and its use is growing.

And so are big feedlot operations, which are either buying small, family run farms or putting them out of business. According to a report by the Center for Agricultural and Rural Development Ames ("Living with Hogs in Iowa: The Impact of Livestock Facilities on Rural Residential Property Values," August 2003), researchers note that "in 1980, approximately 65,000 farmers in the state raised hogs, with an average of 200 hogs residing on each farm. In 2002, the number of farms with hogs had fallen to about 10,000, and the average number of hogs per farm had risen to over 1,400."

The Centers for Disease Control and Prevention (CDC) report that every significant bacterial infection in the world is showing resistance to the most commonly prescribed antibiotic treatments. Diseases ranging from staff to bone infection show increasing resistance to methicillin, our first weapon of defense used against them.

My brother-in-law, Dr. Kim Morgan, a well-known California pediatrician, explains that MRSA (methicillin resistant staphylococcal aureus) is now extremely common in the United States due to our use and abuse of antibiotics. As a result, *traditional* antibiotics provide no protection against this heinous organism that creates skin abscesses and infection in deep tissue and bone. MRSA's ability to rapidly induce resistance requires that physicians use *different* antibiotics in treating their patients. It's succeeded in genetically altering its susceptibility, and has now passed this trait on to its progeny.

In more than one third of the reported cases of salmonella poisoning in 1997, the bacteria were resistant to five different antibiotics currently used to treat it. While the rates of salmonella found in random checks of food carcasses vary, those I've reviewed are unsettling. Not all cases are reported, but experts estimate between almost 700,000 to nearly 4 million cases occur annually. The true number of cases is likely to be far greater.

Antibiotic resistance is spreading *fast*. **Each year, approximately one and a half chickens are killed for every man, woman, and child on earth.** According to the Animal Legal and Historic Center at Michigan State University, that amounts to approximately *8.7 billion* chickens a year, many of them subjected to antibiotics. These resistant bacteria are very quietly infiltrating our lives. With all the resistant bacteria we eat in our food, and antibiotics we use needlessly for colds and viral infections, the percentage of people unable to fight off certain infectious disease is rapidly growing. It's a horror story that's been frequently censored, because some companies and special interest groups fight the FDA to protect their product and profits at your expense.

IN MORE THAN ONE THIRD OF THE REPORTED CASES OF SALMONELLA POISONING IN 1997, THE BACTERIA WERE RESISTANT TO FIVE DIFFERENT ANTIBIOTICS CURRENTLY USED TO TREAT IT.

This story has a familiar ring to it. The forerunner of the company we know today as aspirin maker AG Bayer also has a long history of putting humanity on the chopping block. It's the same company that invented chemical warfare by introducing moisture gas in World War I.[15, 16, 17] IG Farben was accused of aiding the Third Reich, by promoting slave labor and exposing humans to unproven vaccines.[17A] A sister company, Degesh, a subsidiary of IG Farben, reportedly manufactured the poison gas used in Hitler's gas chambers. After the war, the conglomerate was divided up after the conviction of several IG Farben executives for war crimes.

While some companies such as Tyson discontinued the use of arsenic, the practice of using toxins such as this in the production of our food continues elsewhere. According to scientists from the USDA: "Land disposal of animal manure could also introduce pharmaceuticals in surface water." According to a study published in the *New England Journal of Medicine* (October, 2001, Volume 345: 1161-1166, Number 16), "The ingestion of resistant *E. faecium* of animal origin leads to detectable concentrations of the resistant strain in stools for up to 14 days after ingestion. The organisms survive gastric passage and multiply."

As mentioned, arsenic is yet another approved supplement in chicken feed. While the government has established allowable limits for arsenic use in grain-based animal food, they haven't updated them in some time. But the average American's consumption of chicken has risen from 32 pounds to 81 pounds a year since the late 1960s. And the upshot? Tamar Laksky, an epidemiologist at the National Institute of Health (NIH), and her associates at the Food Safety and Inspection Service (FSIS) of the Department of Agriculture report: "If you're eating more than 2 ounces a day, you're eating more arsenic than previously forecasted. Certain groups found to eat even larger amounts of chicken were ingesting ten times the amount of arsenic than we had thought. Will the government take this increased consumption into account and raise the allowable level for safety?"

Because there are many other sources of this toxin in our air and water, fish (particularly bottom feeders like crab), some powdered kelp, and even vegetables sprayed with pesticide containing lead arsenate, why does the government believe legislation of an *allowable* level for one particular food source will protect us?

LABELING: THE TRUE MEANING OF THE WORDS

What do these words really mean? Doesn't the pasteurization process denature our food? Won't high heat kill potential contaminants *as well* as natural nutrients? Isn't milk fortified to add back synthetic versions of the natural vitamins, minerals, and enzymes lost in this process?

Pasteurized chicken is not boiled or heated the way pasteurized milk is. The term "pasteurized" used in this context simply indicates they're raised on sweet wild grasses and bugs on a *pasture*, as nature intended. Unlike cows, chickens are not ruminants and don't graze in the same way cattle do. So, unlike our cattle, chickens are not made to subsist on a diet that's exclusively grass. If permitted to *roam freely* (a simple term that's also not what it appears to be as you'll soon see), 30 percent of a chicken's caloric intake would come from living grasses. And pasteurizing allows birds to have access to just that.

So, it's important that you understand the meaning of labels. What does "Hormone Free" mean? The USDA doesn't allow hormones to be used by farmers on poultry. It's illegal. But as we have learned, it is not illegal to use them to fatten cattle. So, when a label states that no hormones are used, it's just another example of a food giant spinning a truism into altruism.

How about the term "Free Range"? To qualify, the rancher just has to demonstrate to the USDA that they *permitted access* to the outside. The FDA doesn't even dictate the amount of access that's required for them to make this claim. This means producers can legally use the term "free range," even if they do no more than lift the cage door a few minutes each day.

You need to know what's going on down on the farm. When you consider the importance of food in our lives, getting to know your local farmer might be well worth the effort. Farmers' markets are a great place to start. If they raise poultry in what are called "chicken tractors," ask if these pens are being moved around *continuously* to take advantage of natural vegetation. The USDA's definitions may be more harmful than helpful; since all a producer need do is keep the food and water in the hen house, and just lift up the door. If the hen stays put they comply. Be careful of labels that may mean little more than snake oil endorsements. Be certain that their feed is 100 percent organic, as well as pesticide, hormone, and antibiotic free.

Several chicken farmers make products easily available that meet these requirements. Your best bet is to find a producer near you. One producer, Grass Fed Traditions™, offers pasteurized organic poultry fed with organic grain they developed containing coconut pulp (and no soy). Blackwing Quality Meats makes an important distinction between "100 percent organic" and simply "organic."

The word "Organic" means the product comes from ingredients that are at least 90 percent organic, while 100 percent means 100 percent. While a number of suppliers say they use organic grain or soy as the primary source of protein in their mix, I prefer Grass Fed Traditions formula. According to the company, their chickens contain lauric acid–found in coconut oil and human breast milk. It's the primary (healthy) saturated fatty acid found in coconut oil, purported to have important antimicrobial and anti-inflammatory properties. According to the company, *"All natural"* really means *"no additives"* and is based on testimony of the producer.

EGGS

The egg is one of the greatest sources of protein on the planet. For only a few cents, we receive almost 6.5 grams of perfect protein, with all the essential amino acids we require. We also get thirteen essential vitamins, including folate, zinc, and vitamins A and E. Just one egg packs enough vitamin B_{12} to provide almost 87 percent of the average adult's daily requirement. No wonder Americans eat more than 26 million eggs a day; that's enough to go from here to the moon if strung together (almost 10 billion eggs a year)!

In 1972, dietary recommendations urged us to limit our egg consumption to as little as two eggs per week. Those with high cholesterol levels were cautioned to completely avoid them. But why? There's no evidence to support this. After all these years, no study has solidly linked any increase in dietary cholesterol to a corresponding increase in blood serum cholesterol—none. To the contrary, studies have shown eggs balance the inflammatory ratio of HDL to LDL. Apparently, eggs have an anti-inflammatory action independent of their dietary cholesterol. One of the few natural food sources of vitamin D, eggs are chock full of lecithin, a natural emulsifier. They're also a major source of choline, which aids the body in the digestion of fat.

Contrary to popular opinion, eating eggs is heart healthy. Harvard scientists followed the diet of 117,000 public health officials and nurses for several years, and found no significant difference in the rates of non-fatal myocardial infarction, stroke, and coronary heart disease, between those consumers eating one egg per week versus those eating many more. When researchers compared a smaller subset group of those eating more than two eggs per day to those who *never* ate them, there was *no* correlated increase in total cholesterol levels. In "Nutritional Contribution of Eggs to American Diets" (*Journal of the American College of Nutrition,* Volume 19, No. 90005, 556S-562S, 2000), Won O. Song, PhD, M.P.H., R.D., and Jean M. Kerver, M.S., R.D., Michigan State University's Food Science and Human Nutrition Department, reported that people who ate up to three eggs a day enjoyed a *more favorable* cholesterol ratio than those who ate fewer than one egg per day. "No corresponding increase in blood serum cholesterol was found in those eating a large number of eggs on a regular basis. In fact those eating four eggs or more a week showed notable *improvement* in their total cholesterol level." And the scientists continued: "Since eggs are a source of dietary fat and cholesterol, this suggests that egg consumption should be reduced or avoided. Results of our study refute this hypothesis.

The fact that serum cholesterol levels were inversely related to egg consumption supports results of epidemiological studies that show that serum cholesterol levels are not directly related to dietary cholesterol levels. This may explain why increased egg consumption has not been linked to increased risk of CVD." The researchers concluded: "Results of our study indicate that eggs make important nutritional contributions to the American diet, and frequent egg consumption does not associate adversely with serum cholesterol concentrations. Our work repudiates the hypothesis that increased egg consumption leads to increased serum cholesterol concentrations and also adds to the growing body of literature that supports the nutritional benefits of eggs. Although our results suggest that higher egg consumption is associated with lower serum cholesterol, this study should not be used as a basis for recommending higher egg consumption for regulation of serum cholesterol."

A number of other studies support these findings. In 2002, the *American Journal of Clinical Nutrition* reported the results of a study that introduced four egg yolks a week to the diet of 6-month-old infants being weaned. The researchers concluded that "supporting egg treatment had no significant effect on plasma cholesterol, hemoglobin, ferritin, and transferrin but did result in improvements in plasma iron and transferrin saturation compared with no egg treatment."

While eggs do contain 213 milligrams of dietary cholesterol (all in the yolk), there is no solid evidence linking their consumption to an increase in blood serum cholesterol level. Eating eggs, including the yolk, is one of the best things you can do for your health. In addition to their vitamins, minerals, and usable protein, eggs boast the two carotenoids, lutein and zeaxanthin, which have been found to reduce age-related macular degeneration (by up to 40 percent), while lowering the risk of cataracts by up to 20 percent. One of the few natural sources of lutein, with a higher content and far better absorption of this antioxidant than most fruits or vegetables, egg yolks may aid in the prevention of arteriosclerosis (already proven in mice). Elevated levels of lutein in the blood have also been shown to lower the risk of coronary heart disease in humans. In a study reported in the American Heart Association's *Circulation Journal* (103:2922, 2001), subjects with the highest blood levels of lutein had the least amount of thickening in the walls of their arteries.

> EATING EGGS, INCLUDING THE YOLK, IS ONE OF THE BEST THINGS YOU CAN DO FOR YOUR HEALTH.

Can eating eggs improve memory too? Choline is a precursor to acetylcholine, one of the most important chemicals involved in sustaining memory. In an article in the *Journal of the American College of Nutrition* (Volume 19, No. 90005, 528S-531S, 2000), entitled "Choline: Needed for Normal Development of Memory," Dr. Steven Zeisel touts eggs as one of the most important sources of important dietary choline available in our diet. Just one egg supplies almost half of the recommended amount of choline required daily. While there's a close correlation between an excessive intake of certain saturated fats and heart disease, eggs are relatively low in saturated fat. The average egg weighs 58 grams, with 1.6 grams of saturated fat in the yolk. Research shows that eating eggs, yolk and all, may actually help *prevent* heart disease in other ways.

According to the famed "Nurses Study," the blood's level of the amino acid homocysteine is a far more accurate tool to diagnose heart disease than one's total cholesterol *level*; *forty times* more predictive of coronary artery disease. You may wonder why your doctor may have not insisted you take this test? There's little money in prescribing a few vitamins that will correct this problem in just months. Adequate amounts of folic acid alone will get you most of the way there. And the test itself is expensive, because the average lab receives few requests for it. Expensive prescriptions, lucrative charges for office visits, and incentives by major pharmaceutical companies are stiff competition for what you truly require. It's another example of short-term thinking—keeping patients happy and living longer is more than just noble; it's good business as well. Extending a patient's life span builds a successful enterprise, long term.

Today, heart disease claims more lives than cancer, according to data from The National Center for Health Statistics as last reported in 2004 (with 652,486 deaths); closely followed by deaths from cancer (553,888). For those who care about such numbers, note that stroke is the number three killer (150,074 deaths annually). If the government were to track *cardiovascular disease* as a category, deaths from stroke and heart disease would total more than 800,000 a year. Simply maintaining the proper homocysteine level helps you avoid both types of cardiovascular disease (you'll learn the easiest way to do so in Chapter 2).

So what do eggs have to do with homocysteine? Eggs are one of only two animal proteins foods containing choline; the other is beef liver. This choline is derived from betaine, shown to have a powerful effect on reducing homocysteine levels—and eggs have a whopping 251 milligrams of betaine. Like anything else, eat them often but not in excess. Daily consumption can actually create an allergic reaction to egg eating. But eating one or two a day a few days a week is advisable. Dr. Robert Atkins (of Atkins diet fame), a medical pioneer years ahead of his time, wrote an article some time ago that I still recall today entitled "Eggs: The Yolks on You." A true visionary, he had the courage to speak out against the masses at a time that it was unfashionable to do so. He challenged the logic of avoiding this healthy protein. He was right, but few were listening.

It's good to eat eggs. But you may have guessed the rest—eating eggs from *conventionally* raised layer chickens is *not* a good alternative. Fortunately, healthier chickens grown humanely and without antibiotics are becoming more mainstream, and available at a store near you. They'll cost more than industrialized eggs and less than other sources of industrialized protein. If you eat two healthy eggs laid by healthy chicks four times a week, you're spending about 80 cents more weekly than you'd pay for the conventional version (isn't it sad that the word "conventional" is often associated with "tampered with" today?).

What are you getting for approximately 10 cents more per egg? Each pasteurized egg has almost 400 percent more Omega-3 fatty acids, significantly more folic acid, and vitamin B12, 40 percent more vitamin A, 10 percent *less* fat, and for what it's worth, almost 35 percent less cholesterol, and several times the amount of vitamin E. So, while the world is out there boycotting eggs, throwing away nutritious yolks, and dodging bullets from dietary cholesterol, those in the know will be eating the right eggs, yolk and all.

VEGETABLE PROTEIN

While vegetables are an excellent source of important amino acids, no one vegetable is a complete source of protein. Vegetarians *can* abstain from eating meat, and still receive the required amount of protein they need daily. But it's tough. Those who eat several helpings of mixed vegetables throughout the day are going in the right direction. Different vegetables contain different amino acids. Those who approach each day with planning and diligence can indeed achieve this goal. But how many people do so? Even if this could be practically achieved, and sustained, vegetarians would *not* receive the optimum level of certain nutrients without supplementation. A vegetarian diet is not healthful; though I believe the principle source of our diet should come from healthful carbohydrates, balanced with other Synergy of Super-Nutrient (SOS) foods.

Our friend Michael Mina opened up his Salata restaurant in Dallas, Texas, on September 7, 2007. This small but growing chain is one of our favorite places to eat, serving a broad and colorful array of hand-cut vegetables and natural dressings with no additives and preservatives. We saw Michael in Dallas at the end of 2007. He weighed 285 pounds at the time and vowed to embrace a new lifestyle. On January 1, Michael did just that, making a New Year's resolution to eat synergistically. He was going to eat the food he served his guests and truly walk the talk. We were blown away when we recently returned to eat at his restaurant. While the Synergy of Super-Nutrients Program provides *far* more options in foods (snacks and healthy desserts), Michael's diet *did* indeed qualify. Ten months later he looks like a far younger and healthier version of his former self. Incredibly, his ninety-three pound loss (he weighs 192 pounds at the time of this writing) was achieved without a single day of aerobic exercise (he owns three different gym memberships that remain unused)! Of course I stressed the importance of exercise and he committed to do so as well. Based on Michael's willpower, I expect he'll soon look like the next Lou Ferrigno®. His great balance of healthy carbohydrates, fat from nuts, dressing and other foods, and a good amount of protein helped Michael synergistically empower himself.

In his own words: "I felt better every day, my energy level went up, my sleep improved, my work ethic improved, my mind was sharper. Everything became better. I am at 192 right now and have only 12 pounds more to lose. Eating right has literally changed my life." According to Michael, "a typical salad contained a combination of carrots, spinach, greens, romaine (or Salata Mix, which is romaine, spring mix, and cabbage), sprouts, and more. I would typically put 5–7 vegetables in the salad, which made up about 2/3 of my plate, and a small amount of healthy protein. To that I added a small amount of extra virgin olive oil, a tad of natural salad dressing like our ginger lime, almonds or walnuts, and healthy protein like chicken, shrimp, or salmon. I ate this consistently, every day, all week, throughout the weekend. Day in, day out; as the months passed I was losing more and more weight."

> "I FELT BETTER EVERYDAY, MY ENERGY LEVEL WENT UP, MY SLEEP IMPROVED, MY WORK ETHIC IMPROVED, MY MIND WAS SHARPER."

But there's one vegetable that many regard as the king of all protein foods. According to Dean Houghton, writing for Furrow 2, a magazine published by John Deere, we are asked to dream the impossible dream: "Just imagine you could grow the perfect food. This food not only would provide affordable nutrition, but also would be delicious and easy to prepare in a variety of ways. It would be a healthful food, with no saturated fat. In fact, you would be growing a virtual fountain of youth on your back forty. This ideal food would help prevent, and perhaps reverse, some of the world's most dreaded diseases. You could grow this miracle crop in a variety of soils and climates. Its cultivation would build up, not deplete, the land ... this miracle food already exists ... It's called soy."

Made from beans, soy has given birth to a host of fermented and non-fermented by-products. Dr. Andrew Weil is a big proponent of soy and joins a long list of leading authorities who tout soy as the next coming. Many encourage us to add substantially more of this miraculous miracle food as a percentage of our daily protein requirement. In his bestselling book, *Eating Well for Optimum Health: The Essential Guide to Bringing Health and Pleasure Back to Eating* (HarperCollins, 2001), Dr. Weil discussed the *evidence* of soy's health protective benefits: low rates of breast cancer, menopausal problems, and prostate cancer in populations with increased consumption of soy.

What are those populations? According to a large survey conducted in 1930s, 1.5 percent of calories in the Chinese diet came from the consumption of soy, while 65 percent came from the consumption of pork, according to K. C. Chan, editor of *Food in Chinese Culture*. Are we forced to conclude there was a lower incidence of cancers in populations with a higher than normal intake of pork?

The respected Cornell China Study (*American Journal of Cardiology*, 1998) determined that the average woman in China eats only about 9 grams of soy or approximately two teaspoons a day. An annual health survey of Takayama City, Japan, found that Japanese men ate only 5 grams a day and women ate 4 grams a day, which is hardly the 50 to 60 grams a day of daily protein intake we require.

Based on these findings should we start eating oodles of pork? Perhaps we should—particularly if these populations are enjoying lower rates of breast cancer, prostate cancer, and post-menopausal problems as suggested. But, these same populations have a far higher rate of liver, stomach, pancreatic, and thyroid cancer. If soy is the cause-and-effect mechanism that we're told it is, then the evidence would suggest we avoid it.

But it gets worse—strong evidence suggests that soy consumption *leads* to far higher rates of breast and thyroid cancers and other chronic diseases. Crediting soy for curbing breast and prostate cancer without linking it to higher rates of other cancers is misinformed. Certain individuals appear to be at particular risk from eating soy products. Studies show a positive correlation between increased soy consumption and dementia, and for the premature development of breasts and pubic hair in young females before the age of five.

While acknowledging the uncertain effect of soy's phytoestrogens and its potential to interact with prescribed hormones and drugs, Dr. Weil reiterates his recommendation that "the benefits of soy far outweigh the risk." But the information I reviewed suggests otherwise. We've already discovered how some commercially produced protein foods are denatured and combined to the point of posing risk. Certain soybean products may be as well. Like rice, modern industry begins with a known product that once occurred naturally. And if not adding hormones and antibiotics, then high-volume processing plants may add chemicals to increase yield and reduce the time required to produce their versions of these foods. In many instances, what we end up with bears little resemblance to what you thought you were eating. This lack of truthful disclosure appears to be acceptable to most governments throughout the world. Some who take staunch positions with big pharma appear far more tolerant of the major food processors. Drug companies must list the potential side effects and potentially adverse interaction we might encounter through the use of their products. But food companies aren't required to play by these rules. This lack of mandated disclosure is disgraceful—and revealing the process is just as important as disclosing their ingredients.

According to government toxicology experts Doctors Daniel Sheehan and Daniel Dorge, soy isoflavones may be toxic to estrogen-sensitive tissue. Potential risks include abnormal brain and reproductive tract development in developing fetus's. On the other hand, several studies tout the benefits of soy's phytoestrogens. Perhaps that's why these researchers refer to soy as "a two headed sword." So ask yourself this. Would you want your child drinking estrogen? Or your pregnant daughter? While a meta-analysis of 38 controlled clinical trials that appeared in the New England Journal of Medicine found that subjects who replaced animal protein in their diet with soy protein had a positive effect on their blood lipid profile, does that mean eating soy is healthful? Or, that eating commercially fattened feedlot protein is harmful? While you wouldn't knowingly feed your child altered food, if you're feeding your child highly processed soy milk, you may be doing just that. Some producers mix it with other things to get it to look right. In order to rid the soybean of its fiber due to its "mushiness", soy may be mixed with an alkaline solution. Then further separated using an acid wash. If this acid wash is done in aluminum tanks as it often is, this mush or slurry might be loaded with large amounts of aluminum. Nitrites often form during the spraying process, and Lysinoalanine during the alkaline process. Other additives, such as MSG, may be thrown in for flavor. We're led to believe we're eating a miracle food. Again, you be the judge.

Dr. Weil states that "many brands of soy milk on the market are good." For the purposes of our discussion, a little bit of history is in order. In "Tragedy and Hype" (extracted from *Nexus* magazine), researchers Sally Fallon and Mary Enig, PhDs, separate the myth from the legend. Not all that many decades ago, during the time of the Chou Dynasty, even the Chinese felt that soybeans were not to be eaten. Regarded as a sacred grain with strong roots, its most admirable quality was to help fix nitrogen when used in crop rotation. Some time later the means to "ferment" this noble bean was discovered. Prior to that time, the Chinese were concerned about the potential dangers of soy. Full of phytic acid, critics suggest that soy grossly hinders the absorption of important, essential minerals in the intestinal tract such as copper, zinc, iron, calcium, and magnesium—and that soy is loaded with it. Those living in countries with diets high in grain and soy show profound deficiencies of these minerals. Only *very long* periods of fermentation can significantly *diminish* the deteriorating effects of phytic acid, but still not eliminate it. Phytic acid can remain to serve as a potent mineral uptake blocker. And of all of its cousins in the legume world, soybeans boast the highest levels of phytic acid. Yet, leading world trade health organizations are doing everything possible to usher in the use and acceptance of soy protein. Its cost is low and it's readily available. While soy is being touted as a cheap cure for malnutrition, critics argue the reverse is true. Are we malnourishing those we seek to nourish by feeding them a food that hinders the absorption of important nutrients they require? Even when these blocked minerals are made present in the diet, consumption of certain soy and grains can prevent their adequate uptake.

Some suggest that soy's anti-nutrients or natural toxins also inhibit the digestion of the protein itself, blocking the digestion of crucial enzymes such as trypsin. For this reason, some researchers are convinced that the introduction of soy in third-world countries, like Africa, has led to an increase in malnutrition, malabsorption of nutrients, and cancers; particularly those of the liver and pancreas.

SOME SUGGEST THAT SOY'S ANTI-NUTRIENTS OR NATURAL TOXINS ALSO INHIBIT THE DIGESTION OF THE PROTEIN ITSELF, BLOCKING THE DIGESTION OF CRUCIAL ENZYMES SUCH AS TRYPSIN.

Minerals also require fat-soluble vitamins such as A and D to activate their absorption. Soy lacks these important catalysts. The presence of these nutrients is essential to properly absorb water-soluble vitamins, so essential to many in third-world countries. But the lure of an abundant, easily available, inexpensive protein proved too hard to resist. Has its introduction only served to exacerbate the problems it was promoted to solve? Because soy-based products are quickly replacing animal foods in many countries, the only available source of these critical "lost" nutrients may be plant carotenes and sunshine. Other sources of protein are scarce or not affordable. Even in our own country, these sources are insufficient to supply the amount we require. The consumption of soy products actually increases the need for these nutrients. These important fat-soluble catalysts can be found in the high-quality animal proteins that you've learned about -and in butter. This may also explain why vegetarians who depend on soy as their primary source of protein are often deficient in some of these nutrients.

Critics further charge that soy's inhibitors block the adequate uptake of zinc. The brain can't develop or function properly without an adequate supply of zinc. Vital enzymes are unable to carry out important functions. Detractors also suggest that soybeans contain *growth* inhibitors that stunt the proper development of certain organs. In animal studies, soy has been proven to lead to the loss of body weight and bone density. In humans, some argue that consumption may lead to inadequate development that can include deterioration of the brain.[18]

Soy also lacks the important amino acids cystine and methionine, as do other members of the pulse family. And the technique used to process most soy products denatures lysine. Researchers Smirga et al. (*The Journal of Nutrition*, December 2002), found that L-Lysine deficiency increases stress-induced anxiety in lab animals, while Mori Kawada and colleagues (*Journal of Physiological Behavior*, May 1991) showed that it reduced brain growth in lab animals.

In humans, L-Lysine has been shown to reduce stress and inhibit viral growth. It's used in the treatment of herpes, and other viral syndromes such as Chronic Fatigue Syndrome, Epstein-Barr virus, and more. Because lysine is an essential nutrient for optimal bone growth, a deficiency can lead to the type of skeletal deformity we see in people who are malnourished. Many soy products contain hemagglutinin, a clot promoting substance (and growth inhibitor) that causes red blood cells to clot.

As a side note, the book and movie *Jurassic Park* showed cloned dinosaurs that had been genetically altered to stop producing lysine. Scientists had done so to force them to remain on the Island, depending on the veterinary staff to receive supplements of this important amino acid. In reality, lysine is an *essential* amino acid which vertebrates can't produce. It's also unlikely a dinosaur would recognize what "essential" amino acid they lacked in their diet!

Macarulla et al. ("The Effects of the Whole Seed and a Protein isolate of Faba Bean," *British Journal of Nutrition*, 2001, vol. 85, no5, pp. 607-614) discussed the findings of their study. Fava beans, another legume hailed as a cheap miracle food, were given to animals as their chief source of protein. The animals experienced adverse hormonal changes, retarded growth of muscle mass, and decreased ability to gain weight, preventing widespread use of this legume for animal feed.

SILVER BULLET OR BLANK?

Research shows the clear and depressing effects of soy's goiterans on the proper function of the thyroid and debilitating effects on existing thyroid conditions in women. If further research supports these findings, why would we want to feed our babies soy milk? Some soy milk has also been found to contain 100 times the amount of *aluminum* found in unprocessed milk, and 10 times the amount of aluminum found in milk based formula[26]. All infants should drink breast milk. Its protective anti-viral agents, super-charge your child's immunity, reducing their risk for disease, from cancer to asthma, while increasing their intelligence. If you can't nurse, arrange for milk from a healthy mom or from a milk bank near you. At the time of this writing, Israel and other progressive nations are strongly considering a ban on soy in infant formula.If hindering the uptake of important vitamins and minerals (especially the absorption of zinc, which plays a key role in reproduction, and the blood sugar mechanism controlling diabetes) wasn't enough, detractors allege that babies consume large amounts of aluminum through the wholesale consumption of soy. Among other things, a large level of aluminum has been found to be a common thread in the brains of Alzheimer's patients. Many believe it to be a key factor in developing this disease. Aluminum, like mercury, can't be destroyed. It can only change form. So it's basically *in* us, like mercury, *forever.* According to the EPA, we're continually exposed to some degree of aluminum in our air, water, and soil. It's the most abundant metal in the earth's crust, making up about 8 percent of the surface. The mining of ore and the processing of coal-burning power plants (they emit many more toxins than just mercury) adds to the available amount of aluminum ultimately found inside of us.

But manufacturers continue to find new ways to add aluminum to our diet. You can find it in new, "cutting edge" consumer products such as certain antacids, food additives, buffered aspirins (remember this the next time you take one for your heart!), antiperspirants, and now, soy milk. Soy formula is marketed for a *healthier baby*. It's easy to see why we're *Misinformed About Food.* If we must accept the fact that toxic metals such as aluminum and mercury that we've already eaten or otherwise absorbed will remain within us for our lifetime, shouldn't we support makers who have created formulas that reduce our exposure to this poison?

Instead, we've chosen to take the opposite approach. Thanks to approvals from the FDA, the skill of savvy marketing companies, and the opinions of many authorities, we appear to be on a mission to find new ways to add more of this rich source of aluminum to our diet. According to the critics, certain baby formulas, and more than a few childrens' school lunches, contain dangerously high levels of aluminum.

The public relations firms hired by some of the largest commercial soy makers have been enormously successful in introducing their products into the mainstream (in your food and your body). The FDA permits makers to market protein that contains a negligible amount of saturated fat, regardless of the methods used to produce them—and soy qualifies, making it easy for soy lobby groups to continue raising their clients' commercial bar higher. In addition to getting the government to approve the introduction of soy burgers and other soy products into our children's lunch programs, they've continued to find new and inventive ways to put soy in you and your children's diets.

The National Organization of Responsible Doctors has demanded that the U.S. Department of Agriculture allow *soy milk* in the school lunch programs subsidized by the agency. They claim to have made this recommendation to help those children who are allergic to cow's milk. Recommending water, almond milk, or coconut water may have made more sense; there are almost as many allergic reactions to soy milk as there are to cow's milk. But instead, these *responsible doctors* have recommended that our school kids start *drinking* what some suggest is an aluminum-rich liquid, complete with anti-nutrients, toxins, and the power to mimic estrogen.

It's possible that some people, even in light of the evidence, will be reluctant to let go of soy–the miracle food of the new generation. Marketing firms have discovered powerful ways to influence our belief system. You may *still* wonder if there's some truth to soy's much touted ability to prevent or defeat cancers. What about soy's magical isoflavonoids, credited with shrinking tumors, and even preventing their appearance? Actually, some evidence suggests that *fermented* versions of soy, such as tempeh, may have a favorable effect, but typically soy milk and tofu are not fermented. Instead, they are highly processed, heated, and pressurized. Drinking soy milk and non-fermented tofu to get the benefit of the isoflavonoids is like eating cow hoofs to get the benefits of their milk. The isoflavonoids are in a completely different form, known as beta-glycoside conjugates. In this configuration they have little ability to fight cancer. Soy's isoflavonoids and phytoestrogens mimic the effect of estrogen in humans. Classifying soy as a nutritional substance means that it's now unregulated. Unlike estrogen administered by your doctor, anyone of any age can put as much of these estrogen mimicking substances in their body as often as they wish.

In a most unusual move, two of the FDA's own leading researchers wrote a letter to the agency in 1999, citing similar, alarming data and asking that the agency reconsider their opinion. After all, soy has not been granted GRAS (Generally Regarded As Safe) status—shocking, considering its widespread use. The following was written by the FDA experts to their own agency:

DEPARTMENT OF HEALTH and HUMAN SERVICES
Public Health Service
Food and Drug Administration
National Center For Toxicological Research
Jefferson, Ark. 72079-9502

Daniel M. Sheehan, PhD
Director, Estrogen Base Program
Division of Genetic and Reproductive Toxicology
and Daniel R. Doerge, PhD, Division of Biochemical Toxicology

February 18, 1999
Dockets Management Branch (HFA-305)
Food and Drug Administration
Rockville, MD 20852
To whom it may concern,

We are writing in reference to Docket # 98P-0683; "Food Labeling: Health Claims; Soy Protein and Coronary Heart Disease." We oppose this health claim because there is abundant evidence that some of the isoflavones found in soy, including genistein and equal, a metabolize of daidzen, demonstrate toxicity in estrogen sensitive tissues and in the thyroid. This is true for a number of species, including humans. Additionally, the adverse effects in humans occur in several tissues and, apparently, by several distinct mechanisms.

Genistein is clearly estrogenic; it possesses the chemical structural features necessary for estrogenic activity (Sheehan and Medlock, 1995; Tong, et al., 1997; Miksicek, 1998) and induces estrogenic responses in developing and adult animals and in adult humans. In rodents, equal is estrogenic and acts as an estrogenic endocrine disruptor during development (Medlock, et al., 1995a,b). Faber and Hughes (1993) showed alterations in LH regulation following developmental treatment with genistein. Thus, during pregnancy in humans, isoflavones per se could be a risk factor for abnormal brain and reproductive tract development. Furthermore, pregnant Rhesus monkeys fed genistein had serum estradiol levels 50 to 100 percent higher than the controls in three different areas of the maternal circulation (Harrison et al., 1998). Given that the Rhesus monkey is the best experimental model for humans, and that a women's own estrogens are a very significant risk factor for breast cancer, it is unreasonable to approve the health claim until complete safety studies of soy protein are conducted. Of equally grave concern is the finding that the fetuses of genistein fed monkeys had a 70 percent higher serum estradiol level than did the controls (Harrison et al., 1998). Development is recognized as the most sensitive life stage for estrogen toxicity because of the indisputable evidence of a very wide variety of frank malformations and serious functional deficits in experimental animals and humans. In the human population, DES exposure stands as a prime example of adverse estrogenic effects during development. About 50 percent of the female offspring and a smaller fraction of male offspring displayed one or more malformations in the reproductive tract, as well as a lower prevalence (about 1 in a thousand) of malignancies. In adults, genistein could be a risk factor for a number of estrogen-associated diseases.

Even without the evidence of elevated serum estradiol levels in Rhesus fetuses, potency and dose differences between DES and the soy isoflavones do not provide any assurance that the soy protein isoflavones per se will be without adverse effects. First, calculations, based on the literature, show that doses of soy protein isoflavones used in clinical trials which demonstrated estrogenic effects were as potent as low but active doses of DES in Rhesus monkeys (Sheehan, unpublished data). Second, we have recently shown that estradiol shows no threshold in an extremely large dose-response experiment (Sheehan et al., 1999), and we subsequently have found 31 dose-response curves for hormone-mimicking chemicals that also fail to show a threshold (Sheehan, 1998a). Our conclusions are that no dose is without risk; the extent of risk is simply a function of dose. These two features support and extend the conclusion that it is inappropriate to allow health claims for soy protein isolate.

Additionally, isoflavones are inhibitors of the thyroid peroxidase which makes T3 and T4. Inhibition can be expected to generate thyroid abnormalities, including goiter and autoimmune thyroiditis. There exists a significant body of animal data that demonstrates goitrogenic and even carcinogenic effects of soy products (cf., Kimura et al., 1976). Moreover, there are significant reports of goitrogenic effects from soy consumption in human infants (cf., Van Wyk et al., 1959; Hydovitz, 1960; Shepard et al., 1960; Pinchers et al., 1965; Chorazy et al., 1995) and adults (McCarrison, 1933; Ishizuki, et al., 1991). Recently, we have identified genistein and daidzein as the goitrogenic isoflavonoid components of soy and defined the mechanisms for inhibition of thyroid peroxidase (TPO)-catalyzed thyroid hormone synthesis in vitro (Divi et al., 1997; Divi et al., 1996). The observed suicide inactivation of TPO by isoflavones, through covalent binding to TPO, raises the possibility of neoantigen formation and because anti-TPO is the principal autoantibody present in autoimmune thyroid disease. This hypothetical mechanism is consistent with the reports of Fort et al. (1986, 1990) of a doubling of risk for autoimmune thyroiditis in children who had received soy formulas as infants compared to infants receiving other forms of milk.

The serum levels of isoflavones in infants receiving soy formula are about five times higher than in women receiving soy supplements who show menstrual cycle disturbances, including an increased estradiol level in the follicular phase (Setchell et al., 1997). Assuming a dose-dependent risk, it is unreasonable to assert that the infant findings are irrelevant to adults who may consume smaller amounts of isoflavones. Additionally, while there is an unambiguous biological effect on menstrual cycle length (Cassidy et al., 1994), it is unclear whether the soy effects are beneficial or adverse. Furthermore, we need to be concerned about transplacental passage of isoflavones as the DES case has shown us that estrogens can pass the placenta. No such studies have been conducted with genistein in humans or primates. As all estrogens which have been studied carefully in human populations are two-edged swords in humans (Sheehan and Medlock, 1995; Sheehan, 1997), with both beneficial and adverse effects resulting from the administration of the same estrogen, it is likely that the same characteristic is shared by the isoflavones. The animal data is also consistent with adverse effects in humans.

Finally, initial data from a robust (7,000 men) long-term (30+ years) prospective epidemiological study in Hawaii showed that Alzheimer's disease prevalence in Hawaiian men was similar to European-ancestry Americans and to Japanese (White et al., 1996a). In contrast, vascular dementia prevalence is similar in Hawaii and Japan and both are higher than in European-ancestry Americans.

This suggests that common ancestry or environmental factors in Japan and Hawaii are responsible for the higher prevalence of vascular dementia in these locations. Subsequently, this same group showed a significant dose-dependent risk (up to 2.4 fold) for development of vascular dementia and brain atrophy from consumption of tofu, a soy product rich in isoflavones (White et al., 1996b). This finding is consistent with the environmental causation suggested from the earlier analysis, and provides evidence that soy (tofu) phytoestrogens causes vascular dementia. Given that estrogens are important for maintenance of brain function in women; that the male brain contains aromatase, the enzyme that converts testosterone to estradiol; and that isoflavones inhibit this enzymatic activity (Irvine, 1998), there is a mechanistic basis for the human findings. Given the great difficulty in discerning the relationship between exposures and long latency adverse effects in the human population (Sheehan, 1998b), and the potential mechanistic explanation for the epidemiological findings, this is an important study. It is one of the more robust, well-designed prospective epidemiological studies generally available. We rarely have such power in human studies, as well as a potential mechanism, and the results should be interpreted in this context.

Does the Asian experience provide us with reassurance that isoflavones are safe? A review of several examples lead to the conclusion: "Given the parallels with herbal medicines with respect to attitudes, monitoring deficiencies, and the general difficulty of detecting toxicities with long latencies, I am unconvinced that the long history of apparent safe use of soy products can provide confidence that they are indeed without risk" (Sheehan, 1998b).

It should also be noted that the claim on p. 62978 that soy protein foods are GRAS is in conflict with the recent return by CFSAN to Archer Daniels Midland of a petition for GRAS status for soy protein due to deficiencies in reporting adverse effects in the petition. Thus GRAS status has not been granted. Linda Kahl can provide you with details. It would seem appropriate for the FDA to speak with a single voice regarding soy protein isolate.

Taken together, the findings presented here are self-consistent and demonstrate that genistein and other isoflavones can have adverse effects in a variety of species, including humans. Animal studies are the front line in evaluating toxicity, as they predict, with good accuracy, adverse effects in humans. For the isoflavones, we additionally have evidence of two types of adverse effects in humans, despite the very few studies that have addressed this subject. While isoflavones may have beneficial effects at some ages or is some circumstances, this cannot be assumed to be true at all

ages. Isoflavones are like other estrogens in that they are two-edged swords, confer-
ring both benefits and risk (Sheehan and Medlock, 1995; Sheehan, 1997). The health
labeling of soy protein isolate for foods needs to consider just as would the addition
of any estrogen or goitrogen to foods, which are bad ideas.

Estrogenic and goitrogenic drugs are regulated by FDA, and are taken under
a physician's care. Patients are informed of risks, and are monitored by their physi-
cians for evidence of toxicity. There are no similar safeguards in place for foods,
so the public will be put at potential risk from soy isoflavones in soy protein isolate
without adequate warning and information.

Finally, NCTR is currently conducting a long-term multigenerational study of
genistein administered in feed to rats. The analysis of the dose range-finding studies
is near-complete or complete now. As preliminary data, which is still confidential,
maybe relevant to your decision, I suggest you contact Dr. Barry Delclos at the
address on the letterhead, or email him.

Sincerely,
Daniel M. Sheehan
Daniel R. Doerge
Enclosures
cc: Dr. Bernard Schwetz, Director, NCTR
Dr. Barry Delclos

Despite this, soy continues to be marketed as the miracle protein of the new
millennium. Is the FDA fighting for you?

MILK

Can it do the body bad?[19, 20, 21, 22, 23, 24] The research I reviewed raises important questions. Are the benefits real? You decide. We're told it's a great source of
calcium and that we are not getting enough calcium in our diet. Is this true? If so,
is drinking milk the best way for us to receive absorbable calcium? The American
dairy industry wants you to think so. Perhaps they convinced your parents, who
helped them to convince you? Are there other animals that drink milk after their
formative years? Do other species drink the milk of another kind? Does evidence
exist that milk helps builds bone *after* we've grown?

But why? We hear a good deal about our apparent chronic need for calcium.
But, does your body need more of the most abundant mineral in our body?
Can frequent consumption save us from the ravages of osteoporosis? Contrary

to the calcium myth, you can drink all the calcium you want until the cows come home, but you're not going to avoid osteoporosis. This condition is due to a deteriorated matrix of fibrous protein backbone. Getting enough calcium and other minerals before this condition occurs is helpful, but *after* your bones become brittle, it won't correct the problem. It's the foundation that held the brick and mortar of cartilage together that's deteriorated—and no matter how much building material your slather on it, there's no longer sufficient mass to support it. Estrogen replacement therapy has been used to slow or reverse bone remodeling. According to Russell T. Turner, PhD, and Jean D. Silbona of the Mayo Clinic Department of Orthopedics this "is the process by which small areas of bone are destroyed and rebuilt, and leads to an imbalance whereby bone resorption—the part of remodeling consisting of breaking down and assimilating—exceeds bone formation. Osteoporosis occurs when a person has an inadequate amount of bone to provide sufficient strength to perform normal daily activities. Osteoporosis usually is caused by a chronic imbalance in the bone remodeling cycle in which bone resorption is not adequately compensated for by subsequent bone formation."

The loss of estrogen occurs after a woman's child-bearing years. While it doesn't begin after menopause, it does accelerate. Woman who enjoy a healthy balanced diet, and engage in weight bearing exercise, limit their salt, sugar, and cola intake, rarely develop this condition. According to Turner and Silbona, in "Effects of Alcohol Use and Estrogen on Bone," women who drank moderately were found to have higher bone mass than those who abstained. The reverse is true for men. The researchers suggest two plausible explanations: "Alcohol could enhance estrogenic effects by increasing the circulating levels of the hormone or by increasing the number of estrogen receptors in bone cells. Alternatively, alcohol may act directly on bone cells to inhibit the initiation of bone remodeling, thereby reducing the total number of 'weak links' in the skeleton framework."

While osteoporosis has almost nothing to do with a calcium deficiency, there are several ways to prevent it, but drinking milk is not one of them. Neither milk nor other sources of calcium help to reverse it. While osteoporosis is not a reversible disease, slowing loss of bone mass is possible, and helps us prevent further attrition.

There is a disease that results from a lack of calcium. It's a condition known as osteomalacia, otherwise known as rickets, or a softening of the bones. It's primarily found in children, who are either malnourished or lack sufficient vitamin D. The best way to get this important vitamin is by enjoying 20 minutes of sunshine a day. When that's not possible (perhaps during the winter months), take cod liver oil. Skip the supplement on the days that you enjoy that sunshine. Rickets, thankfully, is rare today. It virtually disappeared after foods became fortified with vitamin D in the late 1950s. You cannot overdose on vitamin D from sunshine alone because your body regulates it. But you can overdose if you are also taking vitamin D from prescription retinol and other sources. Other healthy dietary sources that include vitamin D are wild Alaskan salmon, eggs, mushrooms (exposed to just 5 minutes of UV light after harvest), shrimp, baby calves livers, and other foods. Most multivitamins also contain 400 International Units (IUs) of vitamin D; twice the amount required in the latest RDA; which is light years away from the amount required to optimize our health (the ODA). So, why milk? Don't we need *some* tangible evidence that increasing our calcium consumption prevents osteoporosis? Actually, research suggests quite the opposite.

While it varies with age, the Dietary Reference recommendation of calcium for middle-age women in the United States is about 1000 milligrams; but their actual intake is approximately 744 milligrams. Yet, the hip fracture rate in the United States is more than twice that of this same age group in Japan, where the average intake of calcium is only 540 milligrams. In fact, Americans have one of the highest rates of osteoporosis in the world, despite our consumption of large amounts of calcium.

While adequate calcium intake is important, after a certain age rebuilding bone mass can't keep up with those factors affecting its loss. Taking more calcium does nothing to stave off osteoporosis. We need to identify and react to the factors responsible for a decrease in bone density and subsequent bone loss. But increasing our intake of calcium beyond 700 to 1000 milligrams a day has not been shown to improve it; a conclusion that's further supported by one of the largest longitudinal studies of its kind. After twelve years of research by Harvard University scientists studying 78,000 women, the *American Journal of Public Health* stated the following (June, 1997 Volume 87. Number 6): "Data indicates that frequent milk consumption and higher dietary calcium intakes in middle-age women do not provide protection against hip or forearm fractures ... Women consuming greater amounts of *calcium from dairy foods* had significantly *increased risk of hip fractures*, while no increase in fracture risk was observed for the same levels of calcium from nondairy sources." Does eating too much calcium-rich dairy food *increase* your chance of hip fracture? The *American Journal of Epidemiology* supports this same view (Volume 139, No. 5: 493-503, 1994; p. 139): "Consumption of dairy products, particularly at age 20, was associated with an increased risk of hip fractures ... Metabolism of dietary protein causes increased urinary excretion of calcium."

Not surprisingly, one of the chief culprits responsible for reduced bone density and leached calcium is the consumption of excessive amounts of protein. Salt and diets high in processed sugars such as high fructose corn syrup found in soft drinks and other foods further contributes to the leaching of calcium from your bones. Acid from both soft drinks and protein create internal stress that our body buffers by doing just that. Hormonal changes also occur (particularly a loss of estrogen), in post-menopausal women whose levels of this hormone were three times greater during their child-bearing years. Smoking and excessive drinking leach large amounts of calcium from bone. Regular exercise coupled with the reversal of any of the above reduces this loss and helps to protect bone structure from becoming further diminished.

> NOT SURPRISINGLY, ONE OF THE CHIEF CULPRITS RESPONSIBLE FOR REDUCED BONE DENSITY AND LEACHED CALCIUM IS THE CONSUMPTION OF EXCESSIVE AMOUNTS OF PROTEIN.

So, why do we need to drink milk? Other than effective marketing, what makes cow's milk a good source of calcium? Are cows born with more calcium than they physically need in order to sustain themselves? No, they ate it. Some animals are better at processing certain fats and other nutrients than others. Actually, all of our minerals have their origins in *soil*. Cattle, like other animal sources of protein get nutrients such as calcium from the plants they eat, which absorbed them from soil. So, the principle source of calcium for cattle comes from plants. We are capable of eating plants containing nutrients, such as calcium, that *we're* able to absorb. Then, why do we need milk to get calcium? We're literally surrounded by calcium. Our food is raining with it; particularly in our leafy vegetables and nuts. Two cups of broccoli contain as much calcium as a cup of milk. One tablespoon of sesame seeds eaten with the hull contains about 88 milligrams of calcium. Most nuts, vegetables, and certain healthy yogurts (such as Athena brand) are loaded with it. An independent lab measured the amount of vitamin D in a 3.5-ounce serving of Vital Choices' wild Alaskan sockeye salmon and found that it contained 687 IUs! One cup of *fortified* milk contains a paltry 98 IUs. But, is there any real danger in getting some of the calcium we need from milk?

Is milk a veritable cocktail of toxins? According to Robert Cohen, author of *Milk—The Deadly Poison* (Argus Publishing, 1998), milk is a dangerous brew of chemical, bacterial and biological agents. **Cohen suggests that every sip of milk contains 59 bioactive hormones.** Eighty percent of the protein in milk is casein. Casein is a binding agent used in glue and other adhesives and by body builders as an anti-catabolic that inhibits protein from breaking down in the body. It's also been identified as a hazardous substance to be avoided by those with autism. Apparently, their bodies are not capable of breaking it down. There's a high correlation between that inability and autism. Research has shown that some 70 percent of all children diagnosed with Autism Spectrum Disorder experience gastrointestinal problems. Studies by Parracho et al. (July 2005, *Journal of Medical Microbiology*), demonstrate that children with autism have different gut microflora than healthy children do. And, that stimulating more beneficial bacteria may modulate some of the symptoms of autism.

Dr. T. Colin Campbell, author of *The China Study*, found a connection between cancer and casein so powerful that researchers could easily turn **cancer** on and off like a light switch in lab animals; simply by altering their intake of casein. Industrialized milk is just another highly processed, potentially harmful animal food. But it doesn't stop here—bovine growth hormone (bGH) is produced naturally in cattle and controls the amount of milk they produce. But rBGH (the r stands for the recombinant version) is the artificial version that's synthetically derived. We inject this into dairy cattle to produce *more* milk than nature ever intended. Nature gives us plenty of this hormone when we are growing (when we need it most). Monsanto, who produces a synthetic recombinant version of controversial rbST (Recombinant Bovine Somatotropin), commercially known as Posilac, argues that the use of their artificial hormone doesn't change the quality of the milk produced by cows—and they're not alone. The American Veterinary Association, the FDA, and the WHO have issued statements agreeing with them. Canada and Europe however, have taken a strong stand and have completely banned the use of rBGH. America has distinguished itself as one of the few developed nations that sanctions its use.

The University of Chicago's Dr. Samuel Epstein believes that milk is contaminated with a vast array of carcinogens. In a petition to the FDA, he suggests that rBGH may increase udder infections by a whopping 79 percent. Infections often treated with antibiotics. Monsanto's clear statement on their label tells the real story: "Cows injected with Posilac are at an increased risk for clinical mastitis."[27]

While boning up with calcium (from milk) may make bones brittle, precipitate arteriosclerosis, cause cancer in lab animals, and contain 59 biologically active hormones and antibiotics, some people will still insist on drinking it. Those who wish to do so might be interested in a recent study published by the American Academy of Neurology (*Neurology*, 64:1047–1051, 2005). A team of researchers led by M. Park, MD, PhD, and colleagues designed a follow-up study to examine the effect of milk consumption on middle-age adults. Their findings were based on observations of dietary intake for 7,504 men, ages 45 to 68; from 1965 to 1968 data originally gathered in the Honolulu Heart Program. After 30 years of exhaustive follow-up study, this large group of distinguished scientists concluded that milk intake in midlife is directly correlated with an increased risk for Parkinson's disease.

Milk is also required to be pasteurized, which is the process of heating milk at a high temperature for a short period of time to destroy bacteria, viruses, protozoa, molds, and yeast. A practice that generally lasts for 10 to 14 seconds, destroying many of its important nutrients. Beneficial bacteria and all enzymes are also destroyed, that include phosphatase, essential for the proper absorption of calcium. It also destroys milk's *lipase* enzyme, essential for its proper digestion, as well as galactase, which we require to break down galactose. But this assault on milk and its nutrients is not enough for the FDA. Some bacteria and viruses *still* exist, so a new process of *super* pasteurization was introduced to make sure this food was completely dead. Now, it's heated up to a whopping 250 degrees. We're left with a manufactured cocktail, nearly void of enzymes and other important nutrients. This process is known as *fortification*. After they strip off the good stuff, synthetic nutrients such as vitamin D are thrown back in. We're left with a degraded white liquid with diminished value.

The FDA further requires that milk undergoes the process of *homogenization*. This requires the processors to break up the healthful fat found in the cream into minute particles that no longer separate from the milk that remains. Before this nutritionally worthless practice, people judged milk by the thickness of its cream. The thicker the better. A practice that took off in the 1950s, it now allows processors to save money by mixing grade B milk containing small amounts of cream on top with more costly grade A milk. This new cheaper version, less most of the valued cream, could now be labeled grade A since the consumer saw no difference. Through the miracle of mass-market magic (with a little help from their friends at the FDA), producers can now charge more for what used to be called grade B milk. We have chosen to drink milk produced by another species that is so dissimilar to what a cow produced that even their own calves' cells will not recognize it. Research shows that baby calves weaned off their mother's milk and fed today's pasteurized, homogenized version (now void of enzymes and other important nutrients) became ill or died within weeks.

In the end, you can't fool Mother Nature.

END NOTES

1. A kilogram equals approximately 2.2 pounds. Divide your body weight by 2.2 pounds × 0.8 grams of protein daily.
2. For a complete listing, go to Family Education's Web site http://life.family education. com/protein/foods/48678.html.
3. *American Journal of Clinical Nutrition;* Potassium, magnesium, and fruit and vegetable intakes are associated with greater bone mineral density in elderly men and women. 1999;6; Tucker et al.
4. *American Journal of Clinical Nutrition,* Vol. 84, No. 6, 1456-1462, December 2006; Long-term low-protein, low-calorie diet and endurance exercise modulate metabolic factors associated with cancer risk. Luigi Fontana, Samuel Klein and John O Holloszy. "Children who ate the highest protein diets were the ones most likely to get liver cancer."
5. *The China Study:* startling implications for diet, weight loss, and long-term health. Dallas, TX: BenBella Books, Inc, 2005. Campbell TC, Campbell TM II.
6. *American Journal of Clinical Nutrition;* 1999; 6; Potassium, magnesium, and fruit and vegetable intakes are associated with greater bone mineral density in elderly men and women. Tucker et al.
7. *American Journal of Public Health;* 1997; Milk, dietary calcium, and bone fractures in women: a 12-year prospective study. Feskanich et al.
8. *American Journal of Epidemiology;* 1994; Case-Control Study of Risk Factors for Hip Fractures in the Elderly Volume. 139, No. 5: 493-503; Cumming et al.
9. *American Journal of Clinical Nutrition;* Dietary Calcium and Bone Density Among Middle-Aged and Elderly Women in China. Am. 1993: Hu et al.
10. *Building Bone Vitality: A Revolutionary Diet Plan to Prevent Bone Loss and Reverse Osteoporosis--Without Dairy Foods, Calcium, Estrogen, Or Drugs;* McGraw Hill Professional, 2009, Amy J. Lanou, Michael Castleman
11. *The Journal of Nutrition;* Vol. 128 No. 6 June 1998, pp. 1051-1053, Excess Dietary Protein Can Adversely Affect Bone. Uriel et al.
12. lcaanimal.org
13. Environmental Defense Fund; Coal-fired Power Plants Are Big Contributors to Sooty Particle Pollution in Eastern States: "Power plant smokestacks are public health enemy number one for

their contribution to deadly particulate pollution across the eastern United States," said Dr. John Balbus, a physician and head of our health program. "Particulate pollution contributes to tens of thousands of premature deaths annually, heart attacks, strokes and asthma attacks."

14. Other researchers have pegged their atmospheric lifetimes at between 10,000- 50,000 years: Environmental Science and Technology; 2003 Oct 1;37(19):4358-61. Atmospheric perfluorocarbons; Asaim et al.

15. *The Poisonous Cloud. Chemical Warfare in the First World War,* Clarendon Press: Oxford, 1986. Haber, L. F.

16. Bayer and The UN Global Compact. How and Why a Major Pharmaceutical and Chemical Company "Bluewashes" its Image. Philipp Mimkes, Coalition Against Bayer Dangers, July 19th, 2002 www.corpwatch.org

17. *"Bayer AG: A Corporate Profile,"* March, 2002, Corporate Watch

17A. Sci.Tech-archive.net

18. Neurology; 53:337; Characterization of risk factors for vascular dementia. The Honolulu–Asia Aging Study; 1999

19. *International Journal of Cancer:* Volume 93 Issue 6, Pages 888 - 893; Epidemiology and Cancer Prevention Childhood and adult milk consumption and risk of premenopausal breast cancer in a cohort of 48,844 women - the Norwegian women and cancer study.

20. *The American Journal of Clinical Nutrition;* 2004, vol. 80, pp. 1353-1357; Milk and lactose intakes and ovarian cancer risk in the Swedish Mammography Cohort

21. *American Journal of Epidemiology;* Vol. 130, No. 5: 904-910 Lactase Persistence and Milk Consumption as Determinants of Ovarian Cancer Risk; Johns Hopkins University School of Hygiene and Public Health; Cramer et al.

22. *Nutrition and Cancer,* 1532-7914, Volume 48, Issue 1, 2004, Pages 22 – 27 Milk Consumption Is a Risk Factor for Prostate Cancer: Meta-Analysis of Case-Control Studies; Qin et al

23. *American Journal of Epidemiology;* Diet, Obesity and Risk of Fatal Prostate Cancer; Vol. 120, No. 2: 244-250

24. *Israel Journal of Medical Sciences* 1983; 19 (9):806-809 Pediatrics 1989; 84 (4):595-603

25. Life Extension, September 2010. Brittle Bones and Hardening Arteries, The Hidden Link, Dr. Julius Goepp M.D.

26. The politics of breast-feeding, Pandora Press, London, Gabrielle Palmer, 1988, page 304. First published online February, 2006.

27. Center for Food Safety "Petition Seeking the Withdrawal of the New Animal Drug University of Illinois. Office of the Dean. School of Public Health. Center for Food Safety "Petition Seeking the Withdrawal of the New Animal Drug Application Approval for Posilac - Recombinant Bovine Growth Hormone (rBGH)": FDA Docket No. WP-1194.

CHAPTER 2

FATS

No diet will remove all the fat from your body
because the brain is entirely fat. Without a brain you might look good,
but all you could do is run for public office.
—Covert Bailey

F at. This misunderstood word has prompted more fad diets and unhealthy eating habits than any other word in the English language.

Fat is an important part of a healthy diet. A concept that's often misunderstood, the facts stand in stark contrast to popular opinion. A number of the "experts" are misinformed and are misinforming you. If you practice what they preach, your life and the lives of those you love have been compromised. This chapter will help you to separate the *fat* from the fiction by examining solid research from scientists at the forefront of knowledge and change.

Some of you may have discovered that the way you eat is no longer working for you. Dieters often find that while the pounds came off quickly they returned just as fast. Others watch what they eat and exercise only to discover that the slight bulge around their stomach refuses to release its stubborn grip. Some of us experience "brain fog" or a lack of mental clarity. We may find that our occasional lapses of short term memory have become increasingly more common. While many of us simply feel less energetic.

As a result, some of us have grown skeptical. We followed the food pyramid and became fatter. We embraced the Mazola lady, ate bird food, gave up steak and eggs, and still got heart disease. We stuck to pasta, switched to low-or no-fat foods, only to develop type 2 diabetes. After all, they said we should. We ate fish like they told us to, with no knowledge of where it came from, what it was fed, and how it was raised. We turned to soy as a healthier alternative because they urged us to. We took statin drugs to lower our cholesterol level. They told us that our failure to do so makes us vulnerable to heart disease; particularly those with "high" total cholesterol levels (over 200), a level that grows increasingly lower over time. Each week the results of new studies cause us to doubt what we thought we already knew. One headline appears to contradict the next. But if the experts agree on nothing, can we believe anything?

Frustrated, we surrender. At times we strike back with negative affirmations. We may throw in the towel, believing that our attempts to prevent disease are useless, that illness and aging are inevitable, regardless of the decisions we make. After all, what's the use of trying to do the right thing only to find out that it's wrong, or that in the end, it makes little difference? Based on experience, most will wait to worry about their health—until disaster strikes. Only then taking their time and money to fix a real problem that may have been easily prevented long before it occurred.

But there's good news around the corner! For those who have climbed the flagpole of hope only to fall down in despair, this chapter will put you on the right track. You'll learn about the power and value of eating the right fats, to create positive, tangible change.

While growing old is inevitable, aging is not. Living with aches and pains and diminished energy and sexual libido is less than inspiring. Extending a life that feels like slow death, isn't the kind of fountain of youth we had hoped for.

But there's another approach. One based on science, not the next wonder drug, super-food, or green algae miracle.

WHILE GROWING OLD IS INEVITABLE, AGING IS NOT.

It requires commitment, and the knowledge and confidence that you truly *can* effect change.

Multifaceted, it involves a new way of eating, thinking, and behaving. A new way of living that becomes who you are. While you can't grow younger, you can look and feel younger. Though cartwheels may remain out of reach for most of us, you *can* restore the type of vigor and stamina that many of us have turned the page of life on. While some suggest we accept aging, I suggest you don't.

Many "truths" you've come to rely on are about to be shattered. We're told that eating fish is the next coming. But its potential risks are ignored—a powerful recommendation, like so many others that only tells us half the story. Many with little more than opinion to support them. We're inclined to embrace what the media suggests. But much of their information is based on anecdotal evidence from small groups in test conditions that ultimately prove unreliable. Recommendations made by some of the leading experts, based on questionable information, is cause for concern.

Though eating fish may be good for us on one hand, it can be bad for us on the other. Such a wholesale prescription contributes to an already confused and misinformed public. Headlines convince us that the fountain of youth is a pill away. The next fad diet becomes a way of life for the frustrated who are so eager to embrace change; a path that more often than not proves faulty. When someone we've come to respect leads the way we often follow.

Long term, diets are generally unsuccessful. If not, there would be little need for hundreds of new ones each year attracting some fifty million people who collectively spend over forty billion dollars to find the Holy Grail—to find the *one* quick fix that does it all. But 95 percent of those who do lose weight gain it back in one to five years (Grodstein et al., *Archives of Internal Medicine*, 1996). In time, bad advice makes good people with noble intentions lose hope.

We need to be educated, not just enlightened ... *why* should we eat fish? What type of fish should we purchase? What are the important characteristics we should look for? Where should we purchase them? Why? And importantly, which ones must we *avoid*?

Suggesting we eat lean meat falls short of providing us with the information we need to make an informed decision. If it's lean but industrially produced, stuffed with hormones, petroleum-based grain, antibiotics, and viruses, there are better choices. Avoiding egg yolks and other dairy products because they raise our total cholesterol level is misinformed. We need to chase the right bandits before we can hope to solve the right crimes. Like a good detective who interrogates every clue before seeking an indictment, we owe it to ourselves to do so as well. With facts in hand we can build a case and commit to a course of action based on sound judgment, with greater potential for success. Investing the time to do so is time well spent. In fact, your life depends on it.

How can we expect to remain sharp as a tack, when our brains are slowly deteriorating? The connections they require to communicate information are virtually disintegrating over time. Fortunately, we can not only protect and maintain our neural highways required for information to travel on, but we can actually build new ones. While brain fog and forgetfulness are signs that we are aging, they are *not* an inevitable part of growing old. If you've been told that they are, you've been misinformed. Some tell us to accept aging. That it's a fact of life. But it's not. Death is, and growing old is, but what we refer to as aging is not. At least not as quickly and progressively as many experience today. It's possible to grow old, and feel great; just as wonderful as you did when you were young.

This book will not cover every aspect of anti-aging. The balance will be covered in a future work. But here you will learn how to reduce internal inflammation, one of the most significant building blocks of aging. You'll also learn, in this chapter, the importance of eating the right fats to nourish not only your brain, but all of your tissue, by fixing the problem where it began—on a cellular level. All the symptoms we refer to as aging began long ago, precisely there. Like a tiny bubble rising from the depths of the ocean floor, it becomes increasingly visible as it surfaces. Aging is no different. The key is to stop it before it starts, or diminish it before it grows larger.

Throughout this book you'll be introduced to foods and supplements that miraculously protect us on both an inter and intra-cellular level. As well as special nutrients, like a fat-soluble version of the amino acid carnitine, which show promise in their ability to protect and revitalize our important mitochondria, the energy building power plants in our cells. They regulate everything from cell death and differentiation, to cell growth and metabolism. You'll learn not only how to protect them, but how to boost their ability to convert blood sugar to *energy*. That energy, known as ATP, is required by every cell in your body. Protecting our mitochondria is one of many ways we nip the progressive bubbles of aging in the bud before they surface. Dr. Phillip Lee Miller MD, along with the Life Extension Institute (Dr. Phillip Lee Miller, M. D. and the Life Extension Foundation, Life Extension Revolution, the New Science of Growing Older Without Aging, Bantam Dell, May 2006), informs us of this and other important strategies that permit us to turn back time. So do Dr. Barry Sears and others whose mission in life is to provide us with the tools to fight back.

While *Misinformed About Food* provides you with the best and most current information on the finest foods and supplements that allow us to do just that; it's one important leg of a four legged race. Reducing stress, through meditation and exercise, strengthening our muscle and bones through weight bearing and endurance activity and stretching, and restoring "balance" in other important ways, must all be part of the same lifestyle initiative. The closer you come to effecting this change the more you'll enjoy it. You have an exciting opportunity ahead of you that will be evident from the first day you begin the program.

While we can't change our genetic code, we *can* change the way it expresses itself. By following the SOS program, you learn how to turn those genes on and off. Bathing our cells with the right selection and in the right proportion of healthy fats is the first step in helping you do so. After all, two thirds of our brain is fat.

We need cholesterol and other important fats and nutrients to properly maintain neural pathways in our brain. We must provide our tissues and organs with healthy blood flow through vessels transporting the glucose-laden nutrients required to feed them. The sooner we understand this, the faster we can implement a solid program to stop our brains' London bridges from falling down. We can fortify them **before** they begin to self destruct, and restore those that have already begun to show signs of wear and tear.

> *WHILE WE CAN'T CHANGE OUR GENETIC CODE, WE CAN CHANGE THE WAY IT EXPRESSES ITSELF. BY FOLLOWING THE SOS PROGRAM, YOU LEARN HOW TO TURN THOSE GENES ON AND OFF.*

Fat provides more than twice the energy than the equivalent amount of protein and carbohydrate. Nine calories per gram (the equivalent of approximately a quarter of a teaspoon) in fats versus only four calories per gram in proteins and carbohydrates. But isn't a calorie a calorie? As we'll see in Chapter 3, the *type* of food we eat controls the behavior of our organs and glands. The choices you make are that powerful! If your organs are behaving well you're well. If they're out of control, so are you. It's quite literally the responsibility of a lifetime. Each member of your team has a job to perform. Their ability to carry out their designated functions is largely influenced by the decisions we make. Mismanage them and they'll burden you. Overwork them, and they'll quit.

Each choice requires autonomic action from certain organs in your body. Some of these organs are glands that secrete substances known as hormones. The glands required to do so, and the load each must carry, are largely influenced by the choices we make. Enzymes produced by our cells to digest and metabolize this food are required to convert it to useful energy. We hand our organs their marching orders every time we eat. Will *your* team be given a job they're capable of performing effectively? Or will they become slaves to your poor choices, forced to over-extend themselves and ultimately burn out?

Hormones affect every aspect of your health and regulate your blood sugar. If you ate the identical number of calories as your twin brother, but his came from the wrong foods and yours from the right ones, the outcome would differ. Over time he'd gain more weight than you and be plagued by greater health issues. So, a calorie is not a calorie. While a calorie is a measure of the amount of oxidized energy in foods required to produce a certain amount of heat, the *effect* of one calorie can be radically different than another. Those that are created from a meal high in simple carbohydrates will immediately spike your insulin. But calories derived from a balanced meal, such as those suggested by Dr. Barry Sears in his book *The Zone Diet*, won't.

Highly processed sugary foods contain little fiber and force your pancreas to produce additional insulin. The more often we select foods that require our pancreas to work harder—(causing it to usher excess fat out of our blood and into our cells)—the more our cell receptors develop resistance, to the internal mechanism that signals them to open. Doing so too often makes continuing to do so more difficult. Soon, the excess sugar remains in our blood. It has no place to go.

The ensuing insulin *resistance*, which affects the cells of your liver, fat, and muscle, lays the groundwork for diabetes or metabolic syndrome (also known as syndrome X), or a combination of disruptions that leads to the onset of diabetes and heart disease. Now, *more* insulin is required to do the same job it did before. Your pancreas is out of control, working longer and harder. Yet the harder it works, the less it's accomplishing. It's on overdrive now—and so are you.

It took some time before you knew you had a problem. But by the time you did, it became a "condition." Now you're retaining sugar. Your blood vessels are constricting. Your heart must work harder now to pump your blood farther. You're gaining weight from a river of plasma that's laden with glucose. That's in addition to the blood sugar already trapped in your cells. Cells that will no longer open the way they use to. Your circulating blood sugar quite literally, can't find its way out of you.

This resistance results in the mobilization of stored triglycerides by precipitating their breakdown from their interaction with water, a process known as hydrolysis. Now your blood is awash with a greater number of pro-inflammatory fatty acids. It also hinders the uptake of glucose from muscle, since your body is no longer able to utilize insulin effectively.[1] It's a vicious cycle that can simply be avoided by eating the right foods.

Guess which organ is the most demanding? According to Neuroscientist Ian Simpson, the *brain* is the most voracious organ in our body, gobbling up an amazing 60 percent of our blood sugar. Faster and far more powerful than any computer on earth, our brain's ability to multi-task dusts any PC, regulating a complex array of intricate body functions, as well as thoughts and emotions every second; simultaneously processing more than a million point images during that same second transmitted by the retinas in our eyes.[2]

Our miraculous central processing unit weighs in at a meager 2 percent of our body mass, according to Simpson, controlling an array of complex functions and intricate machinations that researchers are only beginning to unravel. While it requires a large amount of fuel, the amount of energy it produces is quite modest. According to Sam Wong and Sandra Aamodt it's a highly efficient organ *(The Times*, March 28, 2008) requiring "less power than your refrigerator light" or "the amount of energy each day found in two bananas."

But deprive this glucose glutton of its food source, and narrow the blood vessels that feed it, and you've laid the foundation for cognitive trauma. Few things in life are as treacherous as an angry brain!

FEW THINGS IN LIFE ARE AS TRECHEROUS AS AN ANGRY BRAIN!

While depression is not listed as one of the symptoms of diabetes, there appears to be a higher than normal correlation between these conditions. Studies show that diabetics have *three times* the rate of depression than that which occurs in the general population. Not surprisingly, too much stress over time prompts the adrenal glands to overwork themselves to the point of exhaustion (adrenal fatigue). Stress comes in many forms that include, but are not limited to, a poor diet from the excessive consumption of sugar (as well as from the excessive consumption of alcohol, negative thoughts, physical or psychological problems, marriage or other interpersonal problems, work related issues, etc). When your adrenal glands are overworked regularly, the cortisol it produces for a flight or fight response (that nature designed to stimulate the flow of glucose into our muscle tissue so we can dodge disaster,) has the *opposite* effect. Adrenaline (which on the short term can actually accelerate weight loss) is overpowered by the continued excessive production of cortisol. Instead of prompting us to action, it increases the storage of excess glucose, depositing it in visceral fat around the belly in particular, and elsewhere.

Today, cortisol is produced by road rage and co-workers; not a chance encounter with a Stegosaurus. Overtaxing your adrenal glands by the excessive production of cortisol can produce a wide variety of metabolic disorders. The next time you fight to win an argument, understand that you lost.

It's also important to note that stress comes in many forms, including intensive *exercise*. Enthusiasts may fail to realize that for some, the more difficult their regimen, the harder it becomes to shed that stubborn layer of visceral fat that's hunkered down around their belly. What we consider a good choice may be a poor one. This underscores the importance of good blood work. It provides a blueprint, a starting point, for a solid program of self defense. There's no substitute for knowing what's going on inside of you.

Further complicating the lives of those who make poor choices, smoking and excessive drinking further restricts the flow of blood by inflaming arteriole walls. Your heart must work harder to pump more blood through an increasingly narrow thoroughfare. Do you really want to do anything to impede your heart's ability to get your blood where it needs to go? According to the Federation of American Scientists, the average heart beats 100,000 times a day pumping blood to "… close to 100,000 miles of blood vessels—about four times around the Earth, or nearly half way to the moon."

If you wish to find ways to avoid these issues, you need to make the right choices. Purposeful eating is just as simple as it sounds. And more powerful than you may think. While 10 pounds of food is 10 pounds of food, the *type* of food, its value, and your ability to digest and absorb it can build you up or tear you down. Sadly, many of us wait for our own personal train wreck before finding a solution to a problem that may have been easily avoided; one that we may not have been aware of until it was too late.

Dr. Ron Rosedale, MD, sites a fascinating study showing that heart attacks are *two to three time*s more likely to occur following a high-carbohydrate meal. A spike in insulin constricts vital arteries, triggering the sympathetic nervous system to cause them to spasm. Importantly, this doesn't occur after eating a meal high in fat. We're not talking about the ratio of carbohydrates to fats on your food plate, but rather the amount of calories from carbohydrates overpowering your meal. Good carbs, such as those recommended in our SOS program, balanced with the correct amount of protein and fat, help us to balance our insulin.

While the type and amount of fuel we eat varies based on the needs of each individual, it appears that eating approximately 2,000 calories a day is the optimum amount required for most adults (currently the average American adult eats almost 3,800 calories a day, mostly from foods with little value). My recommended allocation for each respective food group to achieve this balance on a daily basis is 10 percent healthy fat, 30 percent healthy protein, and 60 percent healthy carbohydrate. The SOS program will show you how you can get there. Understanding and identifying the highest quality foods within each group, and combining them properly (along with the proper selection of the right supplements) is the primary focus of this book.

THE FATS THAT PROTECT AND HEAL

Contrary to popular opinion, a diet high in the right kind of *fat* (not carbs) increases endurance. It's stored in muscle tissue and is readily available. Carbohydrates are stored sparingly, and as the sole source of fuel, they're used up quickly. According to researcher David R. Pendergast, he and colleagues at the University of Rochester have shown that endurance trainers with a diet containing at least 40 percent fat significantly optimized their performance. (*Journal of the American College of Nutrition*, Vol. 19, No. 3, 345-350 (2000); A Perspective on Fat Intake in Athletes).

A second study, following up on the earlier work conducted by Venkatraman et al., showed that low fat diets also compromised immunity and promoted infection in long distance runners. Discussing these findings at the fourth International Society for Exercise and Immunology Symposium, Venkatraman noted that, "Since we have shown that athletes perform better on a higher-fat diet than on a low-fat diet, it was important to determine if the higher-fat diet would further compromise the immune system," she said. "We found that it did not, but the very-low-fat diet did."

Runners on *high fat versus low fat diets* had more than double the amount of natural killer cells the body uses as an important line of defense to guard against infection. In fact, measurements of athletes following these tests found that runners on the low fat diet had a significant increase in the production of pro-inflammatory prostaglandins, known as PGE2.

The right balance of fat in our diet is required to protect us. It also provides insulation for our body. Without a sufficient layer of fat, you'd freeze to death. There are two principle types of body fat: white and brown. Almost 5 percent of a newborn baby's body mass is brown fat. Brown fat helps babies regulate their temperature at birth. Not surprisingly, brown fat also contains a larger number of capillaries and mitochondria (responsible for energy production and cellular respiration) than white fat. The presence of brown fat is one of our body's chief defenses against hypothermia in premature babies. While white body fat or adipose tissue is capable of *storing* a greater amount of heat, brown adipose tissue *burns and heats more* due to its greater concentration of mitochondria. Brown fat actually produces heat in response to cold as well, beyond simply retaining it. And it distributes that heat with greater efficiency, effectiveness, and intensity than white fat due to its dense distribution of capillary.

THE RIGHT BALANCE OF FAT IN OUR DIET IS REQUIRED TO PROTECT US.

Babies are more susceptible to the cold than the rest of us. Their nervous systems aren't fully developed. Their blood vessels don't sufficiently contract to adequately protect them from the cold. Over time, most of our brown fat disappears or changes in function to more closely resemble white fat. Unfortunately, by the time we become adults, the mitochondria largely responsible for the color of brown fat disappears as it takes on the appearance and function of white fat. The result is what we commonly refer to as a *fat deposit*. New and exciting research has begun to examine the switch that trips the molecular structure of brown fat to white fat as we age. Scientists remain hopeful that these findings will allow us to lose weight effortlessly! Today, 60 percent of all adults in our country are overweight, and more than 30 percent of us are now considered to be clinically obese. That makes the prospect of unlocking this mechanism a very exciting one.

Fat also serves to protect our vital organs with padding, insulating our nerve fibers and assisting our body in the transportation and absorption of fat-soluble vitamins E, D, A, and K. These four horsemen are the building blocks of some of the most essential hormones we require to carry out bodily functions. Good fat reduces inflammation while bad fat hastens its formation. Eating the right amount of healthy fat helps to protect us from the ill effects of processed food. Essential fatty acids (EFAs) are those we are unable to produce ourselves but which our body requires nonetheless. Since we lack the ability to create these, we must eat them. And since these hormones affect every aspect of your health, and the food you select affects their utility, the choices you make directly impact your quality of life. Our quest to understand what our bodies require to achieve optimal health is made all the more difficult by some who prefer that we continue to rely on *them* for our health care. In fact, an entire language was created to that end.

Names that sound alike are given to biologically active material that differ fundamentally, making it all the more difficult for us to embrace the notion of caring for ourselves. While *alpha-linolenic* acid (ALA) and *linoleic* acid (LA) are both polyunsaturated fats, the former are Omega-3s while the latter are Omega-6s.

Some fats are manufactured by our body and some are not. The fatty acids we refer to as "essential" are ALA and LA, as well as their descendant fats, which our body cannot produce. They must be gotten elsewhere. Our bodies *are* capable of manufacturing the other fats we need. You'll learn more about these important fats shortly. While we can produce them if we eat the right stuff, our modern diet makes this a challenge. The best foods we require to do so are *less* available now than at any time in our history. But they're still available to those that know where to find them—to those of us who are informed about food.

Myth: Fat is very bad for you.

Truth: Eating the right kind of fat is one of the greatest things you can do for your health. Most of us will or are having health issues largely due to our failure to do so.

Myth: No fat is better than low fat.

Truth: Your body *requires* fat. Deprive your body of fat, the right kind of fat, and you've dealt yourself a crippling blow. In studies mice deprived of fat saw tumor growth mushroom. Their bodies *compensated* for the lack of healthful fat by producing highly toxic fat. But when healthy fat was introduced to their diets, these same mice saw those tumors immediately shrink. Of course, if you find yourself in a situation where you are forced to eat one of the foods we don't recommend, a low fat version may be less harmful than its full fat counterpart.

Myth: Too much fat results in high levels of total cholesterol, a leading cause of heart disease.

Truth: Data from some of the largest longitudinal studies ever conducted suggests the reverse is true. The Greenland study, which focused on the eating habits of the Inuit Eskimos (a people nearly free of heart disease), blew away that assumption. Their diet, which consisted almost entirely of *saturated fat* from whale blubber and other marine animals, enabled them to avoid heart disease. But how can a steady diet of saturated fat prevent heart disease?

Those low-carb dieters whose calories come largely from *healthy* saturated fat enjoy similar results. Many are surprised to discover that their cholesterol levels actually *plummet* when they eat this way. While weight loss and healthy levels of insulin are good things, a balanced ratio of saturated fat to unsaturated fat is equally desirable. Achieving this ratio means you've successfully optimized the absorption of fat in your tissue and minimized the free radical activity of unsaturated fat.

All fats, as is the case with protein and carbohydrates, are classified on the basis of their largest constituent. So a polyunsaturated fat may contain both saturated *as well* as monounsaturated fat. To be categorized as a polyunsaturated fat simply means that food contains a lower percentage of the other two fats.

Extra virgin coconut oil (EVCO) is an example of a saturated fat that contains a lower percentage of unsaturated fat, but it still has a shelf life of nearly a year. Its small percentage of unstable polyunsaturated fats remains balanced and stable. The presence of healthy saturated fat permits the polyunsaturated fat to avoid rapid oxidation. If left standing alone, polyunsaturated fat goes rancid in a matter of hours from exposure to light, heat, and air. Flaxseed oil without additives is an example of an unstable fat.

This same balancing act occurs *inside of* us as well. Understanding the importance of balancing various types of fat gives us the power to use this information to regulate our hormones; enabling us to reverse signs of aging and avoid disease. Something as simple as choosing the right foods can help balance your endocrine system and moderate the action of the organs and glands that produce them. Hormones are the chemical messengers that signal our organs to assist us in regulating important activity-such as eating. Thirty of these hormones control everything from our ability to fall asleep to our capacity to enjoy sex. They also regulate the temperature of our body.

If poor food choices can *interfere* with their ability to perform these important functions, then eating thoughtfully and properly balancing our intake of the right fats should assist them in doing so. Failure to eat properly impedes our ability to produce the hormones we require, seriously compromising our health.

DOES LOW FAT MEAN HEALTHY?

Contrary to what we're told, healthy saturated fat, the primary component of the diet of the Inuits, didn't produce a trace of heart disease in this population. In fact, they were significantly less prone to coronary heart disease (CHD) than the rest of us. But despite this, low-fat diets and low-fat products remain popular. But why? From a health perspective, why are we lining up to buy low-fat tuna, void of Omega 3 fat? After all, the principal benefit is found in its *fat*. If it's fat free, then it's more than likely Omega-3 free. Most tuna packed in water contains relatively little Omega-3 fatty acids. Yet according to the U.S. Tuna Foundation, light meat dominates our grocery store shelves, accounting for some 75 percent to 80 percent of our annual U.S. domestic consumption.

Bad advice from those we respect the most has challenged us. We've been told there's compelling medical evidence to suggest we reduce or eliminate fat in our diet. Yet people on high-fat diets are proving every day that their total cholesterol levels plummet when they make fat an important part of their diet. The facts stand in stark contrast to what we've been told. Does this mean saturated fat in your diet is actually good for you?

Yes, but only the *right* saturated fats and only in moderation. Too much of the wrong ones *are* dangerous. While the South Beach Diet® aids its followers by reducing insulin levels and lowering cholesterol (much to the delight of those that embrace the cholesterol myth), *most* weight loss diets do just that. But I believe any program that suggests we restrict our intake of healthy fats, such as coconut oil and palm oil is, in my opinion, misinformed; laying the groundwork for an unbalanced ratio of saturated to unsaturated fats. This fails to protect us from the free radical oxidation of unsaturated fat. And therein lies the long-term rub. Avoiding this potentially dangerous imbalance requires that our diet contain the right mix of antioxidants as well as a balanced ratio of healthful saturated fat. Suggesting that we limit our consumption of *all* saturated fat is like throwing the baby out with the bath water. And putting coconut oil and palm oil on the same short list of harmful oils to avoid along with corn, peanut, and soybean oils, is misinformed.

Of course, some saturated fats *are* harmful. Some people are dangerous too. So are we to avoid all of them? While Atkins' list of acceptable saturated fats when his diet was first introduced was ludicrous, a wholesale embargo that limits our consumption of all of them is equally flawed.

While *any* diet that limits your calories will cause you to lose weight (at least in the short-term), that alone doesn't make it a healthy program. Dr. Agaston (creator of the South Beach Diet) recommends the use of artificial sweeteners such as Saccharin and NutraSweet®, while blacklisting all forms of butter. His suggestion that South Beach followers use artificial sweeteners, is again, in my opinion, misinformed. We recommend all natural, healthy, Just Like Sugar® (learn more at RKInformedLiving.com).

THE CHOLESTEROL GOBLIN—ARE YOU MYTH-INFORMED?

Authors Fallon and Enig (*Nourishing Traditions: The Cookbook that Challenges Politically Correct Nutrition and the Diet Dictocrats*, 1999) advise us that "when the diet contains an excess amount of polyunsaturated fatty acids, these replace saturated fatty acids in the cell membrane, so that the cell walls actually become flabby. When this happens, cholesterol from the blood is 'driven' into the tissues to give them structural integrity. This is why serum cholesterol levels may go down temporarily when we replace saturated fats with polyunsaturated oils in the diet." In fact, without sufficient amounts of cholesterol we'd have all sorts of problems. But that's not what we're being told and sold.

Myth: We need to rid ourselves of cholesterol and, in particular, the bad type known as LDL.

Truth: This is not true. Cholesterol is vital and sustains our lives. Both LDL and HDL are *required* for our survival. Without them, our brain cells can't communicate and our bodies would be unable to produce bile. In fact, without cholesterol life would cease to exist. It's also important to note that all LDL is not created equal. Fish oil converts damaging hard cholesterol to a second fluffy innocuous form. This isn't a testimonial for LDL. Too much LDL is a bad thing—but only if it's the bad form of LDL—and only if it's not offset with other healthful lipids, such as HDL. Large molecules of LDL are fine, and help transport the same important cholesterol our body needs that HDL does. It's the tiny hard particles of LDL that are pro-inflammatory. It's their make up or density—not their name, that may be cause for concern. But regularly consuming the right fish oil and properly balancing your fats keeps the doctor away. While reducing LDL is a good thing (and a number of safe ways to do so will be detailed shortly), boosting anti-inflammatory HDL and converting hard particle LDL to the soft stuff clobbers its pro-inflammatory potential, eliminating the need for dangerous drug intervention that disrupts the natural order.

Myth: We need statin drugs to significantly reduce our LDL and boost HDL production.

Truth: This isn't true. The good news is that you can lower your LDL with regular exercise, special supplements (pp. 81-82) and the moderate supplementation of natural compounds we'll soon discuss, such as niacin (approximately 500 milligrams for the average adult under the supervision of a health care professional). But a word of caution is warranted. Scientists at Eli Lilly's Research Laboratories and the Oregon Health Sciences University have shown that high doses of niacin may increase your homocysteine level (*American Heart Journal*, Vol. 138, December 1999, pp. 1082-87; Niacin treatment increases plasma homocysteine levels). Should you decide to do so, consider simultaneously increasing your intake of folic acid and TMG. Have your blood tested for your baseline homocysteine levels after consulting with a health care professional, and carefully monitor it.

Another important study demonstrates the powerful LDL lowering ability of natural plant phytosterols, which have been shown to block the absorption of LDL in the digestive track. In a study led by Vivian Lau of McGill Universities School of Dietics and Human Nutrition, she and her colleagues found that: "Plant sterol consumption significantly reduced ($P <$ 0.05) LDL-cholesterol concentrations from baseline in both nondiabetic and diabetic subjects by 15.1 percent and 26.8 percent, respectively (*American Journal of Clinical Nutrition*, Vol. 81, No. 6, 1351-1358, June 2005; plant sterols are efficacious in lowering plasma LDL and non-HDL cholesterol in hypercholesterolemic type 2 diabetic and nondiabetic persons). Dosages are subject to many considerations and high niacin dose therapy should be done only after consulting a physician. Several other studies confirming its efficacy, such as those conducted by Goldberg et al., at the University of Washingtons' School of Medicine (*American Journal of Cardiology*, vol. 97:3, pp. 376-379, Effect of plant stanol tablets on low-density lipoprotein cholesterol lowering in patients on statin drugs) showed this same LDL lowering effect occurred (a 15.6 percent reduction in LDL occurred even for those regularly taking statin drugs-prompted many to suggest that statin drug use is unnecessary).

These studies and others prompted the FDA to authorize foods and products that meet their criteria for making this claim. According to the agency's statement (Press Release: September, 2005; FDA Authorizes new Coronary Heart Disease Health Claim for Plant Sterol and plant stanol Esters): "The FDA has authorized use of labeling health claims about the role of plant sterol or plant stanol esters in reducing the risk of coronary heart disease (CHD) for foods containing these substances. This interim final rule is based on FDA's conclusion that plant sterol esters and plant stanol esters may reduce the risk of CHD by lowering blood cholesterol levels. Scientific studies show that 1.3 grams per day of plant sterol esters or 3.4 grams per day of plant stanol esters in the diet are needed to show a significant cholesterol lowering effect ..." The Cholesterol Education Program Recommends

2-3 grams a day of plant stanol/sterol esters daily. Cognis Corporation's Vegapure® (1.3 g/d) product was successfully used in a number of trials. The company is a world leader in plant sterol esterification, and has begun introducing them in a host of baked goods and other foods. Plant sterol esters are found in fatty acids that closely resemble cholesterol, but foods alone can't deliver the concentration necessary to make a real dent in your LDL. There are several other *natural* products that have demonstrated their ability to dramatically lower our LDL.

Nashai Biotech LLC offers a 375 milligram tablet, marketed under the name of Teaflavin®, containing caffeine free enriched tea extract, was shown to reduce LDL by a whopping 16.4 percent in only 12 weeks. The double-blind, randomized, placebo-controlled, parallel-group clinical study of 240 mild to moderate men and woman with hypercholesterolemia showed that the daily consumption of just one 375 milligram tablet a day lowered LDL by an amazing 16.4 percent, with no adverse effects. In a study designed to test its ability to lower LDL (Cholesterol-Lowering Effect of a Teaflavin-Enriched Green Tea Extract, Archives of Internal Medicine; 2003), scientists demonstrated its power to do just that. This all natural, caffeine-free product is now available to consumers under the name Teaflavin.® (For ordering information on this and other products referenced in this book, go to our Web site at www.RKInformedLiving.com.)

And there's more good news. It's also possible to substantially boost your important HDL with regular aerobic exercise such as walking (40 minutes or more 4 days weekly). According to Mayo Clinic's Dr. Gerald Gau, MD, niacin therapy can also raise important HDL (Mayo Clinic.com, Niacin to boost your HDL "good" cholesterol; March 28, 2008). Eating SOS monounsaturated and saturated fats (such as nuts), extra virgin coconut oil and avocado, my personal favorite, will also boost HDL. Moderate consumption of alcohol (1–2 drinks daily) will also increase HDL; while more may put you in danger, including 2-10 times the risk for liver cancer and 5 times the likelihood for cancers of the neck, throat and mouth, according to the UK's National Health Services. And, women increase their risk for breast cancer by 50%. The more you exceed the threshold the higher your risk. Weight gain (from empty calories), exhaustion, and lack of sexual desire often result from the excessive consumption of alcohol.

IT'S ALSO POSSIBLE TO SUBSTANTIALLY BOOST YOUR IMPORTANT HDL WITH REGULAR AEROBIC EXERCISE SUCH AS WALKING.

While there will surely come a day when big pharma announces the next miracle drug to boost HDL, their attempts to date have failed. Writer Karen Honey, writing for the Journal of Clinical Investigation (117(2): 282-282 (2007). doi:10.1172/JCI31253) tells the story ...

Despite Jefferey Kinder's announcement (the new CEO of Pfizer) that Torcetrapid®, Pfizer's "promising new drug will be one of the most important compounds of our generation." Its development was abruptly scotched just days after his press conference. According to Honey, "preliminary data from a 15,000-patient phase III clinical trial indicated that individuals receiving the drug had higher risks of death and heart failure than did individuals not receiving the drug." As much as I would have hated to be in Kinder's shoes, try being one of the 7,500 persons in the group who would later learn of this. While pharma will surely go back to the drawing board, the means to raise HDL and lower LDL are already here. All we need to do is apply them.

Too little cholesterol will kill us—while too much will allow big pharma to keep dancing in the street. Low levels of cholesterol will put you at great risk for cancer, heart disease, infection and stroke; particularly true for the elderly and statin drug users. The European Heart Journal published the results of a 39 month follow up study on 11, 563 patients conducted by Behar et al. (*European Heart Journal* (1997) 18, 52-59; Low total cholesterol is associated with high total mortality in patients with coronary heart disease). According to the study the low cholesterol group had a 2.27 times greater risk for non-cardiac death, primarily cancer, than the high cholesterol group. And that's just the tip of the iceberg.

Important research underscores the protective value of high cholesterol in the elderly. In fact low total cholesterol is associated with high total mortality in patients with coronary heart disease. Uffe Ravnskov, MD, PhD (The Weston Price Foundation, June 24 2004, The Benefits of high Cholesterol) discusses the work of Yale Universities' Dr. Harlan Krumholz who found that: "old people with low cholesterol died twice as often from a heart attack as did old people with a high cholesterol" (*Journal of the American Medical Association*; 272, 1335-1340, 1990; Lack of association between cholesterol and coronary heart disease mortality and morbidity and all-cause mortality in persons older than 70 years.)

Myth: Statin drugs are good for you.

Truth: Not necessarily, they can also be harmful. Important data suggests that, at best, they're a last resort. While they reduce inflammation (a good thing), their value is more than countered by adverse effects in a number of users. The side effects you may be unaware of, may make your choice to embrace them a poor one.

Think about it. A statin drug doesn't know the difference between the cholesterol needed by your brain to communicate and the cholesterol you're trying to reduce in your blood stream. Read the published warnings. Are you willing to trade off inflammation for muscular degeneration and the reduction of healthy cholesterol? Must we sacrifice our health to get health? Apparently, we must. Just listen to some of the TV commercials marketing the latest and greatest prescription drugs. Play now, pay later. We can dance in the rain but our heads may fall off. And all too often many of us are finding this to be an acceptable trade-off. According to the National Health Accounts (NHA), retail sales of prescription drugs have tripled their share of our domestic gross national product since 1960. But there are better ways to reduce internal inflammation.

Today, statin drug users are actually paying pharmaceutical companies to inhibit their body's important mevalonate pathway, increasing their risk of muscular degeneration, infection and other disease. This is the same pathway responsible for the production of important cofactors such as CoQ-10 (ubiquinone), whose presence is required before important actions demanded by our body can occur, like the proper conversion of food to energy. Not surprisingly, organs with the greatest requirements for energy, such as our heart and liver, contain the largest amount of CoQ-10. Why must we turn to a rapid fire remedy like this, after a condition develops, when so much can be done to prevent it before it does?

Myth: Foods high in cholesterol will cause a rise in your total cholesterol level.

Truth: This is not true. Though we keep hearing it, the data just doesn't support it. In fact, there appears to be no correlation, based on the information I've reviewed, between high blood serum cholesterol and dietary cholesterol— none. Not only is this contrary to what we've been told, what we've been told is also killing us. If you're avoiding cholesterol in foods to keep a lid on the cholesterol in your blood, you may be misinformed. If anything, egg yolks help you lower your cholesterol. Loaded with lecithin, a natural emulsifier, the yolk is chock full of other important nutrients such as folic acid, which is essential for the prevention of birth defects.

Much maligned, there's just no proof that eating eggs causes heart disease. There's also no evidence that eating them raises your blood serum cholesterol.

Like all dairy products (except egg whites), whole eggs do contain arachidonic acid (AA), the constrictor we've already discussed. But for those of you still clinging to industrialized egg whites, take note ... most come from the same industrialized layer chickens living the same miserable lives as those we previously discussed. Fortunately for those that care, there are healthier, organic alternatives. As for me, I'll continue to enjoy my eggs, yolks and all.

Myth: Your total cholesterol level is an important predictor of heart disease.

Truth: This is nonsense. But you wouldn't know it from the president of the American Heart Association (AHA).

After President Clinton's heart attack, in an appearance on *Larry King Live* the president of the AHA had a golden moment to tell a concerned public what we needed to know. Instead, he attributed our former president's problems to his diet. That may have been true. But singling out its effect on his blood serum cholesterol is, as you've seen, quite arguable. He went on to scold Clinton for neglecting to take his statin drugs. By this time, Americans were on the edge of their seats. The former seemingly invincible leader of the free world was apparently brought down, at least in part, for his failure to take his statin drugs. Cable news show ratings went through the roof. After all, our former president, who appeared so healthy and vibrant, had heart disease. A beleaguered public remained fixed as they watched the leading authority on CHD tell them how we might avoid a similar fate. But what we received was little more than the familiar echo of a decades old myth, and this from one of the nation's leading authorities on this subject. The opportunity to tell the world what they really needed to know was gone. At least for the moment. Again, more than 50 percent of those hospitalized for CHD have total cholesterol levels under 200. Think about it.

PIONEERS THAT LIT THE WAY

A brief understanding of the past will allow us to better understand the importance of the right fats in the present. And why we need cholesterol.

Some of our notions about fat began to change thanks to the knowledge and engaging personality of Dr. Robert C. Atkins. He wasn't the first to discover the relationship between the consumption of simple carbohydrates and a corresponding increase in insulin levels. Nor was he the first to understand the relationship between insulin and its role in inhibiting the release of stored body fat. But Atkins *was* the first person to devote his life to furthering these beliefs, doing more to convince a skeptical medical and lay-community than anyone before him.

Dr. Barry Sears has made equally significant contributions, based not only on the research of others, but on his own studies measuring the impact of consuming "healthy" fats on our performance, vigor, and immunity.

In his book *The Omega Rx Zone* (HarperCollins, 2003), Sears brings to light years of research by himself and others on another entire class of hormones known as eicosanoids—a class of super hormones that controls important and complex systems in our body. This family consists of three principal members that work to mediate inflammation. Luekotrienes, a lipid that intervenes in response to inflammation; thromboxanes, a vasoconstrictor that promotes blood clotting by stimulating the production of new blood platelets signaling them to mobilize and aggregate; and prostaglandins that mediate both pain and inflammation. In fact, aspirin works by blocking or inhibiting the cyclooxygenase enzyme required for their production.

Importantly, these hormones are not stored in our bodies but are produced from certain fats as they're required. Their primary influence is on our immunity and inflammation response, which they accomplish through their ability to regulate cells.

The evidence is clear. You *can* control your body's ability to recover from or avoid most major disease. The impact of Omega-3 fatty acids, in particular the new pharmaceutical grade fish oil, makes this fat one of the most powerful links in the puzzle of prevention. Sears celebrates his conclusion that the proper intake and management of this fat, and its affect on good eicosanoids, has the power to prevent or eradicate a long list of chronic illnesses (including Alzheimer's, CHD, diabetes, cancer, and more).

He takes us back to a time, some 550,000 million years ago, when simple single cell algae began to evolve into small multi-cell organisms. Apparently, one of the two mechanisms that permits our brain cells to communicate with each other requires the action of hormones. Eicosanoids, the first hormones developed by living organisms, permitted human cell specialization by catalyzing the transmission of information. To do so, they require Omega-3 fatty acids, like those found in algae. And fish are loaded with them. For those of you that don't believe in miracles, think again. Fortunately for us, we are what we eat ate!

Developing a means to easily access this important food source would prove to be the single most important discovery for mankind—a means that advanced and distinguished our species. As Dr. Sears pointed out, the invention of the fishing pole helped our ancestors to do just that. By unlocking these fats, and by eating the fish that ate the Omega-3 rich algae, our cognitive development took a quantum leap forward. A higher order was born. Dr. Sears does an excellent job of pinpointing this historic place in time, as well as clarifying the cause and effect of this discovery. Its impact on the rapid development of our frontal cortex can't be underscored—endowing mankind with the unique ability to not only think and reason, but to communicate those thoughts as well. It follows that the absence of this important fat diminishes our ability to do so.

FOUR CLASSES OF FATS

There are four classifications of fat: saturated, polyunsaturated, monoun-saturated and trans fat. Let's begin by examining the characteristics of each, as well as the differences among them. A more detailed discussion of fats follows, for those that are interested, at the end of this chapter.

SATURATED FAT—THE CINDERELLA

Some saturated fats are quite different from others. Such differences are a pretty big deal since their unique characteristics result in radically different biological consequences. The same holds true for unsaturated fats. While these broad classifications assist us in our understanding of their unique physical characteristics, they do little to explain the disparity among each of their members. Today, saturated fat remains in the doghouse. But for the sake of your health, it's time we let the *right* ones out. Contrary to what you may have been told, eating the right kind of saturated fat is one of the best things you can do for your health. In *The Oiling of America* (Nexus Maga-zine, 1998), authored by Mary Enig, PhD and Nancy Fallon, note in a 1992 interview (Internal Medicine) with Dr. William Castelli, the director of the famous Framingham Heart Study, that "the more saturated fat one ate, the more cholesterol one ate, the more calories one ate, the lower the person's serum cholesterol ... We found that the people who ate the most cholesterol, ate the most saturated fat, ate the most calories, weighed the least, and were the most physically active."

If saturated fats were half the villain we're told they are, then increasing our consumption of them should correlate with a subsequent increase in heart disease. Yet, between the years 1910 to 1970, the amount of saturated fat in the average American diet actually declined from 83 percent to 62 percent, while heart disease skyrocketed (Weston A. Price Foundation, 2004).

So, what's the deal? Hu et al. conducted a detailed prospective analyses of dietary fat and CHD based on fourteen years of follow-up data from the famed Nurse's Health Study ("Types of Dietary Fat and Risk of Coronary Heart Disease: A Critical Review," *Journal of the American College of Nutrition*, 2001). A vast amount information, meticulously gathered, was based on the repeated assessments of 80,082 women ages 34 to 59. While they found a significant association between CHD and the consumption of trans fatty acids, they discovered a weak, almost nonexistent, correlation between CHD and the consumption of saturated fat. Are you going to believe the anecdotal evidence that supports the wholesale condemnation of this important food, based on hearsay that found its way to headline news on the backs of three blind mice? Or will you believe the largest and most respected study of its kind led by distinguished researchers conducted over many years, that contradict what we thought we knew?

Other studies you're already familiar with corroborate these findings. In addition to the Framingham study, begun in 1948, the Greenland study also showed *no correlation* between the consumption of saturated fat and CHD.

Like other topics you've already learned about in this book, there is more to saturated fat than meets the eye. Indeed, stearic acid (the form of saturated fatty acids you get from meat) does *not* increase your LDL as you've been told. In fact, there is actually more healthy *monounsaturated* fat in beef than *saturated* fat (42.1 percent versus 38 percent respectively). Countless studies give testimony to the benefit of eating *certain* healthful saturated fats. It's just as important as avoiding the wrong ones. The right saturated fat has the *opposite* effect that you've been told it does. Just ask Dariush Mozaffarian and his associates at the Harvard School of Public Health (*American Journal of Clinical Nutrition*, 2004). His analysis of data taken over a three-year period showed that among their participants, those that ate the largest amounts of saturated fat had the *lowest* amount of plaque in their arteries. They studied the foods eaten by 235 postmenopausal women, all 66 years of age and each with some level of plaque when the study began. The purpose was to measure (through the use of X-rays) the effect of a diet high in saturated fat on the subjects' baseline levels of plaque. Results showed that participants who consumed the largest amount of saturated fat also showed the *most favorable* blood concentration of favorable fats.

Not surprisingly, breast milk tops the list of miracle foods containing healthful saturated fat, with one of the highest percentages of both cholesterol and saturated fat found in any food.

But before you go charging into the coconut trees, it's important to distinguish between the saturated fats that are healthful, versus harmful.

EXTRA VIRGIN COCONUT OIL—THE MOST HEALTHFUL SATURATED FAT

This powerful food tops the chart of healthy saturated fats. More than 90 percent of its fat is of the saturated variety. Loaded with lauric acid (which converts to monolaurin when metabolized), coconut oil has powerful anti-viral and anti-fungal power. Not surprisingly, incredibly healthful lauric acid is the most primary fat in breast milk. A mainstay of diets in many third world countries, the lauric acid found in coconut oil has protected millions of people from the possibility of infection, largely due to its ability to inhibit the growth of yeast, fungi, and certain bacteria. It's also been credited with the destruction of the lipid membrane in a host of viruses. The fruit's high content of capric acid stimulates other important antiviral activity as well. Maybe our ancestors knew more than we do today about this amazing fat's important attributes?

Before the turn of the century, coconut oil was American's leading source of fat. But it all but vanished, eventually paving the way for our reliance on other less healthful sources. Not surprisingly, heart disease in this country skyrocketed along with its demise. Was this merely a coincidence? You be the judge.

A "super fat" consisting of medium-chain triglycerides, coconut oil has been proven to lead to an increase in endogenous oxidation of long-chain saturated fatty acids. In other words, *it's the best fat to help you metabolize unwanted fat.* But it won't do this by itself. In conjunction with exercise or purposeful eating, the consumption of coconut oil appears to have a significant impact on weight loss. How can a *fat* help us get *thin*? Coconut oil is composed of medium-chain fatty acids (MCFA). Unlike other lipids that circulate in the bloodstream, these healthy fatty acids don't wander around. They're quickly ushered into your liver where they're instantly converted to energy. This rapid fat burning aids your body in the process known as "thermogenesis," the means it uses to throw off heat by increasing your metabolic rate. At worst, from a slimming perspective, you are not going to gain weight by eating a fat in moderation that our bodies immediately convert to energy. At best, it will assist you in your effort to lose it.

Decades ago, farmers tried to introduce cheap coconut oil into the diet of their cattle in an attempt to fatten up their herd. But the bewildered farmers would soon discover that the opposite was true. They were astonished to see their livestock growing leaner, becoming far more active and hungry. Yet despite this, as a people, we remain misinformed.

Coconut oil all but disappeared from our kitchens when the surgeon general joined the medical community, launching an all-out assault against saturated fat (the cholesterol myth). Ancel Keyes, a prominent member of the Nutritional Advisory Committee of the American Heart Association, showed the world what appeared to be a correlation between coronary heart disease and the consumption of fat in six countries. Eventually other researchers chose to review his findings. Apparently Keyes cherry-picked these countries from the available data. Data from sixteen other countries were apparently ignored. But the damage was done. Unfortunately, Keyes' influence amongst his colleagues on the committee was so pervasive that in 1961, ignoring these findings, the American Heart Association incorporated his notions into their official dietary guidelines—and the rest is history. The Eskimos, Filipinos, and other natives of the Pacific Island, with their radiant hair and glowing skin, must have had a good laugh. As well as the famed Masai warriors of East Africa and Kenyan cattle herdsman whose diets largely consist of saturated fat, such as red meat from game, the whole blood of cattle, and milk. Though based on Mr. Keyes' rantings, the Masai could be no more than obese, coronary time bombs, ready to implode with the next leg of lamb.

When Vanderbilt University Professor George Mann (*American Journal of Epidemiology*, 1972) visited the Masai in the 1960s, he found their cholesterol levels were among the lowest ever recorded in the world. In fact, their total cholesterol level was approximately 50 percent lower than the average American, with no deaths from heart disease. He also learned that despite an average daily consumption of a half gallon of whole milk each day, and 4 to 10 pounds of red meat per person eaten on special occasions alone, the Masai were among the trimmest, most muscular and robust people in the world. As Anthony Calpo points out in "Just the Facts" (*Omnivore*, May 2003), "When given treadmill tests, several of the tribesmen achieved performances superior to those of Olympic champions. Autopsy examinations on deceased Masai males showed an almost complete absence of atheromas, the advanced atherosclerotic lesions implicated in coronary blockage." Cancer was virtually absent in these people, as well as diabetes. Unlike the Inuits, the Masai diet, which includes milk, porridge, beans, maize, butter, and grains, provides an ample source of essential amino acids. (It should be noted that today's Masai have reduced the practice of drinking blood.) And what of the illustrious Mr. Keyes? Some say he was last seen courting the Mazola lady.

These findings were later confirmed over and over again. The long-running Nurse's Study in Framingham, Massachusetts, found that *the more* saturated fat subjects ate, *the lower* their blood serum cholesterol became. But our bias against coconut oil continued, as food companies introduced hydrogenated coconut oil as a hazardous trans fat. Now men were *creating* food in ways they had not done before—rather than *growing* it.

God created coconuts and they were good. Then man tinkered with them. Coconut oil should be the only oil you use for high-temperature cooking. But not all coconut oil is healthful. Most mass producers hydrogenate or partially hydrogenate food using chemical solvents and high heat, making it artificially stable. The result is a product containing dangerous trans fatty acids, processed from what began as a once healthy fat. Use extra virgin coconut oil made from organically grown coconuts for cooking on high heat. It's naturally fermented.

> *GOD CREATED COCONUTS AND THEY WERE GOOD. THEN MAN TINKERED WITH THEM. COCONUT OIL SHOULD BE THE ONLY OIL YOU USE FOR HIGH-TEMPERATURE COOKING.*

Organically grown extra virgin coconut oil continues to be one of the healthiest of fats. Eating it helps to ignite your immune system, providing a healthy glow to your skin and hair. Discover this magical cooking oil, used by some of the most physically attractive people in the world. The daily consumption of this miraculous food is a part of the Holy Grail approach to good eating. By doing so you'll be feeding your heart tissue healthy nourishment while reducing cardio plaque. And you'll feel the difference in short order.

Other great sources of lauric acid include organic coconut meat, milk and water (often referred to as coconut juice). The water found in fresh young green coconuts is the ultimate sport drink, loaded with electrolytes like potassium and sodium which are lost through perspiration during intensive exercise. It's your kidneys' job to maintain a narrow range and continuous flow of these positively or negatively charged salts in the blood. A difficult task, the kidney must work hard to regulate their dispersion regardless of the extreme changes in our body during periods of stress. As blood flows, its electrolytes carry electrical impulses to cell membranes. In doing so it balances voltage delivered there, creating impulses in muscle, heart, lung, and nerve tissue. It's a tough and intricate balancing act, and the failure to do so may result in poor nerve function, fluid absorption and subsequent elimination. While most of us won't deplete our bodies' reserves from moderate exercise, some in the sports drink industry would have us believe otherwise. Electrolyte supplementation is typically required for those who exercise intensely for periods of an hour or more. While individual needs vary (we all perspire at a different rate), other factors such as activity in heat or high altitude and the loss of fluid from diet as well as other stressful events further precipitates the loss of fluid and the amount we may need to replenish. The water (also referred to as juice) of young green coconuts (as the fruit matures, this fluid is eventually absorbed into the white flesh, and becomes "milk") is the finest biologically-pure source available to help us get there. Loaded with important nutrients and void of additives such as high fructose corn syrup, sucralose, sucrose, maltose, sugar substitutes, food dyes and preservatives, the liquid in nature's young green coconuts blows manufactured beverages out of the water. Loaded with lauric acid, (like mother's milk) it's easy to digest.

One serving of my favorite coconut water, Zico®, contains a whopping 670 milligrams of potassium per serving versus just over 32 milligrams in one leading brand. It also contains 40 milligrams of calcium, 17 milligrams of phosphorous and 25 milligrams of magnesium compared to *none* of these important nutrients found in this same market leaders' sports drink. Not surprisingly, it's been used extensively by paramedics as an oral rehydrant during times of epidemic, such as the cholera outbreak of 1977, which effected hundreds of people in the Gilbert Islands. An isotonic beverage, coconut water pinch-hit for intravenous blood plasma in World War ll when supplies of the latter began to dwindle. Because coconut water has the same electrolyte balance as blood (it's "isotonic"), it's also been called "the fluid of life." A sterile fluid that's easily absorbed in our body, its electrolytic balance closely parallels the levels of similar minerals in our blood. A liquid endosperm, it's used extensively for oral hydration at times of epidemic, such as the 1979 cholera outbreak, effecting hundreds of persons living on the Gilbert Islands.[3] Other research suggests that its lauric acid substantially reduces microbial agents from the HIV virus.[4]

If you want to stoke your immune system and bolster your vitality, eat a teaspoon or more of extra virgin coconut oil daily. Regular use will generally produce radiant skin and hair, and increase your ability to metabolize the food you eat.

It's the king of the saturated "super fats." Feed your heart tissue and reduce cardio plaque by eating nature's saturated fats each and every day. On the other hand, show me a tired and frail person with bouts of depression, dry and lifeless skin, cracked nails, and brittle hair, and I'll show you a person who more than likely has a poor balance of lipids. While there may be other causes for all of these things, they are often symptomatic of those people deprived of the right kinds of fat. In my personal experience, after only nine weeks of cooking with saturated fat and eating an additional teaspoon before bed, my energy and stamina increased, and even more surprisingly, a skin condition I've had since childhood known as seborrhea dermatitis disappeared. That's the power of food! Now let's learn more about other healthful saturated fats as well as their evil sisters.

ORGANIC BUTTER—ANOTHER TESTIMONIAL FOR SATURATED FAT

Organic butter is another beneficial saturated fat that bit the dust for all the wrong reasons. According to R. Reiser of Texas A & M University, there is far less cholesterol in an ounce of butter than in a lean chicken breast—approximately one-fifth as much! And since we no longer buy into the cholesterol rhetoric, let's talk more about the wonderful, life-sustaining properties that are found in natural (not processed), honest-to-goodness butter. Because you are what you eat (ate), you need to find butter from cows that have been grass-fed, if possible. While butter produced from raw milk tops our list of powerfully healthy saturated fats, organic butter is a more practical alternative. It's just more conveniently available. You can find organic butter in many health food stores and in the resources of recommended food products posted on our Web site at www.RKInformedLiving.com.

For those of you who continue to eat non-organic butter, what you didn't know just *might* hurt you. The Pesticide Action Network North America (PANNA) listed non-organic butter on their list of the top ten foods containing persistent organic pollutants (POP). Their use is not permitted in organic agriculture, according to the group. The two most pervasive POPs in our food are pesticides DDE and dieldrin, which evolve from the breakdown of DDT. But the United Kingdom's Pesticide Residue Committee, also researching common foods that retained these toxins, found no traces of POPs in *organic* butter.

Dehydrogenated or partially dehydrogenated margarine on the other hand, is dangerous stuff.[5] It's yet another fake, processed alternative to a God-given food.

MARGARINE, ON THE OTHER HAND, IS DANGEROUS STUFF. IT'S YET ANOTHER FAKE, PROCESSED ALTERNATIVE TO A GOD-GIVEN FOOD.

Many are heated up and combined with metals like other man-made foods. Processing vegetable oils at high heat is done to significantly extend shelf life and counteract their unstable characteristics, preventing them from turning rancid in short order. But once inside you, they create chaos. [6, 7, 8, 9, 10, 11, 12, 13, 14] The pro-inflammatory imposters have no purpose in life and your body knows it.[15]

Organic butter is another "super fat" that contains medium-chain lauric acid. In addition to its antibacterial and antiviral properties, butter is full of other immune-building and cancer-fighting fats, such as short-chain butyric acid with antifungal and antitumor forming properties as well as short-chain myristic acid. The latter, such as lauric acid, is absorbed through the small intestine by the liver, where it's immediately converted to energy.

It's loaded with important fat-soluble vitamins, such as vitamin A, and is an important source of vitamins D, K, and E as well. Organic butter is also the single best source of absorbable retinol, the animal source of vitamin A essential for good vision and bone growth. And recent studies have shown that vitamin D, also known as calciferol, plays an important role in the survival rates of cancer victims after surgery or other forms of treatment. In a meta-analysis of vitamin D research (*American Journal of Public Health*, 2005), scientists claimed that taking 1,000 IU (25 micrograms) of vitamin D each day could lower an individual's colon cancer risk by 50 percent and by 30 percent in breast and ovarian cancer! It's also needed for normal sexual development as well as healthy reproduction. But don't take a fat-soluble vitamin such as vitamin D without having your levels checked periodically. Research indicates that dosages are safe up to 2,000 IU a day, or ten times the recommended daily allowance (RDA). But the amount of time your skin's exposed to the sun and other sources of vitamin D should be considered. A study of the food consumption of 16,500 people conducted by Michael F. Holik and associates at the University of Boston School of Medicine showed just how lacking many of these important nutrients

are in our diets today. Young children receive a larger percentage of their recommended daily allowance of vitamin D than adults do. That's largely due to the
reduced consumption of milk as we grow older. But there are far better ways to
get your daily dose of vitamin D. Eating organic butter, and exposing yourself
to sunshine daily, are among them.

A word about vitamin D and the sun... Many of us fail to get even twenty
minutes of sunshine daily. Not surprisingly, the greatest deficiency of this important nutrient occurs in those age fifty years old and older. Of those in this age
group, only 1 percent to 3 percent of women and approximately 5 percent of
men receive their RDA of this vitamin. Even *with* supplementation, Caucasian
males over the age of fifty were found to receive only 35 percent of their RDA.
And the numbers are worse for those with darker skin. Seventeen percent for
Hispanic people and a mere 10 percent for African Americans. The darker our
skin, the greater the barrier to UV light which is required by our body for the
production of vitamin D. And the heavier you are, the more of this important
nutrient is "taken" (or absorbed) from your diet, making the amount you do
produce less available. All too many of us needlessly avoid exposure to sunlight,
leading to record numbers of those of us who have difficulty sleeping. You may
block your body's ability to produce more of this important vitamin each time
you slather on sunscreen. If a deficiency of vitamin D is associated with the
development of certain cancers (and many have this deficiency), why would
you choose to *block* your body's ability to formulate this important nutrient?
Scientists analyzed the rates of cancer in 175 countries and found that those
living the farthest distance from the sun had the *highest* rates of lung cancer.
Five separate studies using global incidence data investigated the relationship
between vitamin D, a specific disease, and the subject's proximity to the equator
(an area and altitude where sunshine and vitamin D are more plentiful than in
other areas that are farther from it). All showed a similar correlation.

Each of these studies was led by the same department at The University of
California, San Diego. The first four of these queries investigated the relationship between different types of cancers and exposure to the sun. The initial
study (*International Journal of Cancer*, September 15, 2006) showed that a
direct correlation did exist between increased exposure to the sun and reduced
rates of kidney cancer; the next study sought to determine if a relationship
existed between the amount of exposure to sunshine and the associated rates of
ovarian cancer (*American Journal of Preventive Medicine*, October 31, 2006).

The third (*Preventive Medicine*, September 16, 2007) investigated if a correlation exists between our exposure to sun and endometrial cancer. The fourth study investigated the potential of this same relationship to rates of breast cancer (*Breast Journal*, May–June 2008). All four studies showed a strong association between the rate of various cancers and the amount of vitamin D received from the sun.

The most recent study, the fifth done by University of California researchers, investigated the incidence of type 1 diabetes in children and their proximity to the equator. And they, too, had similar findings. Other analysis on cross linkage from hospital data banks that tracked the history of MS patients was conducted Dr. M. J. Goldacre of Oxford University's Institute of Health and Health Science. The investigators concluded that "solar radiation may have a protective influence on the development of MS" (*Journal of Epidemiology and Community Health*, 2004; 58: 142-144). Few nutrients have as much scientific data to support their use for the prevention of cancer as vitamin D does.

Do you still think you're better off hiding under a tree to avoid skin cancer? Learn to embrace the sun's ability to heal, while avoiding its potential for damage. Consider enjoying sunshine for twenty minutes a day. Then apply a lotion that protects you against both UVA and UVB rays. While over-exposure can be harmful for those with certain skin types, under-exposure interferes with the production of this important nutrient. The key to good health is balance; moderation, not suffocation. And if you do use sunscreen after those first twenty minutes, remember this–you'll probably fry if you don't reapply.

Fair-skinned persons who burn easily, should cover particularly vulnerable areas. Or, to put it another way, consider only exposing parts of your body less sensitive to the sun. Again, for twenty minutes only.

In addition to organic butter and products fortified with vitamin D such as milk and bread (I don't recommend eating any fortified foods), *baby* calves liver, healthy fish, and eggs are all excellent sources of this important organic compound. While supplements may be required to boost your level, use only when indicated. Too much vitamin D is just as bad as too little. It's a soluble fat that is absorbed as part of your body fat. Don't consider supplementation unless a blood test indicates that a deficiency exists (most do), and then only if your intake and level are regularly monitored. Optimizing your level of vitamin D is one of the key elements in the SOS program, which we will further discuss in Chapter 5.

Reduce your consumption of those saturated fats not mentioned above. Extra virgin tropical oils, such as coconut oil (and natural palm oil), as well as organic butter, are the primary saturated Cinderella super-fats frequently overlooked, and an important part of our self defense.

NATURAL ORGANIC PALM OIL—AN UNSATURATED, SATURATED FAT

While this tropical oil generally contains as much polyunsaturated fat as saturated fat, it remains an SOS food. The majority of its polyunsaturated content consists of healthy oleic acid. The same oleic acid found in extra virgin olive oil. Since it's less stable than coconut oil, EVCO continues to be our preferred choice.

IS CANCER RELATED TO THE CONSUMPTION OF HEALTHY SATURATED FATS?

Studies implicate excessive consumption of meat with cancers of the colon and ovaries. While the Inuit Eskimos had a very low incidence of CHD even after consuming large amounts of saturated fats, they did have an increased incidence of certain types of cancers. Studies at both Harvard and Cambridge Universities found a high correlation between saturated fat intake in post menopausal women (based on questionnaires and diaries maintained by subjects, respectively) and breast cancer. But it's time for us to more closely examine these findings. Could these conclusions have been influenced in whole or in part by important confounding variables—factors researchers may have failed to consider? Does such a correlation exist between saturated fat and cancer?

Even if it did, eating saturated fat from animals wouldn't diminish the integrity of a plant-based saturate, like extra virgin coconut oil. A further look compels us to consider the source.

These animals are often fed foods containing additives and fillers, hormones, antibiotics, and corn-based grains they were never equipped to process. Their lungs can literally deflate from a steady diet of this indigestible grain. Gas trapped in a bloated rumen can lead to suffocation, according to Michael Pollan. Without the use of antibiotics in grain-fed cattle, acidosis can lay the groundwork for a breeding ground for bacteria. A treacherous cycle may ensue where toxins are released, creating havoc in the animal, absorbed into their tissue from a cesspool of gastric juice. New strains of bacteria are occasionally produced that prove resistant to this stomach acid, maintaining their toxic integrity when ingested by humans.[16, 17, 18, 19, 20, 21]

Since grain-fed cattle have an impaired ability to effectively digest industrialized foods; undigested grains reach the colon where they ferment, according to James B. Russell, PhD, a USDA microbiologist and faculty member of the Cornell University section of microbiology (*Science*, 1988). When this occurs, various acids such as butyric, acetic, and propionic acid accumulate in the animal's colon. These are the resistant strains, such as E. coli O157:H7, a deadly variety that's potentially enterohemorrhagic and capable of causing kidney failure. Certain bacteria in grain-fed cattle have learned to thrive in a highly acidic environment and are no longer killed by our stomach acid.

Abdominal pain, diarrhea, and low-grade fever are forerunners of a death rate as high as 30 percent in infected cattle. It's normally present in the intestines of humans (yes, most of us have healthy E. coli in our intestines, not the O157:H7 variety which creates these problems) and more than 20,000 people are infected with heinous bacteria annually.

Not surprisingly, several studies suggest that excessive consumption of the wrong kind of saturated fats precipitate cancer. The U.S. Department of Agriculture's Food Safety and Inspection Service established guideline classifications for inspection of animal protein sources in 1998, then claimed that animals with cancer, infectious causing arthritis, glandular swellings, or lymphomas *did not present a direct public health risk*! These guidelines allow producers to cut off lesions as the animals come down the line, and the remaining carcasses are passed onto consumers.

You can easily eliminate all of these concerns by eating grass-fed beef. It's full of essential nutrients. Jo Robinson (*Pasture Perfect*, 2004) tells us that for those eating the typical amount of beef annually (66.5 pounds), simply switching to the grass-fed variety will save you 17,733 calories a year (approximately 6 pounds). Moreover, grass-fed beef is loaded with conjugated linoleic acid (CLA).

I found no evidence that eating *healthful* saturated fat causes cancer. And as far as the Inuits? The fact that they had an increased risk of cancer seems logical. There was no *balance* in their diet. Eating marine animals and whale blubber may reduce the risk of heart disease, but it creates a dangerous imbalance of fats, important carbohydrates, and other nutrients. No one is suggesting that the Inuits were among the healthiest people in the world, only that they enjoyed a low incidence of heart disease. Again, the key to good health is *balance*.

FISH OIL—THE HEALTHIEST POLYUNSATURATED FAT

All of the oils I have discussed so far have come from plants. But the oil that comes from fish, though derived from the algae they eat, is one of the healthiest oils in the world. Fish oil is unique. It contains a high concentration of important Omega-3 fatty acids EPA and DHA, We've previously discussed the amazing benefits of eating the right type of fish. We also discussed pharmaceutical grade fish oil, the perfect supplement. Fish oil is not a substitute for eating fish. There are likely *other* important constituents of fish that have yet to be discovered. But coupling this *concentrated* source of Omega-3 deals a one-two punch to internal inflammation. According to Dr. Sears (*The Anti-Inflammation Zone*, Regan Books, 2005), eating the right amount will boost Omega-3 EPA and DHA, reducing internal inflammation throughout your body. It actually diminishes the AA that lays the groundwork for pro-inflammatory eicosanoids. In fact, according to Dr. Sears, it can do so in less than a month!

PERILLA OIL—THE OTHER POLYUNSATURATED PATH TO OMEGA-3S

The right fish and fish oil are far better choices to obtain healthful Omega-3 descendant fats DHA and EPA. However, if you can't tolerate fish (or follow a vegan diet and simply won't eat it), there is a powerful plant-based source of ALA that may be of interest to you. More research is required before it can be incorporated as a primary fat in your diet. While not preferable to direct sources of descendant fats DHA and EPA as fish and EPO recommended, *perilla oil* may be the next best thing. Until it's fully researched, use it only in moderation. It's far more stable and less reactive than flaxseed. Indeed, there is no other oil on the planet, unless artificially fortified, that boasts such unique, powerful, and stabilizing antioxidants (olive oil is a close runner-up, and more stable). Often referred to as the "Antioxidant Omega-3," it contains an amazing array of phenolic compounds, including quercetin, catechin, and luteolin. Its high content of rosmarinic acid, an anti-inflammatory, joins a long list of other phenol compounds boasting antibacterial, antiviral, and antioxidant benefit. In human studies, perilla oil was found to substantially reduce allergic reaction, particularly those from shellfish. Animal studies show that significant reductions in the rate of colon cancer occur from a diet rich in perilla oil. Scientists believe this is due to its ability to increase the sensitivity of the colonic mucosa to tumor promoters.

In yet another study, perilla oil's anti-inflammatory Omega-3s protected the lining of the intestine from mucosal damage. Such damage is typically induced by an increase in leukotriene production. These compounds are formed by chemicals released from mast cells, which promote inflammation in the same manner as histamines. Their development is precipitated by allergens and is closely associated with asthma.

Perilla oil may hold hope as a natural alternative, without the potential for serious side effects—and it's affordable. It contains a far better ratio of saturated versus unsaturated fat (19 percent versus 7 percent saturated fat respectively) than flaxseed oil. Perilla seed oil, from the first pressing of the perilla seed plant, also known as the beefsteak plant, contains approximately 55 percent as much ALA as flax. A member of the mint family, Perilla frutescens have a mild, pleasing taste, and unlike other sources of ALA, it's easy to digest. It's been used in Southeast Asian cuisine for many years.

Perilla oil doesn't require cold refrigeration (a moderate amount could provide a handy alternative to fish oil for the traveler). More importantly, it's not processed like flax and most other oils, allowing perilla oil to retain the nutrients that are found in its seed. In contrast to flax, it's as healthy as its seed because most makers avoid pressing the leaves and tops containing toxins. Yet as promising as perilla seed oil may be, I only recommend it in moderation, principally to those unable to tolerate fish and fish oil products.

While excited about these findings, keep in mind that the direct consumption of ALA has shown promise in some areas and potential harm in others. While I believe research will eventually exonerate ALA from perilla oil, due to its unique stability, sufficient studies in humans (difficult to accomplish to be sure) are required before we can trumpet its arrival as a super-fat.

Similarly, while studies on flax clearly demonstrate its ability to reduce tumor regression in rats, the opposite occurred in human trials. In an overview of such research, the Prostate Cancer Forum ("Omega-3 Fatty Acids, Fish or Flax," Vol, 8, Number 7,) reported that of the numerous studies conducted on humans, the majority showed that ALA precipitated progression of prostate cancer. According to the report: "ALA, the major plant Omega-3, increased the risk of prostate cancer by 1.7 fold. ALA from both animal and vegetable sources was associated with an increase in the risk of prostate cancer. Men convert less than 4 percent of ALA to DHA, the Omega-3 fat needed for optimal brain function ..." Why not choose a more reliable source that's already broken down to the descendant fat you really want? I believe the benefit outweighs the potential risk from a negligible amount of ALA. If you choose to do so, take no more than 1 gram a day of the type that's most absorbable. A commercial product called Enterox®, a soft gel capsule is my choice. I take this along with fish oil. The maker claims that its enteric coating allows nutrients to pass through the stomach (without the meltdown normally associated with the stomach's digestion enzymes) to the small intestine for slower more optimal absorption. Clinical trials have shown a far higher integration of their product than in many standard perilla oils, but the studies I reviewed were based on small subject groups.

If you decide to take this in moderation, consider eating it along with of a cup of cottage cheese. Six-time Nobel Award winner Dr. Johanna Budwig's research with flax showed that it only affected the immune system in a positive way when combined with quark. Quark, not easily available in the U.S., is similar to cottage cheese. She found that lipids are only water-soluble and free flowing when bound to protein. Doing so allows the electrons in the fat to be protected until they are required by the body. If cottage cheese is not to your liking, try it with a high-quality yogurt such as Brown Cow™ plain yogurt or Athena brand Greek-style yogurt, which contain living cultures that most other yogurts don't. Eat about one third of a cup with this and all fats whenever possible.

Chia seeds also contain an excellent balance of Omega-3 to Omega-6 fatty acids. Only recently have they begun to receive the notoriety they deserve.

COOKING WITH SATURATED FATS VERSUS POLYUNSATURATED FATS

Public support for *unsaturated* fat is another example of public opinion based on misinformation. Eating certain amounts of a particular unsaturated fat is one of the fastest ways to accelerate premature aging. Certain unsaturated fats are highly unstable and quickly become rancid. Few things are as dangerous as unstable oil that's rancid. As we've learned, unsaturated oils are less stable, breaking down quickly when exposed to heat. Rancid oil and food cooked with unstable fat sets off a small avalanche of free radical activity when they enter you.

But the secondhand consumption of this oil is even worse. Unstable oils are reheated over and over again, a common practice in fast food restaurants.

A recent study (May 4, 2005, presentation, American Oil Chemists Society, annual meeting, Salt Lake City) by scientists at the University of Minnesota found that vegetable based cooking oil reheated for several hours produced a dangerous toxin known as HNE (4-hydroxy-trans-2-nonenal). Cooking with saturated fat did not. According to the researchers, this was particularly true in oils that contain high amounts of LA (linoleic acid) such as *canola*, corn, sunflower, and soybean oils. Please keep this in mind the next time you pull up to that drive-thru window. And they call it a *Happy* Meal.

At home, avoid cooking with most unsaturated fats. They quickly oxidize when heated and are already unstable. Flaxseed oil becomes rancid if not refrigerated in only one hour after sitting out in temperatures under 72 degrees. Imagine how quickly it becomes even more unstable when exposed to higher cooking temperatures. Then we heat it *again* when we eat it. The free radical danger from these highly unstable molecules is formidable. On the other hand, coconut oil has been proven to remain stable for over a year without refrigeration. Don't confuse that stability with its inability to break down inside of you, as folklore suggests. Actually, it's quite the opposite. According to Bruce Fife, N.D. (*The Healing Miracles of Coconut Oil*, 2004), other than breast milk, it's the only food existing in nature whose fat content is 50 percent lauric acid, a rare but important MCFA that allows it to be quickly digested and rapidly converted to usable energy. It easily permeates cell membranes and requires no assistance from your body to produce enzymes. Unlike all other fatty acids, MCFAs race directly into your liver. Almost upon arrival they are immediately converted to energy, not stored as fat, perhaps the opposite of what you've been told. This misconception, that this wonderful stable fat remains as some type of clogging factor inside of you, is just that. This miracle food puts less strain on your digestive tract and helps your body stimulate metabolism. And according to Fife, its ability to do so increases *your* ability to lose weight. The ability for MCFA to be so easily digested also explains why it's an important addition to most baby formulas. Not surprisingly, the only other abundant source of MCFA in nature is breast milk.

But consuming too many bad oils and fats *are* cause for concern, for they create internal oxidation and subsequent inflammation. The effect of internal oxidation can actually be measured by a diagnostic devise known as a BTM (bio-terrain measuring device). Consumption of *unstable* oils such as flax and hemp appear to significantly increase oxidation on a cellular level. But stable fats such as coconut oil actually lower it. The presence of stable fats is also required for the proper absorption and effective utilization of protein and calcium. Stress (and certain soy products) strips calcium from our bodies. But an optimum balance of healthy fat helps us to effectively utilize it. This means that the wrong oils are quite literally aging you while the right fats are required to heal you. I avoid cooking with unstable polyunsaturated vegetable oils. Use extra virgin coconut oil on high heat, natural palm oil, and extra virgin olive oil or organic butter on low heat.

The ratio of good fats to bad fats is radically different in foods such as grass-fed beef and certain other animal meats. They're *balanced*, and therefore are of great benefit. While your dietary cholesterol means little as it relates to heart disease, some of its constituents help fan the flame of internal inflammation. *Oxidized* cholesterol is the leading pro-inflammatory vigilante, catalyzing the production of cardiovascular plaque. It's one of the best reasons to consider the regular and moderate consumption of all recommended healthful, saturated fats.

MONOUNSATURATED FATS: ONE IS A LONELY NUMBER

More stable than polyunsaturated fats, monounsaturated fats have neither the same free radical structure nor the Omega-6s found in polyunsaturated fats. They may lower LDL, but unlike their polyunsaturated brethren, they don't lower important HDL. Recall that fish oil, one of the two polyunsaturated fats recommended, actually converts harmful hard small particle LDL to puffy and fluffy harmless LDL.

We're often told that monounsaturated fats are the real superstars. They're considerably more stable than polyunsaturated fats, due to the balancing action of their antioxidants.

All natural fat classifications have their share of winners and losers. For example, as you've learned, organic or raw butter and coconut oil are incredibly beneficial *saturated* fats. Evening primrose oil and certain fish and fish oils are *polyunsaturated* fats equally worthy of praise. *Safflower* oil is among the least stable cooking oils, with 75 percent polyunsaturated fat, closely followed by corn oil with 59 percent. Both are high in Omega 6 fatty acids. Again, an imbalance of Omega 6 to Omega 3 fats is constrictive.

Monounsaturated fats are no exception. Some have proven to be healthful while others are clearly hurtful. Extra virgin olive oil, avocados, and certain nuts are the standouts. All partially hydrogenated or highly processed oils should be avoided.

Canola oil has had quite an evolution as a man-made oil with several incarnations. If reincarnation were a good thing for an oil, it would be right up with the Dalai Lama, but it's not. It's more like the five faces of Eve. Marketers and scientists have tried to do everything they could to create "the ultimate" monounsaturated oil. As you've already learned, processed food products are far from perfect. More often than not, all that tinkering results in something messed up on some level. While olive oil was known to be incredibly healthful, it was neither cheap nor widely available. The world market cried out for an available supply of affordable oil. So, industry experts created a new class of cheap polyunsaturated trans fatty vegetable oils. They were designed to take over for saturated fat because Keyes said it raised your cholesterol level and caused heart disease. In time, it would be exposed as a charlatan fat. But until that day, many would suffer from a precipitous increase in internal oxidation and inflammation, as we embraced being misinformed.

As a result, companies went back to the drawing board. With saturated fats and fake polyunsaturated fats now in ill repute, the marketing geniuses turned their attention to monounsaturated fat. It was a logical choice. If the world could be convinced to embrace a fake man-made protein like soy milk, it's just possible we could be sold still another fake type of fat.

CANOLA OIL—THE GREAT RAPE-OFF (OF THE MAN-MADE MONO)

We needed an oil we could trust—and it had to be cheap. Rapeseed oil, a monounsaturated fat from the rape plant, had been used extensively in certain third world Asian countries but not as their principal fat. While olive oil contained almost 70 percent monounsaturated fat, rapeseed oil, weighing in at approximately 60 percent, had fatty acids that varied a great deal from its popular, expensive, monounsaturated cousin.

All monounsaturated fats are not created equal.

More than 65 percent of the monounsaturated fat found in rapeseed oil is made up of erucic acid, a 22-carbon monounsaturated fatty acid of the Omega-9 family that Mary Enig claims is associated with Keshan's disease ("The Great Con-ola," www.westonprice.org), characterized by fibrotic lesions of the heart. The remaining monounsaturated fat in rapeseed oil is behenic acid, another fatty acid with 22 carbon atoms. If eating high concentrations of erucic acid can have toxic effects, would a significantly lesser amount prove to be safe? Canadian plant growers weren't about to find out. After all, this was a burgeoning industry. Instead they developed breeding techniques permitting them to create a hybrid rapeseed oil that all but eliminated erucic acid. This monounsaturated fatty acid was largely replaced with the same monounsaturated fatty acid, oleic acid, found in olive oil. But buyers still showed no interest. They couldn't give it away. Would you line up to buy and eat oil from a plant named "rape"? So a new name with a lot more appeal was required.

Time to send for the Smith brothers. The marketing musketeers were up for the challenge. Now a newly introduced oil with a whole new name featuring a significant reduction in hazardous erucic acid, while boasting large amounts of healthful oleic acid, could be introduced. Who ever said what's in a name? And so, what name did the geniuses come up with to entice us this time? LEAR oil (low-level erucic acid rapeseed oil) was the latest incarnation. It was the healthy alternative to saturated fat and trans fats. LEAR had a whole new shtick, a whole new name, and a whole new persona. But "LEAR oil"? Was it a type of motor oil? Back to the drawing board!

Send for the Smith brothers. Could another name do the trick? One more brainstorm and they got it! Third time is a charm. "Canadian Oil" was born. It did have a bit of patriotic ring to it, didn't it? Think of it: an acronym now for Canadian Oil Low Acid. Nice visual. How about simmering some veggies in a few quarts of Canada Oil? The healthy, affordable choice for a new generation of what—automobiles? Back to the drawing board.

But the drawing board had already become a bit crowded. Now it was getting darn right hard to read. But leave it to the Canadians ... send for the Smith brothers again! They had already fooled some of the people some of the time. Now maybe they could fool all of the people all of the time? After all, we went from Rape to Lear without a hitch. Then we wrapped it all up in the Canadian flag. If the average guy failed to connect these dotted lines, what's the big deal if we changed the name just one more time? But this time the name needed to sound really healthy.

After all, after four times, even the Smith brothers might be out! Forget the drawing board. *The Da Vinci Code* had nothing on these guys as they whispered the words that kept them up at night ... Canadian Oil Low Acid. Huh? And then, finally, in one of those moments history will long remember, it came to them. *Canola* Oil! And this time it stuck. They even liked it in Boulder, Colorado, the birthplace of Celestial Seasons™ tea. You can't fool the Boulderites. People there are just plain down to earth. But according to its detractors, *all but* eliminating erucic acid is not the same as eliminating it. The toxin, albeit less of it, is still in there. While I agree with this, I'm not sure I agree with Mary Lou Enig's reasoning as to why that's harmful. Enig claims it's a leading cause of Keshan's disease. The primary cause of Keshan's disease is a deficiency in selenium, also linked to a host of others diseases including cancer. In countries like China, Keshan's and selenium deficiency clearly go hand in hand. Rapeseed oil is used extensively in China and India, countries that have a higher than normal incidence of Keshan's disease. While more studies need to be conducted, it would appear that selenium deficiency provides a pathway for viruses to flourish. It's this virus that produces these lesions on the heart.

Research has begun to validate a link between the viral theory of certain diseases, cancers, and selenium deficiency. Since the introduction of selenium-enriched fertilizers into soils and crops and feedstock as well as table salt, there has been a decline in Keshan's disease, according to the Sam Burcher writing for the ISIS (Institute of Science Society). In an article entitled. "Selenium Conquers AIDS?" (ISIS Press Release 20/07/04), Burcher reports: "A three year study of an entire town in Jiangsu Province where 20,847 residents were given table salt fortified with selenium showed that hepatitis infection decreased to 4.52 per 1,000 compared to 10.48 per 1,000 in communities using regular table salt. The same researchers concluded that a 200-microgram daily dose of selenium-yeast supplement significantly reduced primary liver cancer associated with hepatitis B and C. It appears that death rates from viruses such as hepatitis, Coxsackie B3 and associated heart diseases like Keshan's, can be greatly reduced by increasing dietary selenium intake and would be similarly effective in slowing the progress of AIDS deaths."

But is erucic acid truly toxic to humans? A cause and effect relationship between the consumption of dietary erucic acid found in rapeseed oil and heart lesions in humans has never been firmly established, despite all the hype. It's an assumption, based on a relationship proven to exist in rat studies, which show that the consumption of "high" erucic acid rapeseed oil causes severe cardiac necrosis. Similar research, conducted on pigs and monkeys, failed to support this. Follow up studies on rats using newer "low level erucic acid oil" also failed to demonstrate this relationship. While the original rape oil and canola continue to share some characteristics, producers have done much to substantially reduce its content of erucic acid (now under 2% of the total fat or considerably less). According to Enig and Fallon, breeding methods have also been introduced that virtually eliminate high levels of glycocides, an organic compound found in rape and other plants that its detractors site as being hazardous to our health. Critics also refer to a study showing that the smoke caused by cooking rapeseed oil on high heat causes lung cancer. But I'd venture to guess that inhaling enough smoke from any oil has the potential to do so. Another misconception is that rapeseed is used to produce mustard gas. Though rapeseed is a member of the mustard family, this is nonsense. Mustard gas doesn't contain rapeseed, nor any material from any other plant in the mustard family. This gas got its name due to the odor it emits. Other mistaken notions include that Canola is loaded with 22-carbon long chain fatty acids that may cause degenerative disease if large amounts are consumed. While rapeseed largely consists of 22-carbon long chain fatty acids, morphed canola oil has a fatty acid composition that substantially differs. According to the Canola Council of Canada, it's predominantly composed (over 90 percent) of the 18-carbon unsaturated fatty acids oleic acid, linoleic acid, and linolenic acid. Canola producers have developed a number of methods designed to overcome some of the inherent dangers found in rapeseed oil. They've also sought ways to improve its lipid profile, including the addition of healthy Omega 3 fatty acids. Today, manufacturers are beginning to introduce what they call new, stable, high heat versions, claiming to be "virtually" trans fat free.

... CANOLA OIL IS A MAN-MADE TRANS FAT. THAT'S RIGHT—CANOLA OIL IS EITHER HYDROGENIZED OR PARTIALLY HYDROGENIZED.

I have been less than successful in my efforts to determine what virtually means. In my opinion, any amount of trans fat in the diet has the potential to endanger us. Laws that permit makers to call something trans fat free, that isn't, is absurd. Despite all of the progress of its makers, the information I've reviewed suggests there are healthier alternatives.

Canola is a man-made oil that's highly refined. Most are genetically modified, deodorized and partially hydrogenated, containing man-made trans fats and erucic acid. Exposure of its fat to high levels of heat degrades its value. Polyunsaturated fats already seeking one or more carbon atom become even more unstable when heated. I could find no long term studies in humans showing the long term effect of ingesting Canola oil.

In the end, why would you incorporate this man-made fat into your prescription for good health when there are clearly better alternatives?

EXTRA VIRGIN OLIVE OIL—A SUPER MONOUNSATURATED FAT

Extra virgin olive oil (EVOO) contains 9 percent polyunsaturated fat, 72 percent monounsaturated fat, 14 percent saturated fat, with a 5.8:1 unsaturated/saturated fat ratio (*The Wellness Encyclopedia of Food and Nutrition*, 1992). This is the first of two standouts of the monounsaturated fat family, excluding nuts, which you'll learn about shortly. Boasting a veritable storehouse of antioxidants and nutrients that stabilize this normally unstable family of fatty acids (as well as a 14 percent content of saturated fat), olive oil is a most unusual fatty acid. While less reactive than its polyunsaturated cousins, monounsaturated fats are not normally as balanced. Brimming with healthful monounsaturated fat (72 percent), this oil has healing properties that make it a genuine "super-food."

On the other hand, it's often a toxic carrier of rancid oil capable of confusing your cells and inflaming their membranes. Unless you chose to remain *Misinformed About Food*, it's important to understand which of these two roads you may be traveling. Trusting labels blindly is gambling with your health. A large body of compelling research shows the extraordinary benefits of eating the *right* kind of EVOO. And that, for the purposes of our discussion, is all that counts. If your selection is not educated, then this and other oils will do you more harm than good, as you'll see shortly.

Most studies demonstrate the healing effects when certain bad fats are replaced with this good one. But why? Is it due to the elimination or the reduction of the bad stuff—or the addition of the good? Separate, but equally important, questions concern the studies themselves and are once again the questions that need to be raised regarding the impact of confounding variables. Are the majority of benefits derived from the antioxidants and phenol compounds in the oil itself, or in the monounsaturated fat? So far, the answer is the former. The way this is answered does make a difference. In 2005, in the first of a two-stage health study, subjects received high-quality polyphenol-rich EVOO containing the highest concentration of these antioxidants. In the second stage of the trial, subjects received oil containing only one-fifth of these polyphenol antioxidants. Using a Doppler laser, scientists measured the amount of elasticity in the arterial walls of each subject.

After eating the high-grade, polyphenol-rich olive oil, the subjects experienced increased arterial elasticity. But in stage two, the subjects experienced no corresponding increase in arterial elasticity from the oil with far lower levels of polyphenols. After all, if the right antioxidants are in the oil, that's reason enough to use it, right? The answer is a resounding yes. But only a very small percentage of the olive oil that's purchased today provides high levels of these compounds. Those that do so often lose them quickly, when they're exposed to light and heat. Much of the oil on the market is, in varying degrees, of less or no benefit. Even EVOO may be processed, or blended with lesser grades of oil. Many are highly processed, often with charcoal, degraded or even void of nutrients, and even rancid. Our discussion will be directed to finding the right oil, while hoping to stay clear of the wrong oil. Unlike polyunsaturated fats, monounsaturated fats lower LDL. More importantly, they lower LDL oxidation, a precursor to internal inflammation without lowering healthy HDL. Studies have shown that the right EVOO is actually capable of *raising* the good HDL, which ushers away harmful LDL, reducing internal inflammation. There aren't many natural ways to do that.

Just as important, the *right* EVOO is loaded with powerful, hard-to-find antioxidants that boost your immunity and bathe your tissues with healthful protective fat. You learned earlier that the unstable free radical production from unsaturated fats and the importance of available antioxidants offsets their production and proliferation. But olive oil is an exception. The healthy ones actually counter their own unstable nature and free radical activity. Teaming with a rare mix of important antioxidants, their polyphenolic compounds, carotenoids, and vitamins (such as vitamin E) collectively stabilize their fat, making the right EVOO the single most stable unsaturated fat.

In 2002, the *European Journal of Clinical Nutrition* (56:114–120, April 2002) reported research showing that in just one week, subjects who ate only 2 tablespoons per day of (the right) EVOO had a significantly higher level of antioxidants in the blood and lower oxidized LDL than the control group that did not.[22]

The "more is better" camp may actually be harming themselves. The right *balance* of the right fats and other nutrients is the key to good health. It's really important to find all the right foods as you continue to separate the *fat* from the fiction. Unlike a fine wine, olive oil doesn't get better with age. It breaks down over time, oxidizes, and its healthy chemical balance degrades. Always purchase EVOO in *small* amounts that you can use in one month or less. Stay away from older harvests. Olive oil, like all unsaturated fats, oxidizes rapidly when exposed to heat, air, and light. Store in a cool dry place and buy in dark green or dark brown colored bottles. The best choice is an opaque bottle, but they're harder to find.

Researchers at the University of Bari in southern Italy published their research confirming the destruction that occurs to olive oil's antioxidants when exposed to light (*New Scientist*, August 2005). Their study compared oils stored in darkness and in light. This study showed just how profound this destruction can be in a very short period of time. They discovered that clear bottles of olive oil on grocery shelves lost no less than 30 percent of their tocopherols (vitamin E) and carotenoids in just *days*. After only two months of exposure to light, there was so much free radical proliferation that the purity and grade could no longer be classified as EVOO.

... CLEAR BOTTLES OF OLIVE OIL ON GROCERY SHELVES LOST NO LESS THAN 30 PERCENT OF THEIR TOCOPHEROLS (VITAMIN E) AND CAROTENOIDS IN JUST DAYS.

Olive oil contains an amazingly powerful (and hard to find) array of phenolic compounds (as does perilla oil). Research performed by the Lipids and Cardiovascular Epidemiology Unit in Barcelona, Spain, demonstrated the beneficial effect of olive oil's antioxidants. The "Eurolive" study involved six research centers, investigating 200 men from five European nations and was led by researcher Maria-Isabel Covas (*Annals of Internal Medicine*, 2006 Sep 5;145(5):333-41. PMID:16954359). Using rigid criteria in a large, controlled, double-blind, randomized crossover study, healthy subjects showed marked health improvement that directly corresponded in linear fashion to increasingly greater levels of polyphenols in EVOO. Significant decreases in oxidized LDL were observed in the blood plasma levels of subjects, along with subsequent increases of healthy HDL.

As you've learned, oxidized LDL that precipitates inflammation lays the groundwork for CHD. Three of the most important phenolic antioxidants found in high-quality EVOO are tyrosol, hydroxytyrosol, and oleuropein. Each hunt down dangerous superoxide radicals, clobbering their ability to oxidize LDL and other lipids. These healthful phenol compounds were not only absorbed but actually mirrored in the blood serum of subjects. It appears that the greater the concentration of phenolic compounds in your EVOO, the stronger the protection you'll receive.

EVOO also contains the largest percentage (of any oil) of valued squalene, a lipid also found in a shark's liver (and naturally produced in our liver as well). Squalene, a natural sterol, has been associated with a decrease in the risk of developing certain cancers in animal studies. In addition to abundant antioxidants and important, hard-to-find fatty acids such as squalene, olive oil contains no constrictive Omega-6. This incredibly powerful combination of antioxidants and rare phenolic compounds in EVOO makes finding the right one with the proper characteristics worth the effort. Cold-pressed EVOO contains one of the most powerful, natural, anti-inflammatory nutrients known to man: oleocanthol (a powerful anti-oxidant and anti-inflammatory).

In a study by Gary Beauchamp and other researchers (*Nature*, September 2005; 437, 45-46), the power of oleocanthol was shown. This important lipid actually inhibited COX-1 and COX-2 enzymes from the production of prostinoids (COX-3 is a man-made variant). Cyclooxygenase (abbreviated as COX) is a class of enzymes associated with biological mediation. Inhibiting these pro-inflammatory, pain-producing enzymes can provide relief from internal inflammation and pain. Oleocanthol from cold-pressed EVOO is a natural way of doing so; though the amount found in aspirin and certain pharmaceuticals contains an even larger amount of this inhibiting factor (raw garlic has also been found to have this same inhibiting effect on the same class of pro-inflammatory).

Man-made inhibitors such as diclofenac and ibuprofen, as opposed to oleocanthol, have been shown to increase the risk of atherothrombosis even when used short term. Either can actually double the risk of myocardial infarction. In high doses, both are associated with an increased risk of cardiovascular disease.

COX-1 enzymes have been shown to play a key role in the progression of tumors and in the uptake of certain carcinomas. COX-2 enzymes are more inflammatory than either COX-1 or COX-3. They're only present under certain conditions, and are referred to as *inducible* enzymes. Large concentrations of these are found in our white blood cells at points of inflammation, and are required to assist in the production of arthritis pain and other responses. So, they are useful as warning signs of an underlying disorder but only up to a point.

In this regard, oleocanthol works in the same manner as ibuprofen to stop inflammation in our joints. But ibuprofen has a number of downside risks, including potentially serious blood loss, found in those that use it daily. Oleocanthol is a natural alternative without ibuprofen's' potential danger. You can even tell if your EVOO contains beneficial oleocanthol by tasting it. Like a fine wine, just sip a little into the back of your throat. Oleocanthol has a bitter, stinging, peppery taste. If that tinge is absent, so is the oleocanthol. This is one of the primary tests, allowing you to determine the value of your EVOO. In this regard and in many others, we can see that all olive oils (and EVOOs) are not created equal. One of the problems is the lack of regulation. The U.S. government does not inspect nor require a product labeled "Extra Virgin Olive Oil" to meet any standard whatsoever. But if it's EVOO, how bad can it be?

The first question we must ask ourselves is whether what we think is EVOO is even EVOO? Chances are that it's not—at least not high-quality EVOO with oleocanthol, which we will now call EVOOO to distinguish it from the majority of EVOO, containing little or no oleocanthol. This synonym also recognizes the importance of this organic compound.

In February 2006, federal agents in New Jersey seized 22,700 gallons of Hermes and San Giovanni oil made from soybeans and vegetables that was labeled as extra virgin olive oil. Years earlier, Terry Pristin of the *New York Times* (July 23, 1997) reported that U.S. marshals seized 600 cases of oil from Lionelli Packing. This time the label read "pomace oil," a high-grade variety of olive oil. But upon closer examination, they discovered that it primarily consisted of cheap soybean oil. Soybean oil looks like olive oil, but it's "basically worthless nutritionally (even harmful) adulterated and mislabeled," said Michael A. Chagares, an assistant United States attorney. Sadly, this is just the tip of the iceberg. Olive oil fraud is more rampant in the absence of enforceable regulation, with some of the finer EVOOs costing from $23 to $70 per gallon (approximately 18 cents to 58 cents an ounce at the time of this writing). It's also a big incentive for fraud. In an industry without enforceable regulation and an absence of proper labeling requirements, it's commonplace. Because over 95 percent of the olive oil in the U.S. is imported (California represents less than 1 percent of the olive oil production worldwide), exporters are only regulated by their own local governments and the International Olive Oil Council (IOOC). American makers aren't regulated at all.

> OLIVE OIL FRAUD IS MORE RAMPANT IN THE ABSENCE OF ENFORCEABLE REGULATION ...

Convened by the United Nations, the IOOC, based in Madrid, Spain, was formed in 1959. It set production and safety standards for its members inspired by the International Olive Oil Agreement of 1956. Their annual, coveted Mario Solinas Quality Award is presented by the secretariat of the IOOC, for the best EVOO in quality and flavor among its members (who currently produce 95 percent of all the EVOO in the world). Recipients must pass rigorous health and taste standards. It's a good place for us to search for the "silver slipper." In the world of EVOO, it is as coveted as an Oscar. No EVOO can be submitted that doesn't first meet their standards, flavor, and incredibly high and extensive quality requirements. These include but are not limited to a range of free-acidity (oleic acid content) that's under 0.8 percent, and insoluble impurities of less than 0.1 percent. Their criteria includes everything from maximum allowable levels of iron (required to be less than 3 milligrams), copper, peroxide, water, volatiles, insoluble impurities, halogenated solvents, UV absorbency, and flash point to sensory qualities such as fruitiness and aspect.

Unfortunately, the IOOC appears to have no requirement for their member labeling of important polyphenol content. But the research does show that the lower the free acid found, the higher the polyphenol content that's found in high-quality EVOO. EVOO with over 2 grams of free acid content is generally void of antioxidants. Ten grams of EVOO should contain approximately 5 milligrams of polyphenol. Vasquez showed that 200 grams per kilogram is the minimum content that defines higher quality EVOOs. The altitude the olives are grown and the amount of time required to harvest them, as well as the care taken in processing them further affects the amount and quality of phenol content and their composition (Cinquanta et al., 1997; Kiritsakis, 1998). These factors also affect the color of the olives at the time they're harvested.

In "The Effect of Cultivar and Processing Method on the contents of Polyphenols in Table Olives," Romero and colleagues (*Journal of Agriculture and Food Chemistry*, 2004 Feb 11;52(3):479-84) demonstrate that all other things being equal, olives contain the highest amount of antioxidants when they're harvested just as their color begins to develop. The effect of the additional sun required to fully ripen the fruit *diminishes* the amount of important nutrients that remain. Researchers have also shown that olive juice from table olives further provides an excellent source of tyrosol and hydroxytyrosol. But their concentration was the lowest in stuffed olives, slightly higher in the pitted variety, and the best in those that are plain. The more disturbed olives are by heat, light, toxins, picking, storage methods, charcoal filtering, handling, and processing, the lower the amount of these powerful nutrients.

Extra Virgin *Organic* Olive Oil with Oleocanthol (EVOOOO!) that's cold pressed, with low free-acid content (under 0.8%), is nearly void of harmful metals and toxins and naturally filtered without heat and light.

Admittedly, these criteria are almost impossible to find. But, we have one more requirement. The oil must be made in the U.S. Why? Because of how rapidly the value of this important oil degrades. Between shipping from overseas, handling, light, heat, storage, and time on the counter, finding the perfect olive oil, particularly in this country (where it's not regulated), is tough. Fortunately, the IOOC criterion provides us with excellent data to help us in sort through a long list of candidates for the finest oil available. While the IOOC requirements are a great starting point, this fine organization only considers products submitted by their member nations. There are many other producers in countries such as the United States and Israel, for example, whose excellent products are not eligible for their (members only) consideration.

If you're buying the bad stuff that's masquerading as the good, you may be eating hazardous, unstable oil laden with toxins that may even be rancid. If you're dining out at a fine restaurant, recognize that you may be playing Russian roulette with your selection, and likely eating an unhealthful impostor.

Either take the taste test, as you would a fine wine, or bring your own bottle (small opaque bottle or flask). If you're dining at one of your regular, neighborhood haunts, consider buying *them* a bottle of your choice and ask them if they will keep it on hand for your future use. Too extreme? Think again. For those of us who spent years going out of our way to purchase EVOO or requested a small cupful on the side as I have, it's sad to discover that we may have been doing ourselves more harm than good. Recently, I dined at a famed chef's restaurant in Las Vegas with a friend. I asked the server if the olive oil listed as an ingredient in the dish I was about to order (it did not say extra virgin) was indeed extra virgin. Products labeled olive oil, light olive oil, and pure olive oil are less healthful and more highly processed than EVOO. The waitress was certain it was the real thing, but to her credit she went back to the kitchen for validation. She later returned, hat in hand. It seems she was mistaken. It turned out this high-priced designer restaurant had been using palm oil in place of what the menu listed as olive oil. Well trained by her boss, she nevertheless, although apologetically, defended its use. That's precisely why it's important to know how to determine this yourself.

If you're buying EVOO for your use at home, pay careful attention to the above. If requesting EVOO at a restaurant, take a moment to perform a taste test. Most restaurants will be happy to accommodate you (because in general, they have no clue what you're doing).

The following are recent winners of the IOOC's coveted Mario Solinas Olive Oil Competition. New winners are named each year. First place winners were S.A.R.L. Château Virant, Lançon de Provence, France, (intense fruitiness) and Azienda Agricola Lombardo Francesco, Campobello di Mazara, Italy, (medium fruitiness). According to the competition's rules, winners are allowed to mention their prize on the label of the oil belonging to the same batch as the winning sample. To do so, they have to order the special logo available from the Executive Secretariat.

In addition to the above, the California Olive Oil Council (COOC), Italy (DOP), Spain (DO), or Greece (HEPO) and other national councils also certify high-quality oils from members that meet their rigid standards.

Dr. Barry Sears (www.zonelabsinc.com) offers an organic extra virgin olive oil from select regions of Umbria and Sicily that is labeled in a more reliable manner. Sears, using an independent testing lab, certifies and lists the actual polyphenol and squalene content right on the label. Though this and all EVOOs are subject to the factors previously noted that degrade the oil, it's the first honest analysis and truth in labeling I've found that is verified at the time of testing and bottling.

I encourage all sanctioned olive associations to adopt similar labeling requirements. These same criteria should be embraced by all governing bodies before doling out awards that proclaim they're the finest. While IOOC standards are among the strictest available, they clearly don't go far enough. If a product is consumed because of its potential health benefit, the degree to which these benefits can be found in a particular producer's product should be squarely indicated on its label. Anything less is playing on an eager public's desire to help themselves to the extent they possibly can. It's time for all makers to take the bull by the horns and tell it like it is.

Truthful labeling, like Dr. Sears has done, should be a requirement for not only EVOO, but every product (packaged and bulk) marketed for consumption. If what you eat controls your hormones, why isn't the honest labeling of its contents mandatory? The answer may lie in the number and influence of powerful food companies' whose products might be seen for what they are. The right EVOO is one of nature's most powerful tools of self-defense against the ravages of our modern food system. Fraudulent olive oil labeling, rancid oil, and oils whose nutrients are degraded are nails in the coffins of those who are *Misinformed About Food*.

Olive oil is of such importance to my wife Kelly and me that we've developed our own. And I'm pleased to say, it's the finest EVOOO ever offered, with a phenolic and anti-oxidant content that's off the chart (www.RKInformedLiving.com).

AVOCADO: THE FATTEST MONOUNSATURATED SUPER-FRUIT ON EARTH

Avocado is the second of two rock stars. Weighing in with as much fat as a quarter-pound burger (but loaded with healthful monounsaturated fats, not harmful trans fats and saturated fats), the avocado is close to the perfect food. And it's interesting to note that its name originates from the Aztec word "ahuacatl," which means testicle. Approximately 95 percent of all avocados are grown in California and 80 percent of those are of the popular Hass variety. According to Wikipedia, all Hass avocado trees are related to a single "mother tree" that was purchased as a seedling by a mail carrier named Rudolph Hass. Hass planted the seedling in his front yard in La Habra Heights, California, and patented the tree in 1935. All Hass avocados can be traced back to grafts made from that single tree. Sadly, the "mother tree" died of root rot in 2002 after living a very full and meaningful life.

Avocado joins EVOO as one of the two powerful "mono sisters." They have a content of healthful monounsaturated fats right up there with there with EVOO. It's another example of a monounsaturated fat that's inherently stable due to its wonderfully stable antioxidant content. And, avocados have more essential vitamins than all other members of the fruit family (yes, it's a fruit, not a vegetable). Its twenty-five essential vitamins include incredible amounts of potassium, magnesium, and folate, and it's second only to papaya in folate content among all fruits. Folate keeps homocysteine from building up, helping to protect blood vessels from constricting. Folic acid is an essential nutrient; it aids women in the prevention of miscarriage. It's also a great source of a broad array of other important nutrients (including vitamin B6, vitamin C, and vitamin E), key enzymes (with five different compounds recently found to protect rats against liver damage from known toxins), and antioxidants such as lutein and zeaxanthin. All of these features make the avocado more nutrient-rich than any other fruit.

Here's a classic example of how a food loaded with healthy fat actually helps you lose weight and keep it off. The more of the right fat you eat in reasonable portions, the greater the stability of your body weight. While it's certainly no quick fix, its dense, healthy lipids and high fiber content work to feed your blood sugar slowly, reducing hunger while helping you maintain your body weight over time. We've all heard how important fiber is, but few realize that avocados are the single greatest source of both. Loaded with a whopping 12 grams, its nutrients enter your blood stream *gradually*. The slower a food breaks down the better. Avocado's high concentration of monounsaturated fat (the majority of its calories) feeds your blood sugar on a slow roll without spiking your insulin. While its extra virgin oil has health benefits, EVOO remains my top choice.

What's more, foods that are dense and slow to break down are typically high in fiber. They satiate hunger and all but eliminate your blood sugar's thirst for simple carbohydrates for a sustained period of time. That's why eating the right fat (like avocado), the right nuts, and moderate amounts of coconut oil, coupled with the amazing super-foods discussed at length in this book, will help you stay fit and lose weight. It's not a diet. It's a healthy lifestyle that's easy to maintain, even for those that frequently travel.

Although avocados are high in calories, most come from the right kind of healthy monounsaturated fat. This nutritionally charged, dense, super-fruit is the finest of its kind, with a unique and powerful array of synergistic minerals and nutrients. Work done by Smith and associates (1983) compared the amount of fiber in thirty-four food sources (eighteen vegetables and fruits). Only avocado had the ideal ratio of both; 2.7 percent of insoluble fiber and 2.1 percent of soluble fiber. Soluble fiber slows the rate of entry for glucose in the blood. Insoluble fiber helps keep you regular. The right amount of both types can help manage your insulin level, affording you with additional protection against everything from colon disease to type 2 diabetes.

With approximately 12 grams of fiber, eating one avocado a day provides nearly one half of the recommended dietary requirement of fiber for women (approximately 25 grams), and just over one third of the amount recommended daily for men (approximately 35 grams). Unlike high-glycemic foods laden with glucose that race into our blood stream, that quickly satisfy our cravings and just as swiftly are ushered out, avocado's glycemic load is *zero*. High-glycemic foods such as potatoes rapidly break down and produce excess blood sugar. This signals your pancreas to quickly produce insulin to usher this excess out of your blood stream. The fat-carrying insulin also signals your cell receptors to open up their doors, store the fat, and then close. Incidentally, white potatoes actually rank higher than ice cream on the glycemic index. They raise your blood sugar even faster than candy or sugar. These and other starches have helped usher in a wave of obesity that's reached epidemic proportion. But avocado does nothing of the sort. Nor do any of the recommended SOS monounsaturated fats. So much for the low-calorie, low-fat and no-fat theories.

How many times have you been told to eat a banana (actually the fruit of an *herb*) because of its high content of potassium? But a medium size avocado has *more than twice the amount of potassium* (approximately 1205 milligrams) found in an average-size banana (approximately 487 milligrams). Avocados have nearly *double* the magnesium than bananas do (approximately 78.4 milligrams versus 43 milligrams), more than three times the phosphorus (approximately 82.4 milligrams versus 27 milligrams), many times the folate, more vitamin C, over ten times the vitamin A, and more than six times the pantothenic acid. They also contain more beta-carotene than any other fruit—and more vitamin E. The list of truly amazing benefits of the avocado goes on and on.

The balanced fiber in avocados, along with their large levels of potassium and magnesium, makes it one of the greatest food sources available for added protection against ischemic stroke. A medium-size avocado provides far more magnesium than any other fruit (70 milligrams in a typical California avocado, and an incredible 104 milligrams from an average-size Florida avocado). However, both avocado varieties, as well as bananas, were found by Scranton University researchers to be among the few foods that have a large portion of their important antioxidant phenols in a bio-available *free form*, as opposed to the conjugated form.

Avocados are loaded with glutathione, one of the most powerful antioxidants in the world. It's the second most abundant nutrient in this fruit. Research has shown that this tripeptide antioxidant offers powerful protection against free radical damage on the cellular level. Its reduced form generously donates electrons to reduce disulfide bonds during oxidative stress. In doing so, glutathione works to protect cytoplasm protein from corruption and disruption. Glutathione is also required for the detoxification of methylglyoxal, a normal by-product of our metabolism.

AVOCADOS ARE LOADED WITH GLUTATHIONE, ONE OF THE MOST POWERFUL ANTIOXIDANTS IN THE WORLD.

If all this weren't enough to inspire you to eat an avocado each and every day (consider spreading it on your sourdough toast, keeping guacamole salad on hand in the fridge, or eating one third of a whole one at mealtime), all men should be aware of its proven ability to inhibit the growth of prostate cancer cells. In January 2005, researchers Lu et al., working at the University of California Center for Human Nutrition, David Geffen School of Medicine, published the results of a milestone study (*Journal of Nutritional Biochemistry*, 2005) that examined the effect of avocado extract on just that. Scientists found that the combination of nutrients in avocado inhibited the growth and proliferation of both androgen-independent and -dependent cancer cells by up to 60 percent! The study also showed that exposing these cells to lutein alone (avocados are also the number one dietary source of this important carotenoid) had no such effect on the size or the ability of these cells to replicate. It was the *combined effect of all these nutrients* (their synergistic action, but not lutein alone) that was responsible for this amazing protection. They also noted that this fruit's monounsaturated fat was likely just as important, since it's required to permit absorption of carotenoids and other important vitamins. The whole, in this case, has proved to be far greater than the sum of its parts. This has further implications for nutrients, and the benefit of eating the whole foods derived from them, rather than relying on supplements alone (synergy of nutrients).

In a study reported by the American Society for Nutritional Sciences at Ohio State University's Department of Food Science and Technology and Internal Medicine (*Journal of Nutrition*, 2005 Mar; 135(3):431-6) researchers N. Z. Unlu et al. found that the addition of avocado to a meal (in this case, salads), substantially boosted the absorption of carotenoids (responsible for the pigment in many fruits and vegetables) present in salsa (such as lycopene) and many vegetables found in salads. This includes lycopene, lutein, and beta-carotene, which are all very important. Many of these carotenoids (such as beta-carotene and lutein) have been associated with protective mechanisms that help regulate cancerous cell growth, mortality, and differentiation. Researchers found that in the absence of the avocado, little absorption of these nutrients occurred. Clearly, and in support of earlier research, dietary lipids are required for the effective absorption of carotenoids.

This also helps explain why supplements are not nearly as effective in delivering absorbable lycopene as the food itself (though they're often required; since the amount of certain nutrients required to produce certain proven results can't be practically obtained by eating normal amounts of food).

It also begins to unravel the mystery of why the lycopene in raw tomatoes is not nearly as absorbable as the lycopene in those that are cooked. While exposure to lutein alone may not have been proven to shrink the size of an enlarged prostate (but significantly improves other elements of the urological profile, particularly flow), a study of 480 middle-aged men and women showed that those subjects with the leanest arterial walls over an 18-month period of time had the highest amount of lutein in their blood. Conversely, subjects with the lowest levels of lutein had a five-fold increase in the dangerous thickening of the walls within one of the major neck arteries. Importantly, dietary intake of lutein has a corresponding effect on blood serum levels of these important compounds. The research team, led by Dr. James H. Dwyer of the University of Southern California, demonstrates the protective power of lutein against the progression of atherosclerosis in humans and animals. In addition, their work shows that lutein is significantly more effective than beta-carotene in preventing lipid oxidation on a cellular level. One of more than 600 antioxidant carotenoids, lutein evolved in plants to assist them in the absorption of blue light.

In an *in vitro* experiment (*Circulation*, 2001 p. 103), the volunteers, each of whom had no history of heart disease, had their blood tested for signs of lutein twice at 18-month intervals. Subjects with the highest levels of lutein in their blood were found to have the smallest increases in thickening within the neck artery. Those with the lowest levels had a five-fold increase in growth of their arterial walls after 18 months. The lutein link was supported after factors such as age, smoking, heart medications, as well as the intake of other vitamins, were carefully considered. In still another study (*Journal of the American Heart Association*, June 19, 2001), researchers looked at the lengths of arteries removed during surgery. They found that artery walls pretreated with lutein were less likely to experience a chemical reaction, which is thought to contribute to their hardening. The higher the dose of lutein, the smaller the chemical reaction.

The scientists suggested that lutein intake may partially explain why people who enjoy a high consumption of fruit and vegetables daily, are less likely to develop heart disease. Other good sources of this important pigment include broccoli, lettuce, cucumber, peas, asparagus, beans, brussels sprouts, cabbage, spinach, and watercress.

New research from UCLA (*The Journal of Nutritional Biochemistry*, Volume 16, Issue 1, Pages 23–30) indicates that California avocados are the highest fruit source of lutein among the twenty most frequently consumed fruits. They also found that avocados have nearly twice the amount of vitamin E as previously reported, again making them the highest fruit source of this powerful antioxidant and others you've learned about.[23]

Avocados contain large amounts of beta-sitosterol and glutathione (more of both than any other fruit). In fact, *they contain four times the amount of beta-sitosterol found in oranges*, previously believed to contain the highest levels. Beta-sitosterol may be effective in reducing the incidence of certain prostate problems, though more research is required to substantiate these claims. But data consistently show that marked improvement occurs in urinary flow and in the health of the entire urological system when beta-sitosterol is administered to subjects with benign prostatic hyperplasia; though it wasn't shown to reduce the size of the prostate itself.[24]

It's worth finding creative ways to enjoy this amazing food. Avocados provide a greater variety and larger amount of nutrients and fiber, and a greater potassium-to-sodium ratio than any other fruit known to man. Incorporate EVOO and avocados, two of the healthiest sources of monounsaturated fat, into your life and live longer!

HYDROGENATION—THE SHAKING, BAKING AND MAKING OF A "MAN-MADE" TRANS FAT

We're told that saturated fatty acids, often referred to as SATFAs, are the bad guys. They're typically found in *tropical oil,* red meat, most dairy products, and skin from poultry. One thing inherently wrong with certain plant- and vegetable-based oils (but not tropical oils such as coconut and palm oil) is their unstable nature. Cooking with vegetable oil, illustrates exactly that. Its saturated fatty acids become rancid quickly when they're heated. So, mankind developed a process referred to as hydrogenation, to increase the stability and shelf life of cheap oils so that they might have the shelf life and stability of more expensive ones. Actually, the first object of hydrogenation was directed toward the production of hand soap! Years later, enterprising food companies would find another way to turn liquids into solids. In this case, *hydrogenation* became the chemical process that food companies used to turn liquid vegetable oil (and other oils) into solid fat. In doing so, these new artificially produced fats, known as *trans fats*, bore little resemblance to predecessor oils.

Instead, they became a different brand of bullet that harms us over time. Producers took cheap, highly processed vegetable oil and gassed it with hydrogen atoms to create a solid fat. Then they bombarded these processed oils with metal substrates. By combining these fats with heat and nickel, the industry created a whole new class of long lasting solid fake fats. The process of converting a naturally occurring fat into a man-made fake fat is high tech slight of hand. Because polyunsaturated fats are missing hydrogen atoms, tanks are built to expose them to metals such as cobalt; which are then super-heated and often pressurized to "saturate" them with hydrogen. The result is converting something such as cheap corn oil to something more expensive like shortening. Hydrogen altered that liquid into a fat that retains its shape and lasts far longer on store shelves.

While they're technically saturated, they became that way through a mechanical process which artificially binds its atoms. The result: fake molecules that *react* rather than *interact* at the cellular level—as they interrupt, confuse, and destroy normal metabolic processes, wreaking havoc by confusing and destroying the foundation of every cell in our bodies. This government-sanctioned toxin creates chaos at cell sites and internal inflammation on a scale unlike anything in the history of mankind. It ushered in a new wave of cancer, heart disease, and other biological and immunological disease in short order. Today, a number of children who grew up on partially hydrogenated foods are showing clear signs of heart disease; some by the time they reach their late teens ... if they're lucky.[25]

Beware—although trans fat will continue to be part of our diets for years to come, there's more trouble on the horizon. Industrious food makers are developing still another cooking oil that can find a way to get under the wire. Details are sketchy, but you can count on seeing this soon. While a growing number of researchers believe these man-made fats are little more than bullets of destruction, healthful saturated fats are beginning to again garner the respect they deserve.

While hydrogenation made them stable on the surface, our cells know they're frauds. As the saying goes, you can fool some of the people some of the time, but you can't fool a cell. After all, motor oil is stable too, but you wouldn't cook with it!

As we'll see shortly, there's nothing wrong with certain tropical oils that exist naturally. But today, we've come to regard them as hazardous substances to be avoided at all costs. We're cautioned to remove them from our diets. Tainted now, we tend to associate them with the truly hazardous commercially *hydrogenated* variety; the toxic impostors. Unfortunately, we remain misinformed.

THE GREAT IMPOSTER—THE TRANS FATS

Another one of our four types of fat is arguably the worst: *trans fat*. The U.S. government put saturated fat on its most wanted list and said that eating it caused heart disease. As you have learned, this was based on the since-disproven cholesterol fable that many of us still cling to today. From the time it was popularized, the door was opened for food companies to create their own version of industrialized imposter fats.

Margarine producers had the answer. They developed a cheap substitute that they could claim wasn't saturated. Trans fats were born. Heralded as a means to reduce our consumption of saturated fat, large food companies aggressively marketed what we were told was a healthy alternative. Marketing a potentially dangerous substance as a suitable alternative for a healthy one, is misinformed. And profiting, by failing to disclose important information, is unconscionable.

If substituting fake fats to reduce the consumption of saturated fat wasn't bad enough, the industry had a field day when they discovered that a number of popular mainstream products could now be transformed into longer lasting, aesthetically pleasing versions of their shorter shelf life selves (say that ten times). Not only making them last longer, but less runny and drippy. They accomplished this through the incredibly clever process known as hydrogenation.

Unselfishly, they offered to rescue us, marketing this as a safe and healthy alternative. Now we had products that looked nice, spread perfectly (like margarine), with the texture of plastic butter and the shelf life of a cannonball. The molecules your body formerly recognized had been radically altered. Your cells didn't know what hit them. They couldn't recognize (let alone react to) the invasion of these great pretenders. *Misinformed About Food*, we continued to eat this stuff. Inside of us, a cascading army of unstable fats attempts to engage healthy cells. Confused cells frantically try to communicate with these imposter fats and with other healthy cells. Chaos ensues. While it was you that created this monster, you didn't know it. At least not yet. Disease takes time to show its face in a way you're able to discern. And by the time it does, you'll wish it hadn't. If you think purposeful eating is something you'd rather avoid, think again. Bad habits die hard. So do we.

Margarine ushered in a new generation of heart disease. Shelves at the local grocer were stacked high with vegetable oil, claiming to reduce CHD. Commercial witchcraft found a new way to weave its highly profitable web, making the worthless appear worthwhile. A slight of the hand on the heels of new legislation, and the stage was set. A little good old fashioned American ingenuity, coupled with a dose of public alarm, mixed with a marketing campaign supported by the American Medical Association, and we lined up to buy this stuff. After all, we were told this was nature's oil—low in saturated fat. Maize, corn, mother earth, health, purity ... do you remember the commercials? Corn rustling in the wind, and the Mazola® lady holding the staff of life. This new class of food had a shelf life of its own.

Everyone was happy. From store owners to Wall Street, and from well-meaning housewives to well-meaning docs, the party had just begun. Fake fat was all the rage. We were just misinformed, but it wasn't the first time. Just ask our cells. The introduction of this product marked a particularly shameful period in the life of the FDA—when human life took a backseat to shelf life.

In 2003 the U.S. Food and Drug Administration announced legislation requiring mandatory labeling of trans fats on nutrition labels of packaged foods. The law became effective in January of 2006. Until that time 68 percent of all the fat the average American ate came from trans fat. We gobbled up around 7 to 8 billion pounds of these fake oils each year. Processed food, and in particular fast food, was (and in some cases still is) loaded with this stuff. Manufacturers worked methodically to make this conveniently available to our kids. Trans fats raise your bad cholesterol (LDL) and lower your good cholesterol (HDL). It's exactly the opposite process we need to occur. Since trans fats can't be properly metabolized, they stick to cell membranes, disrupting their ability to communicate. It's like throwing a monkey wrench into a well-tuned engine. Their very presence creates havoc, causing cells to misfire. Almost immediately they induce constriction, quickly causing your blood vessels to tighten.

According to scientists Plotnik and Vogel, it only takes *one* fast food meal (approximately 900 calories and 50 grams of fat) to substantially restrict blood flow for four full hours. That's largely due to a considerable reduction in the amount of nitric oxide produced in the endothelium. An important fact you may wish to consider the next time you pull up to that drive-through window.

THE TEARS OF A CLOWN—THE SUPER-SIZING OF TRANS FATS

How many of your loved ones have already suffered and will continue to suffer from years of eating these toxic fake fats? Please think about this the next time you consider ordering foods that contain them. But you may not be aware of what's in them. You just might be getting fooled by the clown.

Before you applaud the efforts of fast food restaurants that brag about healthy alternatives, understand what they are. Ask for a copy of their nutrition information (the source of the following information). Some are no more than creative versions of old imposters that were previously exposed. More often than not, you can't keep an old trans fat down. Once discovered, their owners may simply morph them.

Take McDonalds® for example, hailed as a more caring company than they formerly were. A company that's rediscovered itself, recognizing its responsibility to a new generation of children—your children, or your grandchildren—and changing their menu, providing you with healthful choices. Before you order their Asian Salad with Crispy Chicken, please note: it contains about the same number of calories as their double cheeseburger (430 versus 440) and an equal amount of trans fat (1.5 grams). Add salad dressing and you're over the top. And their Southwest Salad with Crispy Chicken is even worse (450 calories), with a whopping 970 milligrams of sodium. But if you think I'm just targeting the word "crispy," think again. Their "grilled" southwest salad handily tops their little cheeseburger in calories (320 versus 300) and contains far more sodium (960 milligrams versus 750). Happy they changed the cooking oil on their french fries? A small order alone contains 3.5 grams of trans fat. Are you still smiling? Is the clown? If you're stuck and need to duck in here for a quick meal, consider a *few* side salads. Eating three ought to do it. Combined, they total only 60 calories. Topping with one package of low fat dressing should fill you up with less than a 200 calorie meal (but with more sodium than I'd prefer).

And the King? Their Tendercrisp® Chicken Sandwich has more calories than their Whopper® with cheese sandwich (780 versus 770) and even *more* trans fat (4 grams versus 1.5). It also boasts amazing 1,590 milligrams of sodium. Now that's a whopper!

But don't count the Chihuahua out. Its bite is far bigger than its bark. If you want real junk food just go down to the border. Taco Bell® offers us their Fiesta Taco *Salad*®. This 820 calories "green" option has 36 percent more calories than *two* McDonalds Cheeseburgers (600 calories)! And its 1,790 milligrams of sodium is the giant killer—topping those *two* cheeseburgers with almost 20 percent more sodium than *both* (1,500 milligrams of sodium for two). If you're stuck at this place, I'd opt for two side orders of guacamole, totalling 140 calories and 360 milligrams of sodium.

According to an extensive study of 6,212 youngsters by researchers from Children's Hospital Boston, the Agricultural Research Service of the U.S. Dept. of Agriculture, and Harvard School of Public Health, nearly *one third* of our kids ages 4 to 19 eat fast food each day; packing on an estimated six extra pounds per child per year—further heightening their risk of obesity. Marketing campaigns have succeeded in getting many well-intentioned parents to throw caution to the wind. For a small additional amount of money you can now, quite literally, "supersize" *your children*. Dr. David Ludwig, the lead author of the study and director of the obesity program at Children's Hospital Boston, tells us that fast food consumption has increased fivefold in kids since 1970. In 2004, McDonalds announced they would end supersizing. But the trend has caught on and many other chains continue to offer this popular option.

Even today, trans fats are still found in many fast foods, such as baked products like crackers, bread, cookies, and cakes. According to the FDA's Office of Public Affairs, 40 percent of our intake of trans fat comes from baked goods alone; fried foods and many breakfast cereals that are advertised to be "wholesome" also contain trans fats—like some energy bars. The list goes on. Pancakes and grilled sandwiches often contain trans fats from the margarine that's brushed on the griddle. Many non-dairy creamers and flavored coffees, whipped toppings, bean dips, and gravy mixes also contain large amounts of trans fat. Check your labels!

EVEN TODAY, TRANS FATS ARE STILL FOUND IN MANY FAST FOODS SUCH AS BAKED PRODUCTS LIKE CRACKERS, BREAD, COOKIES, AND CAKES.

Several battles against huge food marketers have been won. Many restaurant chains have replaced trans fats with canola oil (though I would have preferred coconut oil). New York City has asked its restaurants to refrain from using trans fats in foods. But the problem is huge. From vending machines to baked goods, bean dips to fast food, the prevalence of trans fat is that pervasive. The government's labeling requirements were a step in the right direction—but only a baby step. It's unconscionable to simply *limit* a known toxin in our food. The U.S. government must enact legislation to *completely ban* trans fats, and eliminate the coddle talk. But in most states, restaurants are free to do as they please. Many restaurant foods *aren't* regulated by the federal labeling mandate. According to the Associated Press ("Zero Trans Fat Doesn't Always Mean None," August 2007), the U.S. government allows food makers to label their products as zero grams of trans fat, as long as they contain less than 1 gram per serving. But few packaged foods contain only one serving. A single container of potato chips has seven servings. If you ate that container, the governments' regulations would allow the maker to dole out 3.5 grams of trans fat and still label them as absent.

But New York City is not the only one that flew under the trans fat radar. In November, 2006, the Girl Scouts™ of the USA stated that their familiar cookies will contain less than 0.5 grams of trans fat per serving.

Not to be outdone, Governor Arnold Schwarzenegger signed a bill proclaiming the entire state would be the first to terminate trans fats, effective July 25, 2008. The first impact will be felt by restaurants. Eventually all retailers with baked goods will be affected.

As you can see, the FDA's zero trans fat ruling doesn't mean what it suggests. But apparently, the government's priorities remain intact. I call it *coddle* talk. The FDA creates its own language when it needs to—coddling big business in the face of alarming information that compels them to take action. In this case, by declaring a ban and then finding language that allows them to mask something they feel a need to hide. Half pregnant, they're loosely committed to the cause, but not enough to legislate change. But even California's bold initiative exempts pre-packaged foods. Understandably, the governor may have felt that trying to police these foods on grocery counters, from central distribution centers, would have proven costly. My recommendation would have been to bar all such foods, raising revenue for the state by fining those companies that violate this policy.

Michael Mason (*New York Times*, October 2006) interviewed Dr. Walter Willet, a leading researcher at Harvard University. According to Willet, "In the United States, the National Academy of Sciences' Institute of Medicine has concluded that the optimal intake of trans fats is zero." Mason reported that "in early 2006, Dr. Willett and his colleagues at Harvard estimated that if artificially produced trans fats were removed from the American diet, up to 228,000 heart attacks could be prevented each year. By Dr. Willett's calculation, diners are consuming one third to one half of their trans fats in restaurants. New York's proposed ban, he argues, could prevent 500 deaths a year."

New York City's Board of Health *did* take the first progressive step towards banning all trans fats in restaurants. Restaurants had until July 2008 to comply. Hopefully, the rest of the country will follow suit.

But New York City's initiative is not what most of us think it is. In fact, it's darn right coddle talk too. The ban *still permits* restaurants to serve foods containing trans fat that come in the "manufacturer's original packaging." So most *packaged* foods can still contain all the trans fat they wish.

According to the regulation (www.nyc.gov), the law also *permits* partially hydrogenated oils, shortening, or margarine with 0.5 grams or less trans fats per serving. So, while we should applaud all moves in the right direction, we should be aware that many are no more than half-hearted attempts to satisfy an already alarmed public, in a manner that's acceptable to big business and other special interest groups. Unsaturated fats are the precursor fats used to create trans fat, also known as hydrogenated or partially hydrogenated fats. Remember, a polyunsaturated fat lacks multiple (poly) hydrogen atoms and seeks to find them anywhere it can. Your body becomes an open hunting ground to help them to do so. And the state of New York says this stuff is not okay to serve to you (unless we can slip under the legislative wire, with coddle talk.)

CONJUGATED LINOLEIC ACID—THE HEALTHY TRANS FAT

As the name implies, this healthful fat is an isomer of LA, that is more properly categorized as a naturally-occurring *healthful* trans fat. Yes, there is such a thing. Think of it as a mutated form of LA. An isomer is a molecule with the same chemical formula of another molecule but with different characteristics. These characteristics result in different behavior, due to the way the chemicals they share in common are structured.

Recent studies indicate that CLA, principally derived from the meat and dairy products of ruminants, holds great promise in our battle against cancer. As author Jo Robinson tells us in her book *Why Grassfed Is Best: The Surprising Benefits of Grassfed Meats, Eggs, and Dairy Products* (2000 Vashon Island Press), "At this point in time, the research on CLA and cancer is the most promising. When rats are fed very small amounts of CLA—a mere 0.1 percent of their total calories—they show a significant reduction in tumor growth. At 1.5 percent of their caloric intake, tumor size is reduced by as much as 60 percent ... So, is there enough CLA in grass-fed products to reduce *your* risk of cancer? It's highly likely. It's been estimated that people eating ordinary grain-fed meat and dairy products consume about 1 gram of CLA a day. Judging by animal studies, this is one third of the amount required to reduce the risk of cancer. Switching to grass-fed animal products would increase your CLA intake three to five-fold, which could make the all-important difference."

CLA is a rather unique fat molecule. It's part of a group of isomers that share the same molecular characteristics as family member LA (linoleic acid); except for one. Its double bonds of carbon (unlike those in LA) are *joined together*, hence the term "conjugated" CLA.

Foods from plants also contain CLA, but the distribution of isomers differs sharply from those found in animal food, where the microbial product predominates. Animal sources of CLA are more biologically active. The action of this healthful mechanism begins in the digestive tract of ruminants. It's actually incorporated into their cell membranes, fat tissue, and blood lipids after CLA is absorbed in the gut. Mammals secrete large amounts of CLA in their milk. That's why organic milk as well as organic butter and alpine cheese produced from the milk of grass-fed beef are powerful sources of this incredibly healthful fat.

A natural occurring trans fat, not the harmful man-made variety, it actually retains its characteristics, that aren't compromised when it's processed in our food. Oxidative action appears to have little impact on its integrity according to Carol Steinhart, writer for the *Journal of Chemical Education* (1996, 73:A302). Conventional processing doesn't alter its important value, (although its concentration is at times diminished.) Steinhart provides us with a provocative history of this molecule, tracing the discovery of this anti-carcinogen back to research performed in the late 1970s. Apparently we discovered its power some time ago, but failed to properly harness it.

Michael Pariza of the University of Wisconsin's Food Research Institute investigated mutagens in cooked beef. To his surprise, he discovered a fraction from grilled and raw beef that consistently modulated mutagenesis in the Ames (Salmonella) test and frequently showed marked antimutagenic activity. The active material was identified as CLA, and subsequent work by Pariza and his associates revealed its astonishing range of biological effects. CLA protects cell membranes against oxidative attack. Because many antimutagens and antioxidants are also anticarcinogens, Pariza studied the effects of CLA in animal models of cancer.

CLA inhibited cancers of the skin and stomach caused by exposure to carcinogens in mice. It inhibited mammary and colon cancer in rats. Researchers at Washington State University found that physiologic concentrations of CLA killed or inhibited cultured cells of human malignant melanoma, colorectal cancer, and breast cancer. Although the effects of CLA on the immune system and inflammatory response resemble those of fish oil and may be mediated by similar mechanisms, Pariza and his colleague Mark Cook found that CLA is *more powerful* than fish oil in the prevention of growth suppression in mice injected with endotoxin. Similar favorable actions of CLA on the immune system were seen in rats and chickens.

Cook points out that conjugated linoleic acid is the most powerful naturally occurring fatty acid we've discovered, with a proven ability to protect us against cancer. In fact, it's the only known antioxidant/anticarcinogen primarily associated with animal foods. Regular amounts, incorporated into a normal human diet, appear to actually prevent cancer.

SOURCES OF HEALTHY AND UNHEALTHY FAT
ALMONDS: THE SUPER-FAT SUPER-NUT

All nuts share certain, important nutritional characteristics. For example, all are high in fiber and enter your bloodstream slowly, like other healthy, low-glycemic foods. According to J. Salas-Salvano and colleagues, women who ate nuts five times per week were 20 percent less likely than those that seldom ate them to develop type 2 diabetes (*European Journal of Clinical Nutrition*, 2003, p. 57). Almonds also contain copper, which aids us in lowering our blood pressure. Less pressure and an increased flow of blood through your arteries and veins appears to be facilitated by a natural vasodilator found in almonds.

Almonds are also capable of delivering a "one-two punch" in the fight against heart disease. Their high content of the amino acid L-Arginine has properties that enhance the elasticity of these vessels and the subsequent flow of blood to the brain and heart. Research consistently shows that L-Arginine increases the internal availability of a gas known as nitric acid (abbreviated as NO; ironically it's the same nitric acid that's produced as a by-product of the engine in your car). Although its presence in your body is active for only brief periods of time, it's one of the few naturally occurring gases that signal your body to activate important, life-saving mechanisms. The presence of NO sends a signal to the endothelium in your blood vessels to relax. This relaxation response causes your arteries to dilate, thereby increasing the flow of your blood. It's the same concept of expansion and vasodilation that pharmaceutical companies harness to improve erectile dysfunction; through a myriad of consumer products. Pharmaceutical makers use other powerful, man-made dilators that owe their chemical composition in large part to NO. Approximately 40 percent of the chemical composite of NO, a powerful vasodilator, is used to alleviate the chest pain from a heart attack. It's clear why the regular consumption of almonds has been linked to a reduction in coronary heart disease.

The Harvard Nurse's Study (*BMJ*, 1998 Nov 14; 317:1341–5) reported that the incidence of CHD in the 86,000 women studied plummeted 35 percent in those subjects that ate 5 ounces of nuts per week, compared to women who seldom ate them. Eating just 2 ounces of almonds per day produced a meaningful drop in LDL, according to researchers at Loma Linda University who presented their findings at the Experimental Biology 2000 conference. In another study of 31,208 Adventists, also conducted by researchers at Loma Linda University (Archives of Internal Medicine VOL. NO 7, July 1 1992 152: 1416), *subjects that ate nuts more than four times each week cut their chances of heart disease by 50 percent*, compared to those who ate nuts less than once each week. In a study of over 4,000 people, the Harvard School of Public Health found that the risk of a second heart attack dropped 25 percent when subjects ate nuts at least twice weekly. The L-Arginine found in almonds is a natural, gradual means to achieve improved blood flow to the heart, brain, and sexual organs. It's also a powerful anti-inflammatory. Jeffrey Blumberg, Ph. D., the Director of Tufts Universities' University's Antioxidants Research Laboratory Nutrition, and colleagues published the results of an important study. Their findings proved that the regular consumption of almonds reduces C-reactive protein levels in blood plasma just as well as statin drugs do. C-reactive protein is an important inflammation marker. More on this later.

There are other important considerations when selecting almonds. In addition to choosing whole and raw, they should be grown organically, soaked overnight, and lightly toasted. The ultimate almond should be eaten with its skin on. Any good almond worth eating is worth eating with its skin on.

In another study, Blumberg's group found no less than 20 potent antioxidant flavonoids present in the *skin* of the almond. The skin's antioxidant phytonutrients protect cells against free radical damage. Those found include such powerful, hard-to-find antioxidants such as quercetin (abundant in Brazil nuts), kaempferol (found in several healthful berries including cranberry), naringin (found in grapefruit), catchechins (found in green tea), and more. The flavonoids in their skin alone enhanced LDL's resistance to oxidation by 18 percent. But the combined effect of the vitamin E in the almond's meat and the flavonoids in their skin (synergy) boosted LDL's resistance to oxidation by an incredible 52.5 percent!

You want to avoid almonds (and all foods containing L-Arginine) if you have a history of any type of herpes. This includes oral and genital forms of herpes. The herpes virus appears to breed vigorously when a high concentration of

L-Arginine is present. Foods with a large concentration of this amino acid, not surprisingly, appear to exacerbate cold sores. Almonds have also been identified as one of the few foods capable of increasing urinary oxalate. When an excessive dietary oxalic acid found in certain foods like almonds combines with calcium, it may precipitate crystallization and form what we know as kidney stones. Those prone to the production of calcium oxalate stones may want to avoid walnuts as well. Although several foods contain large amounts of oxalate, research has shown that only a few of these actually have the effect of increasing urinary levels. While the majority of oxalic acid found in the urine is produced by the body itself and *not* through dietary intake of any food, studies have shown the value of avoiding them in those so prone. But for most of us, eating a small handful of almonds a day is a natural way to help regulate and maintain blood flow, supercharge your immunity, and maintain your weight.

Glutamic acid, another amino acid, is particularly plentiful in almonds. Glutamic acid is part of the antioxidant tripeptide glutathione, which helps detoxify ammonia in your body. Glutamic acid has an acidic carboxyl group on its side chain, which can serve as both an acceptor and a donor of ammonia, a compound toxic to the body. Once glutamic acid has coupled with ammonia (creating a compound known as glutamine), it can safely transport ammonia to the liver. Once there, the ammonia is eventually converted to urea for excretion by the kidneys. Not surprisingly, a strong correlation between increased glutathione intake and decreased risk of oral and pharyngeal cancer has been discovered. Almonds are also a powerful source of vitamin E, as well as calcium, magnesium, potassium, zinc, phosphorous, and trace element manganese. While far more research is required to confirm its role in preventing cancer, almonds are one of the few whole food sources of amygdalin. First isolated in 1830 by two French chemists, amygdaline, sometimes called nitriloside or "vitamin B-17," has been advanced (but not yet proven) as an anti-cancer compound.

GLUTAMIC ACID IS PART OF THE ANTIOXIDANT TRIPEPTIDE GLUTATHIONE, WHICH HELPS DETOXIFY AMMONIA IN YOUR BODY.

For years, I was convinced that raw almonds, with no salt added, were the healthiest way to eat them. After all, raw is always better, right? If monounsaturated fats are still relatively unstable, why would you ever want to heat them? Surely, any form of heating degrades the antioxidant value, further diminishing their incredible ability to heal and protect us. But researchers at Stanford University have proven otherwise. Gene Spiller, PhD and associates at the Stanford Center for Research in Disease Prevention compared the lipid-altering effect of roasted salted almonds and roasted almond butter with those of raw almonds (*Journal of Nutrition*, 2003). Their results showed that all three significantly lowered LDL. In at least one important experiment, raw versus lightly roasted did not matter (of course, what oil you roast them in does matter). While more research is called for, it appears that lightly roasting almonds in EVOO or coconut oil leaves the fatty acids intact.

There are more advantages to lightly roasting your almonds. Voluntary recalls of more than 15 million pounds of raw almonds were announced by producers. Much of these were recalled beginning in 2004, and were produced on a private label basis for Costco® under its Kirkland Signature™ brand name, as well as for Trader Joe's® and Sunkist™. It began when, in May of that same year, the Oregon State Health Laboratory identified a group of five patients infected with *Salmonella enterica* serotype Enteritidis (SE). Since that time, many more patients, in at least twelve states and Canada, were found to have matching SE isolates, some of which developed as early as late 2003. When something is raw and uncooked, almonds, like any other product, can become and remain contaminated with bacteria. So, lightly roasting whole raw almonds, with the skin on if possible, makes sense. Again, the fatty acids appear to remain intact, and the potential for contamination is significantly reduced.

You now know why almonds should be lightly roasted in EVOO or EVCO (extra virgin coconut oil). Purchase them whole, not slivered or chopped. Cutting almonds precipitates their oxidation.

One last issue remains when searching for the perfect almond. Almonds, and all nuts and grains, contain phytates. These organic nutrients inhibit the uptake of certain vitamins and minerals by binding to them; preventing their absorption in our small intestine. Fortunately, these can easily be broken down by soaking them in water with sea salt overnight. In fact, soaking them actually improves their flavor, increases their nutrient value, and breaks down complex sugars that cause you to have an upset stomach, a technique not unfamiliar to some bean lovers. Think of soaking nuts as you would think of soaking a seed. It brings them to life like a sprout. Eating just a handful per day will lengthen your life. An almond made precisely this way will become available shortly. Bursting with flavor, they're organically grown without pesticides, and actually soaked overnight. Then they're lightly roasted in olive oil and sea salt. Information will be posted on our web site when available, at www. RKInformedLiving.com.

WALNUTS: NOT BAD, BUT NOT THE BEST

Scientists, using carbon dating on petrified walnut shells, have confirmed walnuts' existence some eighty centuries ago during the stone age! But even the most motivated caveman couldn't wait around for Henry Quackenbush to invent the nutcracker in 1909. While Joseph Sexton grew the first walnuts in this country in 1867, who was the guy going to sell them to? He threw a great party but nobody came. Even his closest friends, like the caveman before them, weren't hanging around for Quankenbush's discovery. And while the hammer was invented in 1840, even Sexton's closest friends wouldn't wait another 95 years for a Wal-Mart store to open that sold them. If you think cracking them was a challenge, try growing them. Their roots secrete a toxin called juglone, which clobbers neighboring tomatoes and apples (though it's not been found to be toxic in humans).

Walnuts contain more alpha-linolenic acid (ALA) than any other tree nut, with a ratio of linoleic acid to alpha-linolenic acid (LA/ALA) of 4:l, precisely the same ratio that showed such value in the famed Lyon Heart Study. But due to the inefficiency in converting it to its descendant fats, that's not reason enough to eat walnuts. Walnuts, like almonds, are also high in L-Arginine. L-Arginine increases the production of nitric oxide (NO), which signals the endothelial wall to relax, as you learned previously. This in turn causes blood vessels to dilate, which is a good thing. But because you're already getting NO from eating almonds, it may not be reason enough to recommend walnuts. After all, the total amount of fat you need in your diet is relatively small, which makes it all the more important to be selective.

Walnuts also contain almost three times the amount of unstable polyunsaturated fat than almonds do and almost one third less fiber. Almonds also trump walnuts in vitamin E and magnesium, are lower in calories (164 calories per ounce versus 175 respectively), and have more than *twice* their content of healthy monounsaturated fat. While walnuts may be the only nut with an appreciable amount of Omega-3 fatty acids, but other sources are available with a considerably higher content. Proponents of the walnut still persist, claiming that research shows that regular consumption lowers LDL. But a closer look at the research shows that certain conclusions could prove misleading, or fail to rule out important confounding variables. For the most part, what many of them did prove was that *substituting* walnuts for other harmful fats in the subject's diet does lower LDL. Most of these studies were either were short in duration, or based on less than adequate sample size. Substituting a food that is truly not harmful for an inflammatory food that is, doesn't make the former a health food.

In that regard, Laura M. Tarantino, PhD, Acting Director of the Office of Nutritional Products, Labeling and Dietary Supplements for the Center for Food Safety and Applied Nutrition, provided a thoughtful opinion (FDA Qualified Health Claims: Docket No 02P-0292, March 9, 2004) against the petition, to permit a health claim to be made on behalf of the California Walnut Commission. The claim, if approved, would have permitted labels on whole or chopped walnuts claiming that their consumption lowers the risk of CHD. But after examining the available research, Tarantino concluded that there was nothing unique contained in walnuts based on the supporting evidence in the claim; and that there was no unique property contained in walnuts that could be shown to lower CHD. Only that in short-term studies with small groups showed that "something in a walnut" appeared to reduce LDL *when it replaced harmful saturated fat in the diet* (note the words: when it replaced *harmful* saturated fat in the diet).

In the end, the only claim that Tarantino would allow was a qualified one as follows: "Supportive but not conclusive research shows that eating 1.5 ounces per day of walnuts, as part of a low saturated fat and low cholesterol diet and not resulting in increased caloric intake, may reduce the risk of coronary heart disease." As weak-kneed this claim itself is, prefacing it by saying "supportive but not conclusive research" is about as watered down as a recommendation gets. Walnuts may be touted by many, but the evidence falls short of warranting that eating 1.5 ounces a day, as a stand-alone event, actually lowers LDL. That same amount would equal about 262 calories that are better devoted to almonds, EVOOOO, EVOCO (extra virgin organic coconut oil), and other healthy SOS fats.

PISTACHIOS: RIGHT UP THERE WITH ALMONDS

In addition to almonds, here's a brief rundown on other incredibly healthful nuts:

Pistachio Nuts: Eat them unsalted and plain, not dyed red. They were dyed red by importers trying to cover up their imperfections. Today, most of those we eat are grown in California and are not dyed, although you can still find them that way. The pistachio tree takes 7 to 10 years to bear fruit (the seeds are in the center of the fruit), and twice as long to reach maturity. When the fruit ripens, the shells actually make a popping sound when they open. According to folklore, lovers who were together under a tree when the shells popped found good fortune. Containing almost as much fiber as almonds, pistachios are also lower in calories per ounce than all other nuts. They also trump all other members of the nut family in important phytosterol content, with approximately 60 milligrams per ounce, versus 34 milligrams in almonds. Although almonds, all things considered, remain my top recommendation in this nut family, pistachios are a close runner-up.

Importantly, pistachios contain more potassium than any other nut. Eating foods with high levels of potassium and a low amount of sodium can help offset the growing imbalance of this ratio in your diet, one of the chief contributors to high blood pressure. Salt draws water into your arteries and veins increasing the volume of fluid inside. This requires more pressure and work from your heart to pump more volume through more constricted space (salt is a vaso-constrictor). More than 75 percent of our sodium today comes from fast food and packaged goods. While the typical woman consumes approximately 2,700 milligrams daily, and men 3,900 milligrams, we only need about 1,500 milligrams a day. On the other hand, we need about 4,700 milligrams of potassium a day. Yet according to a report from the National Academies of Science (2004), the average American woman gets less than half of that amount, and men just slightly more. So, in the typical adult diet we're receiving nearly twice the sodium we need and *less than half* the potassium we require.

One ounce of pistachios contains a prodigious 310 milligrams of potassium (the amount found in an entire orange) and only 158 calories, fewer calories than any other nut, per ounce. If the average adult needs about 2,000 milligrams more potassium daily than they're currently receiving in their diet, then 1 ounce of pistachio nuts provides more than 15 percent of your daily needs. A deficiency of potassium may also be related to an increased risk of cardiovascular disease, particularly stroke. In a meta-analysis of thirty-three randomized controlled trials published in the *Journal of the American Medical Association* (Volume 277, No. 20, May 28, 1997), researchers from the Welch Center for Prevention,

Epidemiology and Clinical Research and the Johns Hopkins University School of Hygiene and Public Health concluded that increased potassium intake should be considered as a recommendation for the prevention and treatment of hypertension. Hypertension is a proven forerunner of stroke. The researchers noted that potassium supplementation is associated with a significant reduction in both mean systolic and diastolic blood pressure.

The ability of pistachio nuts to increase blood flow to all body parts might explain why the Queen of Sheba regarded them as an aphrodisiac. You be the judge. Like all nuts, they should be soaked overnight to neutralize the phytic acid and enzyme inhibitors, common to most nuts, grains, and seeds.

MACADAMIA NUTS: THE THIRD MEMBER OF THE NUTTY SUPER-HEROES

This nut's the poster child for "the right kind of fat is truly healthful" hall of fame. Imagine a nut that's high in fat, with the proven ability to actually lower dangerous pro-inflammatory LDL by more than 5 percent, while raising healthful HDL by almost 8 percent (in just 4 weeks)! That's what occurred when lead researcher Garg and fellow scientists studied the effects of macadamia nut consumption on hypercholesterolemic men (with a mean age of fifty four).[26] In only one month the lipid profile of subjects was altered that dramatically. Volunteers consumed between 40–90 grams of macadamia nuts each day for 4 weeks (approximately 15 percent of their energy intake); the equivalent of at least 15 macadamia nuts a day, depending on their total caloric intake. According to researchers, this short term regimen was enough to *substantially* increase plasma levels of important monounsaturated fats; which Dr. Barry Sears tells us it's the best type of fat of them all.[27] And further research has supported precisely that.

Dr. Amy Greil, a former Penn State graduate student and leader in the university study, found that after only 5 weeks, subjects who ate macadamia nuts also enjoyed an 8.9 percent drop in their LDL, a 9.4 percent reduction of their total cholesterol level, and a significant reduction in dangerous triglycerides.[28]

While native to Australia (Aborigines painted their face with its oil and first discovered its healing value), "macs" were grown commercially in New Zealand since 1975. Their popularity has grown quickly in a short period of time. The trees (which take 7 years to bear fruit) were known by farmers as a tough seed to grow that rarely flourished. But a grafting technique first introduced in the late 1920's in Hawaii paved the way for massive commercial planting. High in protein, this nut, one of the healthiest sources of important monounsaturated fat, is a terrific source of protein and fiber. Its Extra Virgin oil is among the healthiest for high heat cooking; containing far less Omega 6's than EVCO. No other oil, not even EVOO, tops its incredible content of healthy monounsaturated fat. So, for high temperature cooking, choose between Extra Virgin Organic Coconut Oil, Extra Virgin Organic Macadamia Nut Oil (EVMOO) or Extra Virgin Palm Oil.

No wonder Dr. Atkins put this nut on the top of his list for health and dieting. According to him "You can eat as many macadamias as you can afford on my diet." The fact is, as expensive as they are; macadamia nuts are the preventative bargain of a lifetime. A different kind of life insurance at a fraction of the price!

HAZELNUTS: IF YOUR NAME WAS FILBERT, WOULDN'T YOU TRY ANOTHER?

Hazelnuts are known by a variety of names such as cobnuts and filberts. The earliest bushes apparently ripened on August 22nd, the same day of the year dedicated to celebrating St. Philibert. Many leading supporters of filberts point to their high content of tryptophan, an amino acid that has been associated with promoting a good night's sleep. But to enjoy this effect, the average adult would need to eat more than 2 grams a day. So, will foods like Filberts, high in tryptophan, truly help us enjoy a good sleep? After all, more than one expert has said so. But a closer look reveals that's quite a stretch.

One hundred grams of filberts (hazelnuts) provide 0.19 grams of tryptophan. So, you'd need to eat more than 10 times that amount (or almost 1000 grams) of hazelnuts a day to receive 2 grams a day of tryptophan. This is not meant to discourage you from eating good sources of certain nutrients. But few of us would attempt to get our total daily requirement from any one source, nor should you. It's only meant to put this type of recommendation, from a study, in perspective. A small handful of nuts, say almonds, is about eleven nuts and weights 13 grams, which is 0.0286 of a pound. To eat 2 pounds, you need to eat between sixty-nine to seventy handfuls. So, it's unlikely that eating hazelnuts will contribute enough tryptophan to put anyone to sleep. This doesn't mean they're not one of many good sources of this amino acid and other nutrients; only that there are better. Almonds, in addition to all their other great benefits, have approximately the same amount of tryptophan as the much-touted hazelnut. Of course, if you like filberts, they're fine. But almonds, macadamias, and pistachios remain the super-nuts of choice.

According to the USDA table of tryptophan content per 100 grams:

Pistachio Nuts	= 0.29
Almonds	= 0.19
Filberts Hazelnuts	= 0.19
Walnuts	= 0.17
Pecans	= 0.09
Macadamia	= 0.07

BRAZIL NUTS: THE NUT OF CHOICE … IF YOU'RE FROM CHERNOBYL!

While Brazil nuts contain more important selenium than any other nut, forget about them. The Federal Register in July of 1990 reiterated what has been consistently found since Turner and fellow researchers first reported it in 1958 (*Health Physics*, 1: 268–275); **Brazil nuts are the world's most radioactive food.** In fact, though tests result vary, they're reportedly 1,000 times more radioactive than any other food! This is not because of the high concentration of radium in the soil as much as the root system's ability to absorb barium, which typically carries radium. (Health Physics, Radioactivity of Brazil Nuts; 14:(2):95-99, February 1968. 95-99; Penn-Franca, et al.). While some may argue the amount of radiation is insignificant, and that *most* of it doesn't stay in the human body, why would we want *any?*[29] Despite its name, the majority of Brazil nuts come from Bolivia, not Brazil.

PINE NUTS: THE HEALTHY SEEDS OF A PINE CONE–THE LAST OF THE FOUR HORSEMEN

Pine nuts, one of my favorites, are also referred to as pignoli, meaning "pine cone" in Italian. With a whopping 31 grams of protein per 100 grams of nuts, they topple all other nuts in protein content. They provide healthy nutrients in foods such as baklava (along with ground sesame seeds) and pesto, which many of us enjoy. They also give salads and desserts a unique flavor and crunchiness. Only 1 ounce of pine nuts has 40 milligrams of phytosterols (almonds contain 34 milligrams per ounce).

In the U.S., the pinyon trees are the most sought-after source. While pignoli is still classified as a nut, they're actually seedlings from the nut, which is a product of the pine cone. Because there is no outer fruit that typically surrounds or borders seedlings on the outside, they remain classified as a nut. It helps us to better understand why they're so costly. A good deal of labor is required to open and harvest them. A healthful choice, they provide a great texture and flavor to salads and taste wonderful in pesto with basil and olive oil.

Our next class of super-foods may really surprise and inspire you, a class of food more nutritionally dense than our highly ranked nuts.

SEEDS ROCK!

More specifically pumpkin and squash seeds, two of the most healthful food sources of protein and nutrients available. With an amazing 0.578 grams of tryptophan (almost three times the amount found in a comparable 100 gram serving of hazelnuts), a 100-gram serving alone supplies almost 30 percent of the daily requirement for this important amino acid. The same size serving contains a whopping 7.4 milligrams of zinc.

For men, the regular consumption of pumpkin or squash seeds (again, unsalted) provides powerful protection against cancer of the prostate. They're also a great source of protein. To put that in perspective based on a 100-gram serving:

	Iron	Phosphorous	Protein
Pumpkin seeds:	15.00 mg	1172 mg	32.97 g
Almonds:	4.30 mg	474 mg	21.00 g
Pistachios:	4.20 mg	485 mg	21.35 g
Pine nuts:	5.53 mg	574 mg	14.00 g
Hazelnuts:	4.70 mg	90 mg	14.95 g
Macadamia nuts:	2.65 mg	198 mg	7.79 g

Of particular importance for women, this same 100-gram serving contains almost 15 milligrams of iron and a whopping 1172 milligrams of phosphorous. Compare that to macadamia nuts, which contain only 198 milligrams of phosphorous.

Perilla seeds are one of the greatest sources of food with ALA. And the important oil from this seed appears to mediate attacks in asthmatics, by inhibiting the generation of leukotrienes that precipitate bronchoconstriction and the ability to breathe (*International Archives of Allergy and Immunology*, Vol. 122, No. 2, 2000, Effects of Perilla Seed Oil Supplementation on Leukotriene Generation by Leucocytes in Patients with Asthma Associated with Lipometabolism). The tremendous potential of the oil from the seed is great indeed, as we have previously discussed. The list of important seeds, and their power to heal us, goes on. Pound for pound, pumpkin or squash seeds (a bit more polyunsaturated than monounsaturated) offer the largest amount of protective armor for the caloric price. But other types of seeds also boast unique characteristics. White mustard seeds are a great source of selenium and magnesium if used in moderation, while fennel seed reduces flatulence and gastric discomfort. Eating a couple after a meal freshens the breath and may improve digestion. Fennel also contains powerful antioxidants such as quercetin. While other seeds show a great deal of promise for the treatment of disease, further analysis is required to determine optimum levels of daily consumption.

Turmeric's active ingredient, curcumin, for example, is a fabulous antioxidant, praised by scientists for its ability to help in the prevention of everything from Alzheimer's disease to oxidation of brain cells. It prevents amyloid protein clumping by activating a neuron protecting gene, that removes debris from the brain. This may explain why elderly Americans have more than *four times* the incidence of this disease as Indians do in the 70-79 year-old age group (Archives of Neurology, 2000;57:824-30). The latter consume an average of 2 to 2.5 grams of turmeric daily from their foods; such as curry, fish soups, and other dishes containing turmeric powder. Studies suggest (*Nutrition and Cancer*, Volume 55, Issue 2 July 2006, pages 126–131, Curcumin Content of Turmeric and Curry Powders) that turmeric powder has a far higher content of curcumin than found in curry powder. Curcumin is a major component of turmeric that gives it its vibrant yellow color, and is used by Indians to season a number of their foods.

Cumin (not to be confused with curcumin) is an excellent source of iron. Cumin has also been shown to prevent tumor growth in lab animals. Dill seeds have been identified as a chemoprotector, protecting your immune system against environmental hazards such as cigarette smoke and industrial pollution. Extracts of certain seeds, such as grape, have been shown to measurably boost the antioxidant levels in the blood serum of the subjects tested. Seeds, like nuts, are also high in fat—generally, the right kind of fat. Even those highest in polyunsaturated fat often contain antioxidants that help stabilize the free radical nature of their lipid balance. Seeds are nature's way of passing on the lifeblood and characteristics of plants, and are teeming with life. Foods such as these are

reducing inflammation and strengthening your immunity.
important tool in your powerful arsenal for self-defense.
salads and other foods boosts their density. Mix them up
ded nuts and eat them daily.

Note: I've reserved the balance of this chapter for those that are interested in an informative but technical discussion of fats, including their unique characteristics; and why certain parent fats fail to elongate to the favorable descendant fats many makers claim they do. Those interested in the birth and not the labor should skip what follows and continue their reading by turning to Chapter 3: Love Story, page 153.

SATURATED VERSUS UNSATURATED FATS (THE NITTY GRITTY)

Fat molecules are organic acids that have long chains or tails, similar in shape to a caterpillar. These caterpillar-like carbon chains or fat molecules are generally classified as either saturated or unsaturated fats. Using the caterpillar analogy, think of the spine as carbon atoms bound by vertebrae on each of its sides, which are hydrogen atoms. They're said to be *saturated* because each carbon atom (again, think of them as vertebrae) are bound together—*solid*, if you will. No room for slipped disks here! If you were to view a saturated fat molecule under a microscope, you'd find no void—there's simply nothing missing.

And *unsaturated* fat is less stable. If you saw one of these under a microscope they'd appear to be *bent*. Scientists refer to this bend in fat molecules as a *cis* formation. While saturated fats are solid at room temperature, unsaturated fats are not. The more unsaturated a fat molecule is, the more its weight shifts to one side. And the more curved they are, the less stable they are.

Saturated fat is the *most* stable. Polyunsaturated fat, missing several carbon atoms, is the *least* stable. Monounsaturated fat, missing one carbon atom, is physically right in the *middle* of both. Though trans fats are physically stable, they're imposters—fake fats that create chaos and are biologically unpredictable.

It's also worth noting that *all* oils are liquid fats; although, not all fats are oils. All oils contain 120 calories per tablespoon. But this doesn't mean that they're all burned at the same *rate*. Some proponents of supplements will tell you that your body burns unsaturated fat more effectively than it burns saturated fat. But there's mounting evidence to the contrary. Extra virgin coconut oil, a very healthful saturated fat for example, is used up by the body and burned as fuel almost immediately and completely when digested.

Interestingly, the first three classifications of fat each have some degree of the other two in them. Saturated fat contains some degree of unsaturated fat, for example. The classification of each type is based on its primary content of fat. But subtle differences in their composition can spell a significant variance in the way they interact metabolically.

As you continue to learn more about saturated and unsaturated fats (as well as man-made "fake" fats known as trans fats), you'll discover their differences are as varied as the proteins we discussed in Chapter 1. Highly processed sources of these fats *can* harm you. It's as true about processed fat as it is about all other processed foods.

POLYUNSATURATED FATS, THE FREEDOM OF A RADICAL

Polyunsaturated fats, one of the two principle types of unsaturated fat, can be found in walnuts, vegetable oils, canola oil, and even fish. They have their origins in both plants and animals.

Most of the plant and vegetable oil derivatives of polyunsaturated fat that provides LA, argued as healthy alternatives to saturated fat, are *not*. In most instances, they're another big fat lie. I call them celebrity fats. They've gained a great deal of notoriety, but few of us really know them at all. A day scarcely goes by that we aren't told to wrap our dietary world around *unsaturated* fat and reminded to avoid the *saturated* variety. Most polyunsaturated fats should be ashamed of themselves, parading around like they were the next coming. While there may be a good side to a couple of them, there's a terrible downside to the rest.

Polyunsaturated fats are the least saturated by hydrogen, containing the smallest amount of paired hydrogen atoms—making them the most unstable. Each missing hydrogen atom represents an unbound electron. So, in its normal state, a polyunsaturated fat is desperately seeking a molecule to latch onto. It must fill the emptiness it feels inside and complete itself. A molecular Velcro of sorts that's dying to stick to anything it can. Liquid at room temperature, they generally originate from plant protein. (Note: while fish and animal protein contains polyunsaturated fat, it *receives* it from breaking down *plants*.) So when you think "poly," think plants. Because unsaturated fats have these voids or openings, they easily combine with other substances in your body. Their ability to be more biologically interactive makes them highly unstable. To what extent do you want unstable fat in your body? Now corrupt it further by cooking it—causing it to quickly oxidize. Now, heat it again when you eat (body temperature). We're left with a rancid molecule with unbound electrons seeking a mate to fill up the emptiness in its life; the very definition of a free radical and precisely what we seek to avoid.

Contrary to popular belief, free radical activity is a good thing as well as a bad thing! Again, it's all about balance. Our bodies produce many of these and require no further assistance from us. Free radicals are a natural by-product of breathing. Too much is a bad thing—and so is too little. Dr. Bruce Ames, PhD, University of California at Berkeley (*Archives of Biochemistry and Biophysics*, 2004), estimates that each cell in your body suffers from 10,000 free radical hits each day. But Ames also reminds us that free radicals *prevent* your immediate death from infection by destroying bacteria. They also work with cytochrome P-450 found in the liver, to help detoxify harmful chemicals, further protecting us. More research is required to better understand how to measure the optimum level to allow these processes to react, without overreacting. But it's clear that the less you create through your diet, the better. As you have learned, an excessive amount of free radical activity accelerates aging, creates inflammation, and precipitates disease. The point here is that we already have too many free radicals. We don't need to find novel ways to invite in anymore (i.e., by supplementing with hemp, flax, etc.).

All polyunsaturated fats are *not* created equal. There are important distinctions among them that should make real differences in the choices you make. Those that are processed from plants and vegetables, such as vegetable oil, contain large amounts of Omega-6s. Potentially damaging and inherently unbalanced, they enter your body (particularly when heated) reasonably unencumbered, free to attack stable molecules until they get what they want. They hammer your insides until they find an electron by attacking an otherwise healthy cell. Unstable polyunsaturated fats invade cell membranes and red blood cells, damaging DNA strands and triggering mutation in your tissue, blood vessels, and skin. Free radical damage to the skin causes brittle fingernails, premature lines, wrinkles, and furrows. Free radical damage to the tissues and organs sets the stage for tumors. In blood vessels, it precipitates the build-up of plaque.

In a 1999 study (*Carcinogenesis*, May 1999, Volume 20, Number 5, Pages 757-763), scientists showed that if left unchecked, an excess of mobilized DNA may not only affect cell proliferation (cancer), but cell survival causing atrophy, premature aging, and even diseases such as dementia and Alzheimer's. Ultimately, it may lead to your death. If you think purposeful eating sounds boring, think again. *Are you dying to eat?*

THE TWO GRANDDADDY FATS IN THE POLYUNSATURATED FAMILY

There are two principal EFAs (essential fatty acids) found in polyunsaturated fatty acids (PUFA). Like the essential amino acids we discussed in Chapter 1, these are nutrients that our body can't manufacture and must be obtained from outside sources.

The first is known as linoleic acid (LA). It is supposed to elongate or change in your body to become its descendent fat (in essence, through a chain of events, a descendent fat is what the parent fat was changed or metabolized into), gamma-linolenic acid (GLA). It's likely that many of the incredible results that were found in the famed Mediterranean Diet were due to the benefits of GLA contained in polyunsaturated fats. This GLA is suppose to elongate also, to a healthful DGLA (dihomo gamma-linolenic acid)—*if you're lucky*. But more often than not *you're unlucky*, and instead it becomes *harmful* AA (arachinodonic acid).

DGLA rocks. As a vasodilator, it's an anti-inflammatory fatty acid we want more of. AA constricts—a pro-inflammatory fatty acid we want less of.

Not surprisingly, healthy GLA is found in breast milk. Though we have more Omega-6s than we need in our diet, DGLA is an exception. It's one member of the Omega-6 family we actually need more of. The question is, how do we get it? As we will soon see, more often than not, it's too difficult to obtain from eating fats high in polyunsaturated fats. DGLA helps control our blood pressure by stimulating the production of important prostaglandins. Prostaglandins are mediators that affect important physiological events and appear to favorably influence mast cells involved with everything from cancer to allergic reactions. DGLA is also required to counter-balance harmful, pro-inflammatory AA excessively present in excess in our modern diet.

But more often than not, the proper elongation to DGLA fails to occur and LA converts to precisely what we hope to avoid—more AA. So we must find ways to avoid more AA and increase our ratio of GLA to AA. Since polyunsaturated oils, such as vegetable, safflower, corn, peanut, soybean, sunflower, cotton seed, and grape seed oils more often than not convert to AA, consider eliminating them from your diet. They will do you more harm than good. In fact products labeled as "vegetable oil" permit the maker, unless specifically stated otherwise, to market any combination of unstable oils such as palm, corn, soybean, or sunflower.

A study in Sweden of 61,471 women ages 40 to 76 (Archives of Internal Medicine, 1998) looked into the relation of different fats and breast cancer. Researchers found a positive association from the consumption of mono-unsaturated fat and the reduction in risk of developing this cancer–and an adverse association between the consumption of polyunsaturated fat (from plant and vegetable oils—sources of LA) and this disease. Clearly, women with diets high in polyunsaturated fat had an increased risk of breast cancer, while those with diets high in monounsaturated fat appeared to enjoy significant protection against it. Interestingly, saturated fats were found to have a neutral effect.

Dr. R. A. Newsholme of Oxford University (Lancet, 1977) was the first to conclude that polyunsaturated fats actually cause cancer. He suggested that the consumption of LA (in particular, that found in sunflower oil) was one of the most powerful ways to *suppress* your immunity.

This was extremely important information. Tissue rejection in the early days of kidney transplants was common. Patients' immune systems, as a means of protecting them from a "foreign invader," rejecting newly transplanted kidneys. For this procedure to succeed, the medical community had to find a way to suppress the immune system so it would stop rejecting a transplanted organ. Newsholme's findings indicated that LA from safflower oil was the most effective way to do so, with the least amount of risk. Doctors regarded this approach as a surprising contradiction, but it proved to be successful. This polyunsaturated oil weakened recipients' immune systems enough for their bodies to accept a donated organ.

But they soon discovered that dosing their patients with safflower oil had an additional, but negative consequence. These same patients began to develop cancers like wildfire.

Fortunately, there is a healthier way to enjoy GLA/DGLA without the risks associated with the failed conversion of LA. First, let's gain a better under-standing of the *second* parent fat, the head of the healthy Omega-3 family, ALA. We want it to elongate to either docosahexaenoic acid (DHA)—the Omega-3 so important in neurological function, or eicosapentaenoic acid (EPA)—the building block of anti-inflammatory eicosanoids. In the case of this parent, *both* of these descendent fats are enormously healthy. As is the case with

LA, an elongation process must occur—and again, it generally fails to do so. Whereas its descendent fats are highly valued, the parent fat often fails to provide us with these healthy descendents. And, according to some studies, may actually be harmful.

While flaxseed, hemp, and other seeds and seed oils contain high amounts of ALA, they're considerably less stable. Eating foods high in ALA, such as flaxseed oil, canola oil, brazil nuts, and walnuts, fail to provide our body, more often than not, with these healthy descendent fats.

... DOSING THEIR PATIENTS WITH SAFFLOWER OIL HAD AN ADDITIONAL, BUT NEGATIVE CONSEQUENCE. THESE SAME PATIENTS BEGAN TO DEVELOP CANCERS LIKE WILDFIRE.

While ALA itself has been shown to favorably impact some conditions, it's also been shown to significantly worsen others. In a fourteen-year study of almost 47,000 men (*American Journal of Clinical Nutrition*, July 2004 80(1); pp.204-216), ALA was shown to stimulate the growth of prostate tumors. However, both LA and ALA's *descendant* fats have consistently proven their ability to heal, without the potential risk from their parent fats.

The famed Lyons Diet Heart Study (Circulation; Advisory 2001, Final report; 1999) was conducted in the 1970s on 600 CHD survivors. A diet rich in ALA was found to significantly lower the risk of a reoccurrence of heart disease. However, the diet also contained *other* important substances such as olive oil and fish. Further research is required to better isolate other important dietary factors that might have influenced this outcome; but the *descendant* fats give us exactly what we need without the potential risk that may occur by eating their parent fats.

Unfortunately, vegetable sources of polyunsaturated fats do not contain the elongated forms your body needs to complete this conversion. As is the case with LA, certain factors inhibit ALA from elongating to important DHA and EPA. These include diet/vitamin and mineral co-factor deficiency, age, and subsequent loss of D6D, and gender. More on the importance of D6D shortly.

In a recent study (*Journal of Lipid Resources*, 2005), researchers found that after supplementation with ALA, only 7 percent was incorporated into plasma phospholipids, and only 1 percent was converted into docosapentaenoic acid (DPA), and subsequently DHA. Other studies have shown conversion rates vary from 2 percent to 8 percent. In a study with young female subjects, the rate was closer to 6 percent on average. According to scientists, the somewhat higher conversion rate may be due to the presence of certain hormones such as estrogen. Still another factor that can influence conversion is the ratio of LA to ALA present in the blood serum. Too much LA hinders the conversion of ALA because both fats compete for the same enzymes required to elongate them into their longer chain fatty acid descendant molecules. This is particularly important for vegans, for example, whose diets often contain a disproportionately high amount of LA. The same holds true for others who avoid fish and animal protein.

As we can see, ALA may actually be harmful while its descendant fats have been consistently found to be healthful. We can be certain we'll obtain the real essential fatty acids we need from ALA by simply eating fish and fish oil. Both fish and fish oil are direct sources already containing their powerful, converted, elongated descendant fats.

The problem with the body's limited ability to convert ALA might also explain why flaxseed's anti-inflammatory ability has not been conclusively proven, but fish oil's has. While numerous studies have shown that fish oil consistently benefits rheumatoid arthritis sufferers, flaxseed has no proven ability to do so.

Now, let's gain a better understanding of why both of these fats fail to elongate into the healthful fats we need.

THE FAILED ELONGATION OF PARENT FATS—LA AND ALA

Several factors inhibit the elongation of LA to desirable GLA. Among these factors is *aging*. As we grow older, the production of certain hormones required to complete this conversion diminishes. In addition, too much insulin in the body from low-fiber carbohydrate diets; the presence of trans fatty acids; deficiencies of certain vitamins such as C, E, and certain B vitamins; and the lack of certain minerals all act to inhibit the activity of delta-6 desaturase (D6D), the enzyme we require to make the important conversion from LA to GLA. The elongation to healthy GLA is further compromised by the consumption of alcohol, sugary foods, and prescription medications. While certain foods may be healthful, they're poor choices to rely on for the important GLA we require.

How much LA is really essential for us to obtain from outside food sources? The answer is *none*. Simply supplement with evening primrose oil (EPO). Though borage oil contains the highest amount of GLA (18 percent to 26 percent versus black currant seed oil's 15 percent to 20 percent, and EPO's 9 percent), EPO is the supplement of choice to enjoy the healthy benefits of important GLA. While both borage oil and black current oil will cost you less for the same amount of GLA, according to famed author, nutritionist, and lecturer Dr. Udo Erasmus, PhD (www.udoerasmus.com), borage leaves, the seeds, seed cake, and the unrefined borage seed oil can contain pyrrolizidines, which are toxic. While the process of refining removes the majority of them, it also damages the oil molecules. Instead, he recommends EPO, because it's naturally free of toxins. EPO is available from organically grown seeds that are mechanically pressed. As you've learned, most polyunsaturated fats are highly unstable and easily oxidize, enhancing free radical activity when exposed to light, heat, and oxygen. While many authorities recommend borage oil or black currant seed oil to supplement GLA availability, organic evening primrose oil is the *only* one of these three sources that is both naturally free of toxins and does not require the damaging process of refining.

Makers of borage oil, such as Bio Original, have challenged these findings with lab essays showing that their product demonstrated the absence of pyrrolizidine alkaloids at a limit of detection of 4 µg/kg. Dr. Erasmus provided this response to their information: "First, note that only refined borage oil was tested. Refined oil is oil that has been destructively processed, using harsh chemicals ($NaOH$, H_3PO_4, bleaching clays), and then, to get rid of rancid odor developed by the chemical treatment, is heated to frying temperature (deodorized). During this processing, 0.5 percent to 1 percent of the molecules is damaged and made toxic … In either case, thousands of consumers have been misled for many years. When oils are treated with $NaOH$, H_3PO_4, then bleached, and then deodorized, damage is done to the oil." According to Dr. Erasmus, "1 Tbsp. contains about 6 × 1019 damaged toxic molecules that can do harm to health."

Once again, we see that regardless of all the smoke and mirrors, industrialized processing of essential nutrients hinders your ability to properly utilize them. And cooking them on high heat strengthens their ability to further weaken you.

Another reason EPO gets the nod over borage oil and black currant seed oil is that its GLA is more efficiently absorbed. Despite the fact that it contains less GLA on a percentage basis, the balance of other fatty acids in the borage oil hinders its uptake. An expanding body of research suggests that GLA plays a strong role in regulating the growth of cancer cells and reverses nerve damage. It also effectively mediates or dramatically influences the progression of rheumatoid arthritis, diabetic neuropathy, cardiovascular diseases, and even healthy skin. Without sufficient DGLA, the body cannot produce the prostaglandins it needs, a sub-class of eicasonoids that are required to catalyze important hormones as we've previously discussed. For all of these reasons, supplementation with EPO is a smart choice. And now it's also an informed one.

The amount you take depends on your condition. Most EPO supplements contain relatively small amounts GLA. Research has shown that rheumatoid arthritis sufferers experience a marked reduction in swelling and soreness of their arthritic joints with regular use. In one study, this occurred in just 26 weeks after taking a dosage of 1.4 grams of GLA from EPO daily. Premenstrual headaches, bloating, and even irritability have been shown to be significantly reduced by supplementation of EPO.

A company named Bio-Alternatives® (www.bio-alternatives.net) offers organic, cold-pressed EPO and claims it's free of additives, solvents, and preservatives. Their oil has a 9 percent content of GLA (GLA content in EPO is typically from 7 percent to 10 percent). Regardless of which EPO formula you use, always take it with food. And never consume any unsaturated oil without at least minimal dosages of important antioxidants. Consult your physician to determine the right dosage for you, since no optimal dose for the general public has been clearly established. The recommendations are varied. But fortunately, even in high doses, no toxicity has been reported in any of the research reviewed here. Based on this information, I take 500 milligrams of GLA from EPO daily in gel form with food for daily maintenance. Again, consult your health care professional to determine the dosage that's right for you.

We can't count on getting GLA without daily supplementation. So, forget LA and consider the health benefits of its descendant fat. Obtaining GLA in moderation (after all, it's beneficial but still not stable) through the consumption of EPO is the only logical choice as a source of GLA and AA (Omega-6) from a plant-based polyunsaturated fat.

END NOTES

1.   According to Neuroscientist Ian Simpson in an interview featured by Research Penn State (Feeding the Diabetic Brain): "The hallmark of diabetes is this: The blood is too rich in glucose and yet muscle cells are stressed and starving. The muscle cells can't get enough energy because the diabetic body can't properly provide or use insulin—the hormone that stimulates the uptake of

glucose into muscle cells. And when diabetics take insulin for treatment, they often get "too much stimulation and too much uptake," says Simpson, which leaves them with too little glucose in their bloodstreams.

2. While the brain trumps computers handily in broad based processing, the computer appears to win in straightforward single task computation. But does it really? According to Library Think Quest; Computer versus the Brain: a think quest project. "The brain is made for general purposes, not specifically just for computational jobs. In theory, the brain could be as quick as a computer in computational and recording jobs but in real life, it will never be possible because the average human is constantly distracted by his overwhelming senses, his emotions and his own thoughts."

3. *American Journal of Tropical Medicine and Hygiene*; Cholera in the Gilbert Islands. II. Clinical and laboratory findings; 1979 July;28(4):685-91

4. *Journal of the American Oil Chemists Society* 1984;61:397-403.

5. The industry has begun introducing margarines with reduced or with zero amounts of trans fat. The potential problem here is two fold. First, as you'll understand shortly, a product can be legally labeled free of trans fats, but still contain a small amount of them. Makers are permitted to use one half a gram of trans fat per serving size, and still label their product as though it contained none. Since no amount is healthy, how are we to know if the product we wish to purchase does or doesn't? The other problem is that over-processing of even a healthy fat can substantially degrade its nutrient content.   While extra virgin palm oil or extra virgin coconut oil are healthy fats (when pressed or squeezed), the newer margarines featuring palm oil often use a method known as fractionalization; involving heating at high temperatures to separate the solid, non-organic palm from the seed oil. Those I've seen to date, use cheaper palm oil seed, or even less expensive palm kernel oil, which is typically fractionalized; a process that involves the use of a solvent to extract it from the pit. Don't be fooled.

6. *Circulation*, 1994; 89:94-101.Trans-fatty acids intake and risk of myocardial infarction. Ascherio et al.

7. *New England Journal of Medicine*, 2006: 354, 2006."Trans fatty acids and cardiovascular disease." Mozaffarian et al.

8. *Journal of Nutritional Biochemistry*; Dietary Trans Fatty Acids Modulate Erythrocyte Membrane Fatty Acyl Composition and Insulin Binding in Monkeys. Journal of Nutritional Biochemistry 1:190-195.

9. *Mayo Clinic Medical Update*; 1994: Is butter really better? Trans fat in margarine may be more of a risk for disease, July 01, 1994

10. *The American Journal of Nutritional Science*, March 2005, 135:562-566

11. Atherosclerosis, Thrombosis and Vascular Biology, July 2001, A scientific study comparing trans fats to saturated fats.

12. *Nutritional Epidemiology*; 2005, Consumption of Trans Fatty Acids Is Related to Plasma Biomarkers of Inflammation and Endothelial Dysfunction; Lopez-Garcia et al

13. *American Journal of Clinical Nutrition*, June 2001 A study looking at the increased risk of trans fats and the development of type 2 diabetes in women

14. Nutritional Effects of Isomeric Fats: Their Possible Influence on Cell Metabolism or Cell Structure," Dietary Fats and Health, (E. G. Perkins and W. J. Visek, eds), American Oil Chemists' Society, Champaign, IL, 1983, pp 391-402; Kummerow

15. *New England Journal of Medicine*. 354: 2006. "Trans fatty acids and cardiovascular disease". Mozaffarian

16. *International Journal of Cancer*: Volume 93 Issue 6, Pages 888 - 893; Epidemiology and Cancer Prevention Childhood and adult milk consumption and risk of premenopausal breast cancer in a cohort of 48,844 women - the Norwegian women and cancer study.

17. *The American Journal of Clinical Nutrition*; 2004, vol. 80,pp. 1353-1357;Milk and lactose intakes and ovarian cancer risk in the Swedish Mammography Cohort

18. *American Journal of Epidemiology* ;Vol. 130, No. 5: 904-910 Lactase Persistence and Milk Consumption as Determinants of Ovarian Cancer Risk; Johns Hopkins University School of Hygiene and Public Health; Cramer et al

19. Nutrition and Cancer, 1532-7914, Volume 48, Issue 1, 2004, Pages 22 – 27, Milk Consumption Is a Risk Factor for Prostate Cancer: Meta-Analysis of Case-Control Studies; Qin et al.

20. *American Journal of Epidemiology*; Diet, Obesity and Risk of Fatal Prostate Cancer; Vol. 120, No. 2: 244-250

21. *Israel Journal of Medical Sciences* 1983; 19 (9):806-809 Pediatrics 1989; 84(4):595-603

22. According to John McDougell, "When a large amount of one type of nutrient is given, then it displaces the metabolism of other similar type nutrients. For example, high doses of eicosapentaenoic (fish oil) given to Westerners also lower levels of dihomogammalinolenic acid (DGLA), a substance with a wide range of desirable cardiovascular and anti-inflammatory actions" ("Prostaglandins Leukotrienes and Essential Fatty Acids," 1991 Jan;42(1):31-7).

23. J.M. Fielding and colleagues at the School of Nutrition and Public Health, Deakin University, Malvern, Victoria, Australia (*Asia Pacific Journal of Clinical Nutrition*, 2005;14(2):131-6), proved that adding olive oil to diced tomatoes while cooking significantly boosts the bioavailability of the lycopene, in contrast to cooking tomatoes without it. While more research is required, it's clear that the proper and most effective absorption of nutrients is boosted by the presence of the right lipids. Adding avocado to your intake of complex carbohydrates makes them work together far more effectively.

24. In January 1987, the *New England Journal of Medicine* published the findings of a study conducted jointly by the Schools of Medicine of the University of California San Diego and Cambridge University. Researchers Connor and Khaw et al. examined the relationship between potassium intake and stroke in 859 men and women, ages 50 to 79. They discovered that an incredible 40 percent reduction in risk was associated with a daily increase of just 400 milligrams of potassium, the amount of potassium in only one third of an avocado. In fact, just one average-size avocado contains a whopping 1,204 milligrams of potassium.

25. According to researchers at the University of Maryland (Feature Story, Trans Fats 101, May 4, 2007), "Children who start at age 3 or 4 eating a steady diet of fast food, pop tarts, commercially prepared fish sticks, stick margarine, cake, candy, cookies and microwave popcorn can be expected to get heart disease earlier than kids who are eating foods without trans fats ... Some of our research here at the University of Maryland has shown that kids as young as 8, 9 and 10 already have the high cholesterol and blood fats that clog arteries. By starting healthy eating habits early, parents can help their children avoid heart attacks and stroke."

26. *Journal of Nutrition*. April 20 133:1060-1063, Macadamia Nut Consumption Lowers Plasma Total and LDL Cholesterol Levels in Hypercholesterolemic Men

27. Living in the Zone: http://www.prosperitypromises.com/drsears.htm

28. *Nutrition Research Newsletter*, June, 2008 Macadamia nuts for a healthy heart.

29. *Health Physics*; Retention of radium due to ingestion of Brazil Nuts; 1969; 16: 812-813; Gabay et al

CHAPTER 3

LOVE STORY

"All I ask of food is that it doesn't harm me."
—Michael Palin *(Monty Python's Flying Circus)*

It's motherly nature to delight in giving children whatever they want. Coming home to the scent of freshly baked cookies is the stuff childhood memories are made of. Buttery popcorn, soda in the fridge, and birthday cake topped with a fat scoop of slowly melting ice cream is the special handiwork of loving moms. And how many dads, the keepers of special treats, softly request us not to tell Mom while "sneaking" us a piece or two of our favorite candy? Not to be outdone, holidays are special events for grandmas too, who show their love by creating food feasts and bake-offs as part of their desire to smother us with affection. Piles of buttery mashed potatoes dripping with gravy, bread smothered in margarine, and baked beans adorned with bacon are packed with Grandma's special need to be heard.

Love has no boundaries.

Going overboard with eating happens in everyday life. Well-respected moms have well-stocked homes. Kitchens bulge with secret somethings hidden behind closed doors—a jar brimming with cookies in easy reach for privileged children. Don't forget the cold cuts in the fridge. Bologna makes children smile. A cute kid on TV sings a song that his bologna "has a first name."

But cold cuts take a back seat to Jell-O™, a favorite food of many school and hospital dietitians. These professionals are charged with making important decisions regarding the selection of proper foods for your kids during their formative years. They also design meals for patients who are physically or behaviorally ill. The principal ingredient in Jell-O™ is gelatin. Gelatin is made from the skin, connective tissue and bones of animals, according to the Gelatin Manufacturers' Institute of America. The parts are ground and treated. Kraft, the maker of the Jell-O™ brand, insists they don't use hooves ... just the bones, skins, and hides, which are boiled down to release collagen. In the end, all these parts are boiled and filtered. Collagen is extracted, further processed, and dressed up with artificial colors and sweeteners, such as red dye 40. Also known as "allura red," it is banned in several countries, such as Switzerland, Germany, Denmark, Sweden, and Austria. But in our country, it's no problem. It's found in many red-colored processed foods in the United States (even in other colored foods and beverages such as orange soda). According to Carolyn Wyman's book *Jell-0: A Biography* (Harcourt, 2001), more than 758,000 boxes are purchased each day in the U.S. alone. The physical reactions, in children, include temper tantrums, aggressive behavior, hyperactivity, and more. Kids with attention deficit hyperactivity disorder (ADHD) often benefit from the elimination of this and other dyed and preserved foods from their diets.

Breakfast is another area where families fill their stomachs with everything from sugary cereals to frozen waffles. Many moms feel that cereals are a good thing. But processed cereals are high on the glycemic scale. Processed puffed rice cereals and flakes made from corn are quickly broken down to blood sugar. Researchers at the British Consumer Center (Health Warning to Government, March 31, 2004 press release) found that one serving of some common breakfast cereals contained four times the amount of salt as a 25g bag of roasted peanuts. One of those tested was actually a high-fiber "healthy" cereal.

MANY OF THESE "NATURAL" GRANOLA BARS CONTAIN RED DYE 40, YELLOW DYE 5, YELLOW 6, HIGH FRUCTOSE CORN SYRUP, MALTOSE CORN SYRUP, AND SUGAR.

The worst processed foods are the masters of disguise. These wolves in sheep's clothing make a conscious marketing effort to fool you. On a recent trip with my wife to the store, I looked at a few labels down the breakfast aisle. What I found was startling—granola bars with "nature" in their name had introduced a new "sweet and salty" product. Don't we have enough sugar and sodium in our diet? What started out as a natural oat bar has been kidnapped by these masters of spin. "Natural" conjures up thoughts of a lush green meadow, blue skies, and song birds. Many of these "natural" granola bars contain red dye 40, yellow dye 5, yellow 6, high fructose corn syrup, maltose corn syrup, and sugar.

Another curious food product can be some makers' fruit roll ups, often found near cereals and marketed as a healthy food for kids. The label, again, tells the real story.

Some foods with artificial ingredients cause problems for kids who count on us to protect them. Sugar races into their bloodstream, signaling their tiny pancreas to produce insulin (it's also charged with producing somatostatin, gastrin, and glucagon). Trans fatty acids accelerate their risk for heart disease. Preservatives, artificial additives, man-made sugars, white carbohydrates, and processed foods add fuel to this internal fire—the building blocks for cellular multiplication, irregularity, and degeneration. We know the enemy. From generation to generation, we unwittingly transport our own brand of toxic waste, providing our kids with a solid foundation of bad habits and apathy. Like wildfire, it quietly burns its way through a corrupt food supply. We eat it without hesitation. We would rather pay to play.

Our brains have learned which foods provide a quick fix for their insatiable souls. The simplest of carbohydrates that break down rapidly are the foods our brains crave the most. Today, Americans are the most overweight people on earth. Over 60% of us are actually classified that way, by definition. In a major study of trends in weight and obesity for Americans (Overweight and obesity in the United States: prevalence and trends, 1960–1994 January 1998, Volume 22, Number 1, Pages 39–47), lead researcher Dr. Katherine M. Flegal and her colleagues at the National Center for Health Statistics, and Centers for Disease Control and Prevention, discovered that from 1976 to 1980 and 1988 to 1994, the prevalence of obesity increased markedly in the U.S. But why did we witness such a surge in the rate of obesity during these particular points in time?

Is it coincidence that high fructose corn syrup (HFCS) was first introduced commercially in 1977? At that time, farmers were stuck with low-priced corn and financially dying on the vine. That year, the Secretary of Agriculture signed legislation that allowed processors such as Archer Daniels Midland Company (ADM) to market HFCS to makers of commercial foods. Before the 1970s, HFCS represented less than 1 percent of all caloric sweeteners (*American Journal of Clinical Nutrition*, 2004). By the year 2000, HFCS represented an incredible 42 percent of all sweeteners. Some suggest that this single stroke of a pen ushered in a new wave of obesity from 1976 to 1980. But what about the subsequent increase in obesity in the United States that began in 1988? In 1987, just months before the next spike in obesity, the United States government approved an even cheaper version of HFCS. This allowed food processors to produce HFCS at lower cost, permitting them to use it in a growing number of foods. Known as "crystalline fructose," it's produced by allowing the fructose to crystallize from a fructose-enriched corn syrup, according to the folks at www. sugar.org. ADM's own information shows that their popular CCC® brand of crystalline fructose contains no more than 1 milligram of arsenic/ per kg, as well as lead, chloride, and up to 5 milligrams of heavy metals.

ACCORDING TO THE DATA, 184 MILLION CHINESE PEOPLE ARE OVERWEIGHT.

We've successfully exported obesity to the farthest corners of the earth. Ancient Chinese ways have given way to type 2 diabetes. The Chinese were formerly among the leanest people on earth. But now, almost one-fifth are classified as either obese or overweight. Based on the size of their 1.3 billion-plus population, they've already surpassed us in terms of overweight people. Today, 184 million Chinese people are *overweight*. At the time of this survey (*BMJ*, January 1998, Volume 22, Number 1, Pages 39–47), only 31 million Chinese were classified as *obese*. But that was several years ago. The rise of obesity and heart disease directly corresponds to the availability of fast and processed foods. It's also worth noting that according to *Circulation* (2001, p. 131), the Chinese have the largest cigarette habit in the world. *One in every three* cigarettes manufactured in the world is consumed in China. Three in every five Chinese smokers began smoking between the ages of 15 to 20. If left unchecked, it will "kill one in three Chinese men who are now 29 years or younger" (*Join Together*, "China Tries to Cope with Smoking Epidemic," January, 2007).

Advertising, along with celebrity testimonial, gives credibility to junk food. While targeting impressionable kids should be a crime, it's hard to show your anger to a smiling clown. We send our children off to school with still more good intention—lunch money with a little bit extra to buy dessert. Vending machines reach to grab your kid's quarters with promises of a quick sugar fix for those that didn't have the time to eat (or a parent to cook) a real meal. From artificially flavored cheese crackers, to pastries filled with HFCS, and juices with more sugar than soda, we've engineered a life for our kids where it's become necessary for them to go out of their way for a wholesome meal. Sadly, few families regularly enjoy dinner together. Our priorities are reflected in our diet, and the lack of time we now spend honoring this age-old tradition. According to Michael F. Jacobson PhD, writing for the Center for Science in the Public Interest ("How Soft Drinks Are Harming Americans' Health," 2005): "Today soda pop provides the average 12- to 19-year-old boy with about 15 teaspoons of refined sugars a day (57 pounds of sugar a year) and the average girl with about 10 teaspoons a day (38 pounds annually)." And that's just from soda pop—if your kid is "average."

Fermalab, a government nuclear laboratory that smashes atoms, found that Twinkies™ remain intact when exposed to the same amount of centrifugal force a spacecraft undergoes when it's launched into orbit. That would come as no surprise to Roger Bennatti, a teacher who shared his passion for things he loved with his students. According to a story that appeared in *USA Today*, the retired science teacher kept a Twinkie on top of his blackboard for most of his thirty-year career. "We wanted to see what the shelf life of a Twinkie was," said Bennatti. "The idea was to see how long it would take to go bad. It's rather brittle, but if you dusted it off, it's probably still edible." As of 1954, it adorned his board; and although a bit moldy, according to Bennatti, "It never spoiled." Imagine that, after 30 years! According to Hostess®, over half a billion Twinkies™ are sold each year.[1]

Why do we insist on feeding our loved ones like cows with multiple stomachs? Parents are guardians who are supposed to guard and protect, not win popularity contests. We're supposed to be able to say "no." In a world where the majority of us spend more time investigating the purchase of a TV or a microwave oven, than we do the food we eat—why do the issues of life, premature death, and the future suffering of our children from avoidable diseases, take a backseat?

Previous generations used the "ignorance is bliss" excuse to justify why they smoked. They lived in a world where habits like this began before they knew what they were getting into.

But after reading this book, you must ask, "What's our excuse?" Vending machines and drive-thru restaurants dole out quick fixes. Fake foods loaded with dangerous preservatives have permitted food producers to keep tasty junk on the shelf far longer than ever before. McDonalds® tugs at the heart of every small child to enter the world of a friendly clown with tasty treats and yummy meats. If clowns, bargains on toys in a meal, and eye popping foods bursting with sugar and trans fats weren't enough, there are games for parents too, with prizes that reward them for bringing kids back for more.

According to the Centers for Disease Control and Prevention (*International Journal of Obesity*, January 1998, Volume 22, Number 1, Pages 39–47) almost 31 percent of kids ages 6 to 19 are overweight. Another 30 percent are dangerously close. Their conclusions were based on a report from data gathered in the year 2000. By now, it's likely that over 60 percent of our children in this age group are officially classified as overweight. Obesity rates have doubled for preschoolers and adolescents, and tripled for children ages 6 to 11 in the last few decades. More than 30 percent of our children are overweight, and more than 15 percent of those ages 6 to 19 are obese. And rates are expected to grow even higher in years to come.

Researchers Shapiro et al. drew the following conclusion after an extensive study of 450 children ("Obesity Prognosis: A Longitudinal Study of Children From the Age of 6 Months to 9 Years," *American Journal of Public Health*, 1984 September; 74(9): 968–972): "There is evidence that impending or actual obesity begins at ages 6 to 9 years with some predictability provided as early as age 2 years for girls, age 3 years for boys." And childhood obesity rates are clearly on the rise. Obesity has even been found as early as six months of age. But how can six-month-old children become obese? At a recent obesity seminar, a handout from Patrika Tsai, MD, MPH (slide courtesy of M. Walker), suggests one possibility. Similac Isomil, a powdered feeding formula, contains 43.2 percent corn syrup solids, 14.6 percent soy protein isolate, 11.5 percent-high-oleic safflower oil, 10.3 percent sugar, 8.4 percent soy oil, and 8.1 percent coconut oil (we'll hope it's extra virgin). You already know how damaging processed oils can be. And certain processed soy products. To put the former in perspective, Mary G. Enig, PhD, tells us ("Soy Infant Formula Could Be Harmful to Infants: Groups Want it Pulled," *Nutrition Week*, Dec 10, 1999;29(46):1-2):

"The amount of phytoestrogens that are in a day's worth of soy infant formula equals five birth control pills." Fortunately, nature has provided the answer.

Children that are fed breast milk appear to have a lower incidence of obesity not only in childhood, according to scientists at Cincinnati Children's Hospital Medical Center ("Study Detects Protein In Human Milk Linked To Reduced Risk Of Obesity," 2004, May 3, as reported in *Science Daily*), but later in life. Parents with good intentions are loving their kids to death. Maybe it's time for a little tough love?

OUR BRAINS—WE'RE HERE TO DO THEIR BIDDING

Our incredible brains developed the means through our evolution to harvest blood sugar. Legs and arms developed in ways that allow us to effectively hunt, gather, and cook food to satisfy our gluttonous brains. Teeth developed to help us properly grind and digest the nourishment required to sustain them. Taste buds signal us to use our hands and limbs to do their bidding. We gather this stuff, break it down, and feed them. Today, there are other ways to secure our food. Hunting has been replaced by commuting. Our means of securing a steady supply of food for our brains is by earning enough to buy it. Behavior is shaped by what we perceive to be its consequences. Eating is a perfect example of shaped behaviors that are reinforced in a number of different ways by food makers. Visually pleasing food provides immediate gratification, appealing to some or all of our senses as we *perceive* they will eliminate our hunger (though empty calories do little to sustain us, and when they do it's short-lived). We've come to learn that sugary foods are quick fixes. They provide us with immediate gratification by satisfying our hunger and our brains' craving for glycogen. In essence, feeling secure in life means having enough financial wherewithal to secure the food our brain requires to survive.

In modern society, eating is often a cultural or social event as well as a personal activity. The more we see foods and the easier they are to obtain, the more we eat them. The more we eat them, the more we *need* more. Our brains are pigs. As the largest organ in our nervous system, the average adult brain contains over 100 billion neurons *each* linked to as many as 10,000 other neurons through as many as 7,000 synaptic connections. With all this potential to process life's experiences, nature had the foresight to insure that the brain itself experienced no pain. While it knows where injury is sustained elsewhere, it can't feel when damage has been done to itself. You see, the brain is actually void of sensory nerve endings. According to a special report by Helen Phillips for the news service NewScientist.com (September 4, 2006): **Our brains form a million new connections for every second we're alive.** And they've tripled in size in the last couple of million years[2] (*Journal of Evolution and Technology*. 1998. Vol. 1) to process an expanding array of new stimuli it's bombarded with, and to accommodate or store that growing body of knowledge. In the course of our life the brain will capture about 50,000 times the amount of information that's found in all the books in the Library of Congress.[3] According to author Rene Marois this is "more than five times the amount of the total printed material in the world." Professor Alan Dix of the computer department at Lancaster University believes the brain's capacity is "equivalent to a billion bibles, about the number which stacked floor to ceiling would fill a medium sized church." It processes data from light that's captured by our retina; a tiny converter box of sorts that's found in the back of the eye. This small (less than one square centimeter) but incredibly dense nerve tissue, featuring approximately 100 million rods and 75 million cones, transforms light into images made of chemical energy (like the film in a camera). It then transmits this data through the human-like transmission cable we refer to as our optic nerve, which in turn delivers it to the deepest portions of our brain.

We're conditioned creatures, and the food companies know it. They've got our number and understand precisely what it is that makes us tick—they've analyzed what ingredients triggers our brain to purchase their products and how to inspire its loyalty. Adding the scent of buttered popcorn to a favorite American classic, then heating and salting it slightly and slathering it with melted oil (it's seldom real butter) is enough to bring out the kid in most of us. Pavlov and his dog had nothing over the sound of fresh popcorn popping with all these special effects. In the end, your brain knows where its bread is buttered.

But often the butter-like taste in certain store-bought popcorn comes from what the industry calls a "flavor vapor." The popularly known diacetyl is under investigation for its potential role in causing lung disease and other respiratory illness. The National Emphasis Program, a 2007 initiative, was launched by OSHA after the agency reviewed studies implicating diacetyl for its role in causing hazardous respiratory illness. Not surprisingly, in 2007 ConAgra Foods® owner of popcorn brands ACT II® and Orville Redenbacher's, announced they had reformulated their products with a new butter flavoring that eliminated diacetyl. This was seven years later when, in May 2000, "an occupational medicine physician contacted the Missouri Department of Health and Senior Services to report eight cases of fixed obstructive lung disease in former workers of a microwave popcorn factory," according to the Morbidity and Mortality Weekly Report (*MMWR Weekly*, April 26, 2002/51(16); 345-7). Again, the food companies have mastered the science of *us*.

Our sense of smell signals our brain to trigger eating-related behavior as well. An article in *Food Quality News* (October, 2004), aptly states: "Smell is intimately related to how human beings taste food but has long remained the most enigmatic of our senses. The average human nose can detect nearly 10,000 distinct scents, a feat that requires about 1,000 olfactory genes, or roughly 3 percent of the human genome."

The tactile power of food, and the visual ability of food to elicit a cognitive response, was demonstrated by Marie-Pierre St-Onge et al. *(The Journal of*

Nutrition, 135:1014-1018, May 2005.) In a small study, researchers introduced foods, and then scanned the brain of volunteers using an MRI machine after each item was seen and touched. Each scan was then compared to MRI images following the introduction of non-food items. They found that five areas of the brain were stimulated for the presentation of food and or the tactile sensation of real food by subjects who were fasting. These areas correspond with those you might expect to effect the behavior of eating and are as follows: memory (hippocampus and parahippocampus), cognitive control and decision making (cingulate gyrus), association and interpretation (superior temporal gyrus), and food-related interest (insula). According to the study, "These findings support the claim that the presence of food (either seen or felt) elicits a unique cortical response that is differentiated from nonfood items." Our brain signals us to eat foods that provide blood sugar as quickly as it requires it. Especially foods that are visually appealing, tactilely attractive, and aromatically pleasing. And purveyors understand this. They continue to make food easily accessible. Fast food at drive-up windows, or even faster food from vending machines, is within easy reach when our brains need them. Day long journeys to hunt and gather, have been replaced by the push of a button and the convenience of a drive up window. Food companies shape our perceptions and learned behavior, with suggestive marketing; and reward us with a strategic array of ingredients that titillate our senses. Understanding this phenomenon allows us to take control, to break the chain of events that produced a vicious cycle we're all too often unaware of.

A cycle that finds most of us, quite literally, *Misinformed About Food*.

INSULIN: THE KEY TO A LONGER LIFE

Disease occurs when something inside of us begins to go wrong. A chain of events is set in motion that eventually plays itself out. At some point, symptoms become observable, and acute enough to notice. It may start out as fatigue, sleeplessness, irritability, or anxiety. Eventually, it may evolve into physical pain. In time, it will blossom into a constellation of symptoms we can label. At that point in time, we typically treat the symptoms with pharmaceuticals. If successful, the symptoms are no longer observable, and acute. But the internal events that created those symptoms remain.

Maintaining an optimum insulin level is one of the most important factors required to maintain good health. And eating properly is the best way to do so.

What we eat immediately affects the balancing act of our hormones. An invisible war takes place, and while we don't see it being waged, it's played out at every meal. Each time you eat food, internal events take place that impact your life. This internal tug-of-war with homeostasis helps determine the bumps in the road of your own mortality.

But there's hope. You can begin reversing this hazard as soon as you eat your next meal. It's that true. It's that simple. Carbohydrates, also known as "saccharides," are sugars. Some break down slowly while others are quickly digested. The slower they're synthesized, the better. If carbohydrates carry little or no nutrients, you should avoid them. It doesn't matter how quickly they break down.

While your body can actually acquire all of the energy it needs from fat and protein (technically making carbohydrates non-essential), they're also needed to build body tissue and cells—and are better off being left alone to do so. While your brain craves glucose and can't burn fat, it can get all the glucose it needs from protein. But again, protein is required elsewhere; we need to do what we can to let them focus on getting there. That's why carbohydrates are often referred to as "protein sparing." They make themselves available to be broken down to satisfy the body's requirement for glucose, thereby "freeing up" protein molecules so they can focus on building tissue, enzymes, cell structure and immunity.

The important role that high-fiber carbs play in optimizing health can't be underscored. Some types of fiber are required to usher excessive amounts of cholesterol out of your bloodstream and waste material out of your digestive tract. As you've already learned, their resistance to digestion allows glucose to enter your system slowly, enabling your blood to maintain the narrow range of intake that's so important for well-being.

Feeding our body's requirement for blood sugar *gradually* is an essential building block for both vigor and immunity. Consuming healthy carbohydrates that break down slowly is like building a drip system that feeds your blood with nutrients. The more slowly they're absorbed into your blood, the better. And, of course, the higher quality your food choices are, the better. Your ability to do so will permit you to achieve longer life and avoid most diseases.

POOR CARBS = EXCESS INSULIN = POOR HEALTH

There are good carbohydrates and bad carbohydrates. Those with the highest amount of fiber are good for you. Those with the least amount of fiber generally are bad for you. Most white carbohydrates generally lack fiber and are often the worst. Complex carbohydrates typically contain the greatest amount of fiber and are the best. The more fiber a food contains, the longer it takes your body to break it down. That's precisely what we want. Carbohydrates are broken down by enzymes in our blood to form glucose. The longer it takes to do so, the less insulin is required.

Glucose is transported through the bloodstream to cells and relied upon by your body as its chief source of energy. When we need energy from blood sugar that's not readily available, our brain signals our appetite centers to go out and find it. The best source for blood sugar is carbohydrate. Complex carbohydrates are those foods that contain a good deal of cellulose fiber and long-chain sugar molecules that resist immediate digestion. Eventually, the liver breaks them down into shorter molecules that slowly feed the brain. Typically, these complex carbs are found in natural foods.

On the other hand, *simple* carbohydrates are generally found in sugary processed foods and are quickly broken down. Like honey and other simple sugars, they're immediately absorbed through the wall of the stomach. From a glucose load perspective, it's the equivalent of shooting yourself up with corn syrup.

One danger of simple carbohydrate consumption is pancreatic burnout; caused by nutritionally-void foods lacking fiber that break down rapidly. When white carbohydrates of no real value are eaten, they're broken down like greased lightning. Glucose races into your bloodstream. Your pancreas rises to the occasion by pumping out insulin produced by its beta cells. Insulin ushers that excess glucose out of your bloodstream, and carries it into your fat cells where it's stored. Up to a point, storing glucose is a good thing. If energy wasn't stored, our species would have died off after our ancestors had their first bouts with hunger. Excess glucose, swept out of your bloodstream, is stored in receptor cells found in your liver and muscle. This stored glucose is referred to as "glycogen."

When glucose can't be found by breaking down food, and energy is required, the pancreas signals the release of a second hormone known as glucagon, produced by its alpha cells. It's glucagon's job to break down the glycogen reserves and release them into the bloodstream in an effort to maintain homeostasis.

When glycogen reserves are full and excess glucose remains in the blood, it's immediately stored in plumped-up fat cells. The fat that gets tucked away is not just any kind of fat, but the worst kind of fat. The doors of your receptors are now slammed shut and locked tight. The excess sugar is left to circulate in your bloodstream.

Soon, you're tired. That burst of energy is gone as quickly as it came. A quick surge of sugar only briefly satisfied a demanding brain; not the ideal slow roll we hope to achieve—that gradually breaks down into glucose. In only a couple of hours you're on the prowl for more quick hits from simple sugar and you're hungry again. While the simple carbohydrates you ate provided your brain with a few seconds of glucose, the rapid spike in excess blood sugar was ushered out of your bloodstream and into your fat cells by insulin from your pancreas.[4]

... INSULIN AND GLUCAGON, ARE DOING THEIR BEST TO BALANCE OPTIMUM LEVELS OF BLOOD SUGAR. THEY'RE THE LEADING PARTICIPANTS IN A HORMONAL TUG-OF-WAR.

A destructive cycle has begun. Your brain again signals your appetite center to find more magic bullets. You're on a dangerous teeter-totter. The more of these empty carbohydrates you eat, the more you crave them.

At the same time, the two pancreatic endocrine hormones, insulin and glucagon, are doing their best to balance optimum levels of blood sugar. They're the leading participants in a hormonal tug-of-war. The pancreas is at the center of this fight. When your glucose level is too low, the pancreas produces glucagon. When your blood sugar is too high, it produces more insulin. Your hormones are now out of kilter.

If it's *continually* low, you may be hypoglycemic. If it's consistently too high, you may have hyperglycemia, the immediate precursor to type 2 diabetes.

Your pancreas is about the size of your hand, looks like a squashed banana, and is found just behind the lower portion of your stomach. This organ battles to help your blood sugar maintain its equilibrium. And your pancreas is now on overdrive—*all the time.*

The risk of type 2 diabetes is just the tip of the iceberg. An excessive amount of insulin, the regulating-hormone circulating in our blood, has also been linked to everything from heart disease to breast cancer and even renal cell carcinoma. Fats, known as "triglycerides," build up in the blood plasma of type 2 diabetics. These triglycerides are not necessarily formed from the consumption of fat as you might expect. They result from excess sugar in the liver. High triglyceride levels, accompanied by low HDL in type 2 diabetics, are predictors of everything from ischemic stroke to heart disease.

According to Gaziano et al. (*Circulation*, 1997 96:2520-2525), "People with the highest ratio of triglycerides to HDL—the 'good' cholesterol—had 16 times the risk of heart attack as those with the lowest ratio of triglycerides to HDL in the study of 340 heart attack patients and 340 of their healthy, same-age counterparts."

Again, the first line of protection against a high triglyceride level is neither a low or no fat diet, nor the use of statin drugs. The solution may surprise you. Eat more of the *right kind* of fats discussed in Chapter 2, along with the right kind of proteins and high-fiber carbohydrates (eating fruit and fats in moderation). Substitute sugar, with Just Like Sugar® (RKInformedLiving.com). Increase HDL by walking 40 minutes or more daily, minimum 4 days weekly.

In his paper entitled "Insulin and its Metabolic Effects" (Designs for Health Institute's BoulderFest Seminar, August 1999), Dr. Ron Rosedale, MD, explains that all centenarians (people who live past the age of 100), though different in almost all aspects of their dietary and living habits, share one particular thing in common—they all have relatively low insulin levels. While some had low cholesterol levels, other had high levels. While some smoke and drank, others abstained. But in the end, even the 122-year-old woman from France, Jean Calumet (a smoker and drinker), shared this one discernible characteristic with her fellow centurions.

As Rosedale suggests, "Insulin is the common denominator in everything … The way to treat cardiovascular disease and the way I treated my stepfather, the way I treated the high-risk cancer patient, and osteoporosis, high blood pressure, the way to treat virtually all the so-called chronic diseases of aging is to treat insulin itself."

Dr. Rosedale reiterates insulin's evolutionary role, with power well beyond its ability to lower blood sugar. Its role is to store *other* important excess nutrients as well. If cells become insulin resistant, they won't open up to store these nutrients. Chief among these substances is magnesium. If you lose intracellular magnesium (whose job among other things is to relax muscle), your blood vessels constrict. This increases your bloods pressure. It's tougher for blood to flow in narrow corridors. So another damaging cycle has begun. Without a sufficient amount of magnesium, insulin can't get into tissue, so its level increases. This causes you to lose even more *magnesium*. And losing magnesium is a very big deal.

According to Dr. Mildred Seeling (*American Journal of Clinical Nutrition*, 1964) **80 to 90 percent** of the adult population in the United States is already magnesium deficient. A sudden death in an athlete may be the result of an enlarged heart caused by a magnesium deficiency. Those that sweat profusely through endurance training deplete magnesium reserves in their tissue.

Researcher C. J. Johnson and associates (*American Journal of Clinical Nutrition*, Vol 32, 967–970, May 1979) found that subjects with ischemic heart disease had significantly lower levels of myocardial tissue magnesium. Stress and alcohol further perpetuate a magnesium deficiency. Now that less insulin is produced, your blood sugar continues to escalate and your level of magnesium plummets. Increased insulin means a greater retention of sodium. Constricted blood vessels and excessive amounts of sodium in the blood result in greater retention of fluid. These imbalances work together to collectively lay the groundwork for congestive heart failure. *Balancing* your insulin is *that* important.

The next time the child you love with all your heart wants a piece of cake with frosting, think twice. While you won't win a popularity contest with this kind of tough love, you and your children *can* stop dying to eat.

SUGARS—ALL ARE NOT CREATED EQUAL

As we've previously discussed, sugar is the basic building block of carbohydrate. A simple sugar is known a "monosaccharide." *All* carbohydrates consist of *units* of sugar known as "saccharide units" (from the Greek word *saccharin*, meaning sugar).

There are three principal types of simple sugars or monosaccharides: glucose, fructose and galactose. The two most infamous monosaccharides are fructose (fruit sugar) and glucose (blood sugar).

Glucose, as we've already discussed, is the *only* sugar that circulates in your bloodstream, providing important energy and nourishment to every cell in your body. Fructose and galactose *do not*. Fructose is the major sugar component of most fruit. It's also the sweetest naturally occurring sugar. While a small amount of fructose may assist our body's ability to process glucose, less is best. Fructose (unlike table sugar) is processed in the liver; too much overwhelms it, causing the liver to produce dangerous fat molecules such as triglycerides. The excessive consumption of table sugar is equally dangerous. While moderate amounts are sustainable in a healthy individual, *table sugar* makes the pancreas work harder.

The glycemic index (GI) of the monosaccharide fructose is a mere 22, while table sugar (a disaccharide known as sucrose) is 64. More on this later, but remember, the GI does no more than tell you how quickly a 50-gram serving raises your blood sugar. While a rapid rise isn't healthy, it's only one factor that helps us determine the true value of a given food. Our goal should be *to create the perfect drip system.* This allows blood glucose to flow as consistently as possible and carry nutrients to each of your cells continuously. Carbohydrates that lack nutrients are worthless and may be harmful, *regardless* of how low their respective GI and glycemic load (GL) indexes may be.

While fructose has a slower feed of only 22, *it's just as damaging as sucrose* (table sugar), but for reasons that differ.

Unlike certain sugars and fats that are carried into cells by insulin, fructose makes a beeline for your liver. It doesn't require insulin to sweep it into fat cells, it's the sugar of choice for many diabetics. But while an excessive amount of glucose is swept out of your bloodstream by insulin, fructose doesn't pass go. Eventually, it's metabolized into a compound known as "acetyl-CoA."

According to Dr. Robert H. Lustig, professor of Pediatric Endocrinology at University of California at San Francisco (UCSF) and director of the Weight Assessment for Teen and Child Health (WATCH) (ABC interview, July 9, 2007), acetyl-CoA also produces compounds of free fatty acids that ultimately damage the liver. "Acetyl-CoA damages the liver the same way alcohol does," says Dr. Lustig ("Drinking juice is no better than drinking soda," Obesity Discussion, August 7, 2006). "First, excess acetyl-CoA can produce a compound that is toxic to beta cells in the pancreas. Some think this may be what triggers type 2 diabetes. In addition, acetyl-CoA also is converted to form free fatty acids, which enter the bloodstream and promote atherosclerosis (cholesterol deposits in the arteries). The free fatty acids can also build up in the liver and cause liver disease similar to what is seen in long-term alcoholism."

Simply put, the excess consumption of fructose may cause a condition known as nonalcoholic fatty liver disease (NAFLD). Fat accumulates in the liver causing inflammation, which may ultimately result in cirrhosis.

"People think fruit juice is healthy, but it's not," says Dr. Lustig. *"Drinking juice—even if it says '100 percent natural'—is no better than drinking soda* … In my practice, I've had a 15-year-old boy who needed a liver transplant from drinking soda—his condition of NAFLD was that bad. I've also had a 6-year-old morbidly obese patient who drank a gallon of orange juice a day," says Dr. Lustig. But you don't need to drink a gallon of juice a day to create an excessive amount of glucose. *"Moderate"* consumption of the *right kind of whole fruit* and fruit juice is healthful. All of life and nutrition is a matter of degree and balance. One of the most healthful parts of fruit is its pulp. Pulp is by definition soluble fiber suspended in water. Yet, for a profit, many TV juicing evangelists have convinced thousands of us to pay for juicing machines that separate the pulp from the juice. Juicing also makes it tough to eat the pectin found in the inner lining of the skin in many fruits. Pectin and pulp are both among the healthiest parts of any fruit. Pulp helps us achieve the ultimate drip system. Why would anyone design a machine to eliminate it? You already know the answer. We believe what we are told. And what we are told, we are often willing to pay for.

Fortunately for all of us, mastication type juicers like the Vita-Mix 5200® allow us to blend whole fruits and vegetables in their entirety. This is the only method of what some call juicing that I suggest (note: see chapter 6 end note #8). The juice contains all of the pulp, as well as the skin and seeds. Studies have shown that the skin of certain fruits and vegetables contains an even higher content of important nutrients and metabolites than the foods themselves. The fiber allows us to slow the emptying of fructose in our liver, helping us better balance our blood sugar. Though I am no fan of fruit juice, mixing in a little with plenty of water using this type of machine allows us to enjoy the good stuff, rather than separating and eliminating it. I'm particularly excited about blending *vegetables*. It's an easy and healthy way to enjoy the amount and variety of vegetables we require daily; allowing our organs to devote their time to other important duties, since less of their time is required to predigest our food.

It's also easy to mask healthy vegetables (and fats) that your children may have otherwise avoided. Jonny Boden, PhD, C.N.S. (the 150th Healthiest Foods on Earth; Fair Winds Press; 2007) has an outstanding suggestion: "reduce the glycemic load by adding fish oil to your fruit juice." The fat makes the carotenoids in the vegetables and fruits more bio-available—or usable—to the body, says Jonny. "And fat lowers the glycemic load. Plus I get the benefit of the incredibly valuable anti-inflammatory Omega-3s from the fish oil."

Other fats such as avocado, and acidic foods such as lemon, lower the glycemic composite of companion foods.

Now, you can enjoy far greater absorption of important nutrients from the world's greatest foods by breaking them down *easily*—while reducing the impact on your blood sugar. For more information on masticating machines see this and all resources I've suggested on our web site.

Galactose, the last of three simple sugars, combines with glucose to form *lactose*, known as "milk sugar." The *only* significant carbohydrate we can obtain in any meaningful amount *from animals* is milk and the dairy-related products derived from milk. While whole milk carries a reasonably low glycemic load of 27, there's little reason to drink it—and more good reason to avoid it. Simple sugars break down in your bloodstream rapidly. They taste sweet. Fruit becomes a natural yet simple carbohydrate when its sugars are used to make juices, sodas, and other beverages. Simple sugars represented by mono- and disaccharides make up the first of three different types of basic classifications of carbohydrates. They're sweet and easy to digest because they lack fiber and are generally high in both their GI and GL.

The primary source of sugar in such altered sweeteners is high fructose corn syrup (HFCS), which began life as corn syrup, before it was combined in an amazing array of processed milling wizardry. Critics suggest a link between the growth of this processed sweetener and obesity. But the American Medical Association says there's insufficient evidence to limit its use.[20]

Manufacturers enjoy far lower product costs and far higher gross margins utilizing HFCS among other inexpensive highly processed sugars, regardless of its alleged potential to damage your health. According to Kim Severson's article, "Sugar coated: We're drowning in high fructose corn syrup. Do the risks go beyond our waistline?" (*San Francisco Chronicle*, February 18, 2004), "A single 12-ounce can of soda has as much as *13 teaspoons of sugar* in the form of high fructose corn syrup. And because the amount of soda we drink has more than doubled since 1970 to about 56 gallons per person a year, so has the amount of high fructose corn syrup we guzzle. In 2001, we consumed almost 63 pounds of it, according to the U.S. Department of Agriculture." Severson further cautions us that even low-fat, fruit-flavored yogurt (only eat plain yogurt) can have as much as *10 tablespoons* of fructose-based sweetener. Today, the average American's daily dose is more like 35 teaspoonfuls of fructose—most of it coming from soft drinks. Are we properly informed about food?

CARBOHYDRATES: THE STARCH FAMILY

Complex carbohydrates require considerably more time to be broken down and digested than simple carbs. While the first group of carbohydrates were simple monosaccharide sugars, the second and third group, starches and fibers, are *complex* carbohydrate polysaccharides. When you eat a starchy food an enzyme found in your intestines and saliva, known as "amylase," breaks apart its simple sugar units, which are easily absorbed in your blood. It's used by bakeries to break down the complex sugar found in the starch and flour. Yeast is then added to feed on the now simpler sugar.

Starch is the second major classification of carbohydrate and again, is a polysaccharide. Polysaccharides are tougher to break down into fuel than simple monosaccharides. However, all foods within a broad classification are not necessarily alike. Selecting the right foods should therefore be based on particular characteristics. Some starchy carbohydrates contain more fiber and more nutrients than other starchy carbohydrates. They may also raise blood glucose and insulin levels faster or slower than other starches. One member of this group may be far more bio-available than another. Cooking time, processing, and the method used to prepare foods can also alter their value.

The longer you cook a starch, the greater its surface area. Heating puffs them up, making them an easier target for digestive enzymes to quickly convert them to blood sugar. Certain starchy foods, such as pasta, have a lower GI when undercooked (*al dente* style). It's the same principal as puffing up rice to form rice cakes; a hazardous form of adulterated high-glycemic food. In general, the denser the food, the less it spikes your insulin; feeding your blood more gradually than a low-fiber selection.

Starch comes from plants. Energy, created by the process known as photosynthesis, is stored in plants as starch. Beans, bread, pasta, cereal, rice, and potatoes are the best known examples of starchy carbohydrates. Classifications of carbohydrates overlap in the same way as fats and protein do. A food classified as a polyunsaturated fat generally contains some degree of monounsaturated and saturated fat.

GLYCATION

Significant chemical reactions occur within, as we grow older, that accelerate the process of aging itself, degrading both our quality and quantity of life. While the damage caused by some of these actions can be reduced and even reversed, in others the damage is done and can't be undone.

Glycation occurs when sugar molecules get caught up in a fat or a protein molecule's underwear. Simple sugars such as fructose, glucose and lactose combine with lipid or protein molecules to form warped biological structures with significant potential for destruction. And the process is irreversible. In time, these aberrant glycated molecules mingle and eventually combine with others to form dangerous sugar laden debris which cling to special cell receptors, inflaming their membrane. Once activated, this glycated cellular "gunk" begins to produce a variety of damaging pro-inflammatory compounds known as *advanced glycation end products* (AGE—not to be confused with the same acronym used to refer to healthy aged garlic extract).

The more blood sugar a person has, the greater their likelihood of damage from glycation. Not surprisingly, diabetics are particularly prone to the ravaging effects of this non-enzymatic *cross-linking* (the bonding of these garbage molecules occurs without the action of an enzyme). So are all those people with high blood sugar from a diet laden with foods high in glucose, fructose or galactose. Among other things, it's a warning to soft drink, candy and fruit juice lovers. It's also one of the many reasons I avoid eating a good deal of fruit. While I'm not suggesting you avoid *all* foods containing simple sugars, you need to be aware of them.

Milk, garbanzo beans, and celery (yes) are among the foods high in galactose.[5] Carbonated beverages, *honey*, raisins, dates, and figs top the list of foods with the largest amount of fructose. While some authorities have implicated the poor watermelon as a food high in fructose, they're misinformed. As a percentage of its weight, watermelon is one of the lower fructose-laden fruits, with just over 3 grams per 100 grams of "weight" (dates have a whopping 32 grams). Consult a food's GL and GI ranking (more later) to determine its impact on your blood sugar (glucose). While all carbohydrates contain glucose, some are worse than others. Rice cakes, corn flakes, and starchy foods such as white potatoes and white pastas are particularly poor choices.

Glycation (which may be likened to the caramelization of food) has been implicated in most chronic disease. It's also a primary cause of aging in skin and other tissue. Author Ben Best (Mechanisms of Aging) tells us that the production of free radicals is *50 times greater* in glycated versus unglycated cells!

Cooking can cause foods high in sugar to combine with fat or protein to generate substantial reactive glycation. When egg whites were cooked with fructose, researchers Koschinsky et al. found that they were 200 times more immunoreactive (Proceedings of the National Academy of Sciences of the U. S,. June 10, 1997 vol. 94 no. 12 6474-6479; Orally absorbed reactive glycation products (glycotoxins): An environmental risk factor in diabetic nephropathy).

Exogenous (or outside of the body) pre-formed glycations are often formed by highly heating foods containing protein or fat that are burnt or browned with sugar (watch that marinade!) Donuts, french fries (some fast food makers add sugar—so hold the ketchup!), toasted breads, cakes and grilled meats are all heavily laden accidents waiting to bond with similarly distorted protein or fat molecules inside of us.

... ADVANCED GLYCATION END-PRODUCTS ARE A PRIMARY CAUSE OF AGING SKIN.

Among other protein molecules that cross link with simple sugars, AGEs easily destroy those associated with youthful skin—such as collagen and elastin. These important proteins are cross linked with sugar molecules to form onerous glycated compounds that impede their ability to function. According to authors Daniel Schmid, Retto Muggli and Fred Zulli (Collagen Glycation and Skin Aging-Paper-Mibell AG Cosmetics) advanced glycation end products are a primary cause of aging skin. They indicate that the most profound alterations occur in the dermis, the underlying layer of skin, where collagen and elastin give the outer layer or epidermis its strength and resilience.

AGEs are implicated in everything from Alzheimers disease (increasing the production of amyloid proteins), to diabetes, and cause damage to the nerves in the peripheral system known as neuropathy, when toxins from AGEs destroy the insulating phospholipid layer known as myelin. Cancer, vascular destruction of the retina (ultimately causing blindness), deafness, atherosclerosis, and heart disease are part of a long line of illnesses that may also be attributed to AGEs. In fact, they can potentially destroy all organs that have Receptors for Advanced Glycation End products to bind to (known as RAGE). Yes, AGE can indeed cause RAGE!

But glycation is no laughing matter. Along with methylation, and oxidation, it's a primary cause of premature death and all age related illness. The more we live and eat, (the more data, so to speak, we put in our hard drive) the sooner we overload it, and crash. Without defragging (which I liken to the elimination of waste in humans at the cellular level—physiologically through calorie deprivation, and cognitively through meditation) the greater our potential for glitches and errors.

Fortunately, you *can* do something about it. While glycation will remain a fact of life, particularly for those that weren't aware of it and eat large amounts of sugary foods, you *can* shift glycation into low gear and substantially reduce its presence.

Begin by immediately reducing your intake of sugar. Less obvious offenders, fructose-laden foods (honey and certain fruits), should be avoided. (The Dangers of Honey, http://drmericle.blogspot.com/2005/04/dangers-of-honey.html)

500 milligrams daily of alpha-lipoic acid, the master antioxidant we'll discuss in more detail in Chapter 5, helps put the brakes on; though I only suggest 100 milligrams a day for regular "maintenance." Unless you've regularly consumed high levels of sugar-or have other sugar related problems, stick to the SOS recommended dosage in Chapter 6.

The most powerful glyco-buster known to man, and one of the most important anti-aging nutrients in the SOS arsenal, is the naturally occurring amino acid, carnosine. Found in meat protein (vegetarians please note), the amount required to protect ourselves from glycation exceeds the amount we can typically obtain from our food. Supplementing our diet with this important nutrient is one of the most powerful things we can do to optimize our health.

Dr. Phillip Lee Miller couldn't agree more. In his book (co-authored with the Life Extension Foundation) *The Science of Growing Old Without Aging* (2005, Bantam Dell), he discusses the importance of increasing the free *carnosine* that circulates in our bloodstream and states that "carnosine may be one of the most potent anti-aging compounds available today."

Miller suggests daily supplementation of 1000 milligrams (divided into two doses of 500 milligrams a day due to its short lifespan) and notes that we'd need to eat two pounds of cooked ground beef to receive the equivalent amount from our food. In addition to its role in preventing glycation, he cites its amazing ability to restore the vitality and increase the life span of aging cells in animals and in animal tissue cultures. Carnosine-revitalized aging cells "restores their appearance and function to that of more youthful cells." In fact, they lived three times longer than those cells receiving none. He also cites research showing its ability to protect us against a host of glycation related diseases; from cataracts (in rabbits and dogs), to brain damage from toxic metals. Overall, it has the power to protect the integrity of our skin by preventing the loss of collagen.

A study by Gille et al. (*Mutagenesis*. 1991; 6(4):313-8. Effect of antioxidants on hyperoxia-induced chromosomal breakage in Chinese hamster ovary cells: protection by carnosine) showed that out of all antioxidants tested, only carnosine significantly reduced damage to chromosomes when exposed to pure (90 percent) oxygen (inducing hyperoxia, or oxygen toxicity that creates free radicals).

Like so many important nutrients, hormones and enzymes, our level of carnosine declines dramatically as we age. According to a study by Stuerneberg et al., carnosine levels were found to be 63 percent lower in the muscle tissue of subjects between the ages of 10 to 70 (*Archives of Gerontology and Geriatrics* 1999. 29: 107-113; Concentrations of free carnosine a putative membrane-protective antioxidant in human muscle biopsies and rat muscles).

Are you prepared to accept aging gracefully as some suggest; or fight back! Now that you know what glycation is, it's time to stop one of the most heinous effects of sugar in its tracks. Miracles can occur if we're aware of the problem, and take the appropriate steps to reduce or avoid it.

CARBOHYDRATES/STARCH: BEANS RULE!

Certain beans are starchy super-foods. They're the only starchy carbohydrates that contain high protein as well as fiber and fat. Scientists have discovered that in addition to the high dietary fiber found in legumes (beans, lentils, and peas, for example), certain members of this family contain a third type of starch known as "resistant starch" (RS); far more of it as a percentage of their dietary weight than is characteristically present in grain-based foods.

Researchers at the University of Illinois (*Journal of Nutrition,* 2001;131:276–286) constructed the first database showing the percentage of starch and fiber in processed flour.

This RS is broken down by friendly bacteria after finding its way to the colon with little degradation. It *resists* digestive enzymes as its name implies in much the same way dietary fiber does, slowly feeding your blood glucose while carrying important protein, vitamins, and nutrients to your cells. Gallantly fighting enzymes in your saliva and stomach, it makes its way past your small intestine to your colon, where it's attacked by bacteria. This encounter produces a substance called "butyrate," a desirable fatty acid that's been shown to deter or prevent colon cancer.

Beans also lower the pH of feces, by reducing the amount of bile acid. A lower pH in feces is associated with a lower incidence of colon cancer in several populations. While bile acid is required to break down fat, excessive amounts of this bile acid can actually create cancers in the large intestine and elsewhere.

Beans reduce internal inflammation as well. In a study conducted by James W. Anderson, MD, and colleagues ("Hypocholesterolemic Effects of Oat-Bran or Bean Intake for Hypercholesterolemic Men," *American Journal of Clinical*

Nutrition, 40:1146–55, 1984) male subjects who were hypercholesterolemic enjoyed a whopping 24 percent reduction in LDL serum cholesterol when supplementing their diets with beans. As you've already learned, beans are loaded with resistant starch in addition to their protein, nutrients, minerals, and fiber content. This RS helps balance your blood sugar while causing the production of disease fighting butyrate.

If you have a problem tolerating beans, wash them thoroughly prior to cooking or soak them overnight. This helps break down the indigestible sugars that cause gas. Soaking them also improves them nutritionally, by cutting down the amount of time required to cook them, thus permitting them to retain more important nutrients.

The chart below, developed by George C Fahey with his colleagues at the University of Illinois (*Journal of Nutrition*, February, 1997), provides the first comparative database showing the percentage of RS. It also indicates the amount of starch that actually reaches the colon, as well as its fiber content. Thirty-nine different carbohydrates were tested:

Percentages of Key Components Identified in Illinois Study			
Selected ingredients	**Resistant starch (RS)**	**RS reaching colon**	**Total dietary fiber***
Legumes			
Black beans	26.9	62.7	42.6
Red kidney beans	24.6	57.7	36.8
Lentils	25.4	47.7	33.1
Navy bean	25.9	52.5	36.2
Black-eyed peas	17.7	32.8	32.6
Split peas	24.5	37.9	33.1
Northern beans	28	56.1	41.1
Cereal grains			
Barley	18.2	33	17
Corn	25.2	32.3	19.6
White rice	14.1	14.8	1.5
Brewer's rice	3.5	4.1	2.1
Brown rice	14.8	16.8	5.7

Percentages of Key Components Identified in Illinois Study			
Selected ingredients	Resistant starch (RS)	RS reaching colon	Total dietary fiber*
Wheat	13.6	26.8	17
Mlllet	12.6	14.6	5.4
Oats	7.2	16.6	37.7
Sorghum	36.1	45.6	4.6
Flours			
Corn	11	13	2.8
Wheat	1.7	2.5	12.1
Rice	1.6	1.8	5.1
Potato	1.7	2.1	2.1
Soy	0.6	10.9	15.4
Barley	1.2	1.7	22.9
Sorghum	1.6	1.8	1.3
Grain-based food			
Macaroni	6	8	5.6
Spaghetti	3.3	4.5	5.6
Corn meal	5	5.7	4.4
Rice bran	3.4	11.9	28
Rolled oats	8.5	15.2	10
Hominy grits	8	12.3	11.4

The above table shows that the amount of RS *in beans* that reaches your colon is *far greater* than the small amount that's found in starches and fibers. With the exception of beans, most other foods we classify as a starch should be avoided.[6]

CARBOHYDRATES/ STARCH: THE UGLY FAMILY?

The frequent consumption of certain nutrient-void white carbohydrates is hazardous to your health. But not all white carbs are created equal.

Most processed flour (unless it's fortified) is made of empty carbohydrates void of nutrients that race into your bloodstream. Mechanical processing generally converts what began as whole grain into high-glycemic white flour, by removing its outer sheath. Stripped of its bran, this fiber-barren flour breaks down to glucose with lightning-like speed. Modern technology subjects grain to a progressive series of rollers that crush it to a fine white powder bearing no resemblance to its coarse stone-ground ancestry. This worthless, dull-looking white stuff, is now gassed in ovens with chlorine dioxide to remove the smell. At the same time, it's bleached like laundry detergent for whiter and brighter whites. Any healthy fats once present in the original grain are either removed through sheathing or crushing, or placed in a high heating system and later, prolonged storage. Depending on the processor, trace amounts of fat that may have survived are generally rancid. Our desire for profit and convenience once again appears to have trumped our quest for wellness. Not long ago, bread was referred to as "the staff of life," boasting whole grains and stone-ground goodness.

The modern day industrialized miracle we're left with is a cheap white powder void of nutrients (other than synthetic vitamins that may replace natural compounds lost in processing). This impostor is difficult for your body to absorb. It's the perfect cheap and worthless food and an exciting prospect for commercial makers. What remains is a glue of sorts that binds together chemicals, preservatives, and sodium, with the shelf life of a petrified rock.

In a study of over 1,800 women in Mexico, Isabelle Romieu and colleagues from Instituto Nacional de Salud Publica (*Cancer Epidemiology Biomarkers & Prevention*, 2004) showed a direct correlation between breast cancer and a high-glycemic diet. In fact, these researchers observed an astonishing *220 percent higher risk* of breast cancer in women who received at least 57 percent of their dietary intake from low-fiber carbohydrates. They also discovered that these high rates were substantially reduced when these women received a corresponding increase of dietary fiber.

If all of this weren't bad enough, Swedish researcher David Sharp led a study (*Lancet*, 2003 (361) 9355 :361–362) which showed that dangerously high levels of *acrylamide*, a powerful toxin, exists in bread and other popular processed foods regularly eaten in North America. These include almost all baked goods that require high heat to process them.

Topping the list of tested foods showing the largest amount of contamination are french fries, potato chips, breakfast cereals, pastries, breads, and rolls. A large order of french fries, for example, was found to have *hundreds of times* the amount of this dangerous poison (between 32 to 89 micrograms) than the EPA's maximum allowable limit of 12 micrograms in an 8-ounce glass of water.

Acrylamide has been shown to increase the risk of endometrial, ovarian and kidney cancer in humans[7, 8] and has been linked to serious birth defects in animals. Heating these foods at home further increases the presence of acrylamide. In fact, toasting bread even *lightly* increases the level of this toxin. The crust contains even more than the softer part of the bread. Breads containing the *largest amount of protein* appear to also contain the largest amount of acrylamide. This makes even whole wheat and rye a poor choice. While 100 percent whole-grain breads are generally better alternatives for balanced blood sugar than those containing less or no grain, think again. They're actually poor choices based on their acrylamide content. While there's a good deal of debate on how much is too much, any amount of a potential human carcinogen is more than we need. All become part of the battery of toxins we're exposed to each day.

A good rule of thumb is to try to avoid all processed foods including breads, flour, and their by-products. This includes most baked goods, particularly those made from bleached white flour.

But what if they're fortified? When foods are fortified, they've been stripped of key nutrients through processing. But it's not just synthetic vitamins that are added back artificially—preservatives, additives, dyes, and fillers are also thrown in. Many synthetic vitamins are tar-based and lack the cofactors that are required to duplicate the behavior of those that occur naturally.

We've been fooled again by big business who have taken nature's grain and de-natured it. This enables them to process what began as a healthful food at high speed and low cost, leaving little in common with its source. You're left with a hunk of broken-down starchy powder that temporarily satisfies your craving. It quickly spikes your blood sugar and increases the potential for insulin resistance. The subsequent hormonal imbalance creates internal inflammation, the foundation for most disease.

Processed flour is only one of the many building blocks of inflammation and subsequent aging that we eat regularly, with little regard for its consequences. Celebrity chefs show you how fun and easy it is to flavor and fashion your own personal time bomb.

CARBOHYDRATES—LOW FIBER: THE POTATO

The best time to plan for a longer life is before it's cut short.

White potatoes are one of the starchiest foods of them all. Mashing them permits their starch to break down even faster, increasing the surface area to be attacked upon entry. Even a baked potato has a GL of 26 (anything over 20 is considered high). Once a favorite food of mine, I abandoned them. But the Chinese are clearly embracing them. Today, China is the largest producer of potatoes in the world. In fact, an incredible 80 percent of all global production is in Asia. But we still eat our fair share, a whopping 130 pounds of potatoes a year eaten by the average American, and almost 17 pounds of these are in the form of french fries. The same french fries that topped the list of foods we just discussed that are most contaminated with acrylamide.

Sunfresh of Florida Marketing, a cooperative of farming families who have grown potatoes for many generations, have purchased the exclusive rights from Netherlands-based seed potato company HZPC to market SunLite™ all-natural low-carb potatoes. Members of the group originally approached Dr. Chad Hutchinson, program leader at the University of Florida's Institute of Food and Agricultural Sciences Research farm in Hastings, Florida, to help them find a healthier and more flavorful potato. According to the co-op, "Hutchinson and his team screen about 400 new varieties of potatoes a year for taste, shape, color, and skin quality." After further testing, they discovered that one SunLite potato contained 25 percent less calories than a Russet (87 versus 117), and 30 percent less carbohydrates (18 grams versus 27 grams) for one potato. You can order from the company's Web site at www.sunfreshofflorida.com.

Another exciting development for potato lovers may soon become commercially available. It's already getting the attention of large food makers such as Frito Lay™. Agriculture Research Services geneticist Charles R. Brown has worked for the past several years on cross-breeding a new kind of potato with an antioxidant value that rivals the Oxygen Radical Absorbance Capacity (ORAC) score of kale and brussels sprouts! According to Kathryn Barry Stelljes, staff writer for ARS Information Services: "Brown has developed orange-fleshed potatoes with up to four times the antioxidants zeaxanthin and lutein as white potatoes … Some of his experimental breeding lines may be ready for commercial testing once enough seed is available." Only time will tell if Brown can succeed in also lowering the amount of carbohydrates in this new cross-bred potato.

WHAT TO ADD SO THEY'RE NOT SO BAD

While most processed flours and breads made from them are rapidly converted to glucose, it *is* possible to eat bread that's less harmful if you must. And a particular bread that's actually healthful.

Sourdough bread is a good alternative. The high-acid content of this bread gives it a tolerable GL. The fiber slows the uptake even further. Consider topping it with EVOO or organic butter; which improves the flavor *and slows down* the transformation of the bread into blood sugar. You can even reduce the rate that sugar in alcoholic beverages is absorbed. Just add a twist of lemon or lime, or eat cheese, nuts or other protein foods. Eat nuts between sips. ***This helps reduce the rate of absorption of the alcohol in your blood.*** Of course, the drier your vino, the less carbs it contains. Red wine is better for you than white. Stay away from beer; its maltose sugar is the worst of the worst.

Want other good reasons to combine foods properly when we eat? Adding certain acidic ingredients to beans after they're thoroughly cooked, like tomatoes and vinegar, prevents beans from becoming tough. The acid reacts with the starch in the beans, preventing them from swelling. These same acids further slow the breakdown of all carbohydrates. Enjoying healthy fats and protein, as well as acidic foods with any carbohydrate, slows down its entry in your bloodstream. Another healthy topping you may wish to consider is organic cottage cheese. But toppings aren't the only way to slow down this stuff. Just combining them at mealtime with the right foods does the job.

If you don't like sourdough, try 100 percent whole-grain breads made from real whole wheat flour, low in carbohydrates (though you won't avoid the acrylamide—unless you buy stone ground). Carol Ness, staff writer for the *San Francisco Chronicle* (February, 2004) in her article "Taster's Choice: Among lower-carb breads, one brand stands alone" ranked the Oroweat™ brand on top. If you wish to order, go to their Web site at http://www.oroweat.com. We've tried it and see why.

Certain varieties of bread, such as wheat, can be just as worthless and damaging as white bread. "Wheat" bread is *not* the same as whole-wheat bread. It's a marketing ploy. Wheat bread is made from wheat flour, like white bread and most other breads. It just hasn't been chlorinated white.

Whole-wheat bread is made from whole-wheat flour, flour containing the entire wheat kernel. True whole-wheat bread is a nutritional titan compared to wheat bread, which is not. Next time you're faced with the choice of eating white or wheat, you'll know it's the lesser of two evils. At least wheat bread isn't chlorinated white. Ask if it's *whole*-wheat bread when dining out. If the answer is yes, ask if it's *100 percent* whole-wheat. Unless the package clearly states its *100 percent whole-wheat,* food processors can put any amount in it that they wish to. Occasionally, they get caught. The FDA has been known to call makers on the carpet, audit them, and fine them if evidence suggests they were making false claims.

I'm never embarrassed to ask a waiter or waitress to check something out in the kitchen. I learn a great deal. More often than not, the servers do as well.

Remember, breads and pastas are man-made foods. Sourdough won't spike your insulin the way other commercially available breads do. Some varieties of sourdough have GL numbers as low as 6. Topping them with the right protein or fat can lower that number. But there's another bread that is actually *healthful,* which we'll discuss shortly. So healthy, that it's best reserved for our discussion on fiber that follows. We've even introduced healthy pasta!

CARBOHYDRATES: THE FIBER FAMILY

You've learned a good deal about simple sugars and starchy carbohydrates. Now let's examine generally healthier high-fiber carbohydrates. As you may know, there are two types of fiber: soluble and insoluble. *Soluble fiber dissolves in water. Insoluble fiber does not.* Neither is digestible. Great soluble sources of fibrous carbohydrates include organic steel-cut oatmeal; you'll taste the difference. It's usually available in the bulk food section at Whole Foods® Market. My favorite is McCann's Irish Oatmeal. David Mendosa, one of the most knowledgeable and passionate advocates for low-carbohydrate foods (www.Mendosa.com; Living with Diabetes), couldn't agree more. In an article entitled "My Favorite Low Carb and Low GI Foods" (www.mendosa.com/low_carb), Mendosa highly endorses the wonderful flavor and value of McCann's. He also sites another McCann steel-cut oatmeal devotee ... Marrion Burro proclaimed McCann's to be the best of the best, after evaluating oatmeal producers for The *New York Times* (January 5, 2005). *Rolled oats,* in contrast to steel-cut oats, are simply whole oats that are *flattened* out. According to McCann's, rolled oats are steamed first, then rolled, then steamed again, and then toasted. Far more processed than steel-cut oats, flattened rolled oats have a thinner surface area that breaks down more rapidly into blood sugar. In contrast, *steel-cut oats are only cut,* and only in two or three pieces. They're denser, more nutritious, and high in fiber. According to McCann's, one cup has *twice* as much fiber than Cream of Wheat™. You can taste the difference that gentle, minimal processing makes.

Organic oats, oat bran, and other whole grains such as rye and barley are also healthful. As Mendosa reminds us, *barley* is the lowest glycemic grain, even lower than oatmeal. His favorite barley-based cereal is Whole Control's™ Golden Barley Cereal. You can order from their Web site listed along with all resources in this book. I buy their 40-ounce bag. Most breakfast cereals that aren't made from whole-grain nutrients should be avoided, including those that boast a high content of fiber, if they're *fortified* with vitamins and preservatives.

IT'S IMPORTANT THAT WE TRY TO EDUCATE OUR KIDS TO MAKE SMART FOOD CHOICES.

Some will continue to throw caution to the wind. TV evangelists and food marketeers prompt us to forget what we already know. Cereal companies, who spend almost a billion dollars annually marketing to children, can be formidable adversaries. It's important that we try to educate our kids to make smart food choices. It takes real courage to walk this talk.

For a high-fiber, low-carbohydrate, great-tasting bread, try Food for Life's® Baking Company's Ezekiel 4: Sprouted Grain bread. One slice contains 15 grams of carbohydrates, but 3 of these grams are fiber. So, you're left with only 12 carbohydrates from a blood sugar perspective, per slice. The company's products are alive, freshly sprouted whole organic grains that include sprouted wheat, organic sprouted barley, organic sprouted millet, malted barley, organic sprouted lentils, organic sprouted soybeans, organic sprouted spelt, filtered water, fresh yeast, and sea salt. They make a low-glycemic sprouted pasta, too. You either love it or you don't. I don't. Mendoza is also a fan of Trader Joe's® Low Carbohydrate Pecan Spice Bread, with only 6 grams of available carbohydrates per slice (actually 8 grams of carbohydrates, of which 2 grams are fiber).

But none of these breads were what I considered to be truly healthful. Fed up in my quest to find a bread that was loaded with value, I created my own. I found nothing on the market that accomplished what I sought. In my quest to find the healthiest bread, I tasted many that were gluten-free. Most tasted like a sole on a pair of old gym shoes. So I set out to do something about it. To my knowledge, it's among the healthiest available.

It was initially inspired by Bruce Fife's excellent cookbook, *Cooking with Coconut Flour* (Piccadilly Books, 2005). The book had a basic recipe for coconut bread that started me on my journey. Now, I eat my low carb bread teaming with fiber that fills me with health and vitality. Bread that's actually *good* for me to eat, great tasting, loaded with nutrients and gluten free.

Few people are truly allergic to wheat. For those that are, it's a serious food allergy. But celiac disease, also known as gluten-sensitive enteropathy, presents far greater risk for those that suffer. Unlike a food allergy to wheat, celiac disease is a lifelong autoimmune intestinal disorder. An adverse reaction occurs in those genetically predisposed to this condition when they eat gluten. Gluten is a *protein* found in all forms of wheat and the portion of wheat that gives bread that sticky feeling. Bakers rely on it to hold bread together. It's produced by the baking process whenever yeast is used to leaven dough, which causes sugar to ferment. That process itself creates carbon dioxide. ***The gas that is trapped by gluten causes the dough to rise.*** It's created by the buildup of trapped CO_2 from the yeast. Typically, the fluffier a baked food, the larger the amount of gluten. So, the amount in a cake would topple the amount in a bagel. Its presence in cereals, breads, and other products (including certain lipsticks, toothpastes, stamps, envelopes, and even children's stickers) makes them hazardous to those genetically vulnerable. Eating gluten triggers a chain reaction in those individuals, prompting the body's immune system to begin to attack normal tissue. This is particularly true in the lining of the small intestine. There, it destroys finger-like projections called "villa," whose job is to expand the total cellular surface area; an area required to be large enough for the proper absorption of nutrients. The ensuing malabsorption often leads to a wide range of other disorders, including osteoporosis and deficiencies such as iron. This affects approximately 1 in every 250 people, and often goes undetected (so the incidence is likely far greater). But most of those adversely affected by wheat have wheat or gluten *intolerance*. A smaller amount are allergic to wheat, while others have celiac disease. It's important to understand the differences in these conditions.

Unlike other breads, very few people are allergic to coconut flour, one of the amazingly healthful ingredients in our Informed Living™ Coconut Bread. It's wheat free, gluten free, and *organic*. It's loaded with fiber and lower in carbohydrate, with more non-digestible carbohydrate and less digestible carbohydrate than any other bread we've discovered. Though coconut oil is a saturated fat, it's a rare medium-chain triglyceride that's uniquely processed by your body. It's a fat that's burned, almost upon entry, as energy. As Fife points out, it's not stored as fat in your cells the way other fats are. With 61 percent of its content coming from calorie-free fiber (versus a measly 27 percent for wheat bran, and only 8 percent in buckwheat flour), its unusually high percentage of non-digestible carbohydrate trumps the comparatively small amount found in other flours. This fiber passes through the body undigested, gradually breaking down into glucose. It also absorbs a great deal of water, helping slow the emptying of your stomach. We feel fuller longer and desire to eat less. Fife cites several studies that show that populations relying heavily on coconut as a food source don't struggle with weight loss or obesity. They also have far lower rates of heart disease and other illness.

David Mendosa also suggests a high-fiber, low-carbohydrate alternative to what we know as bread: La Tortilla Factory's whole-wheat, low-carbohydrate, high-fiber tortillas (www.latortillafactory.com), each with only 3 grams of available carbohydrate (12 grams, but 9 are fiber). Replacing high-carbohydrate foods with healthy and great tasting low-carbohydrate alternatives is easier than you think; and an important step toward balancing your insulin and blood sugar. Chose Just Like Sugar® rather than sugar or sugar substitutes (diabetics, take note). All natural, it's loaded with fiber and natural pre and probiotics (approximate 50 pounds equals one calorie). Replace that white pasta with our Informed Living 100 percent hard durum wheat semolina pasta, infused with EVOO, fresh herbs and spices (www.RKInformedLiving.com).

In addition to steel-cut oats and other whole grains, soluble fiber is found in the legume family in foods like lentils and beans. Peas can be eaten as well, but you might want to dip them in EVOO. They're a high-glycemic food that's best to avoid unless you properly *top* them. Blueberries and apples are an *excellent* source of this important fiber. Apples have gotten a bad rap because they have a GI of 38, but one medium-size apple has a GL of only 5. Moderate consumption has almost no effect on your blood sugar. Eat them with their skin on and really harness the power of this amazing fruit. But the next time you pour yourself a glass of apple or any other juice, do the math. It takes a good deal of fruit to produce it. Since most juice is void of fiber, you're far better off eating the fruit itself. You'll feel fuller from the fiber, and get far less calories from sugar. But only eat moderate amounts of the right fruit in moderation, for the reasons we've previously discussed.

While strawberries are also a good source of soluble fiber, blueberries and black-berries may be better choices. Strawberries are one of the most heavily laden fruits grown with pesticides, so only purchase fruit whose package states that they are pesticides-free. Pears are another great source of soluble fiber and contain only 26 grams of carbohydrates. Eating a single pear provides you with 24 percent of the dietary fiber you need daily, and a whopping 41 percent of that fiber is pectin!

When it comes to soluble fiber, my top recommendations are psyllium seed husk, nuts, seeds, steel-cut oats/oatmeal, lentils, blueberries, apples, and broccoli. Psyllium husk is part of my regimen, but only in moderation when the need arises. Use 1 tablespoon to top a full 8-ounce glass of water with lemon just before bedtime. Never eat psyllium on an empty stomach, and don't start with even this small amount. Begin with less, gradually building up your intake over time. While psyllium may cause uncomfortable bloat, eating reasonable amounts periodically is one of the best ways to keep "regular." And it's great for those that travel. Moderate consumption provides added protection against heart disease and irritable bowel syndrome. *Excessive* use of this or any fiber can rob you of essential friendly bacteria. It's important to replace them with a good probiotic containing acidophilus. Intemperate consumption can also hinder the absorption of important nutrients, such as iron.

While there are many sources of *insoluble* fiber, my top recommendations include wheat bran, cauliflower, bulgur, couscous, sesame seeds, and the other seeds we'll discuss in this chapter. Cooked tomatoes (cooking allows absorption of lycopene, the now infamous anti-carcinogenic), barley, carrots, and zucchini top the list. Others sources (though not on our top foods chart) include cucumbers, whole-grain breakfast cereals, and *100 percent* whole-wheat breads (made from stone ground flour). And of course coconut bread. Coconuts are a wonderful source of important insoluble fiber, and a host of other important nutrients.

Whether soluble or insoluble, *all fiber* is simply non-digestible polysaccharide—that portion of a carbohydrate that can't be broken down. **Bacteria lack the enzymes necessary to do so.** From a caloric point of view, fiber is *empty*. You can't get calories from the portion of foods that can't be broken down. A calorie is a measure of burned energy and there is none from fiber itself, which escapes digestion.

> ... ALL FIBER IS SIMPLY NON-DIGESTIBLE POLYSACCHARIDE— THAT PORTION OF A CARBOHYDRATE THAT CAN'T BE BROKEN DOWN.

Why would we eat a food with no caloric value? Well, the food carrying the fiber typically does have calories that provide us with a useful source of energy. The indigestible *portion* of that food containing the fiber itself does not. An intake of 25 to 30 grams of fiber per day for an adult is an important step toward optimizing your health. One important study by the *New England Journal of*

Medicine (2000 May 11;342(19):1392–8) showed that subjects with type 2 diabetes showed marked improvement in their blood sugar levels when they did just that. Other studies have shown far lower rates of colorectal cancer. Despite its significance in our lives, the average adult intake is less than half that amount, or a mere 12 grams a day. Noted authorities, such as the National Academy of Sciences' Institute of Medicine, believe it's even worse. Their studies reveal that the average American is getting only 5 to 7 grams of fiber daily. Our children appear to be getting even less. ***By the time they reach the age of 9*** (children ages 2 to 3 appear to do better, due to diets typically rich in apple sauce and other high fiber foods), ***they are at considerable risk for heart disease and type 2 diabetes.***

Now that you've learned about the three types of carbohydrates—sugars, starches, and fiber—let's understand the important characteristics of specific foods themselves. We'll identify those with the greatest value that will help reverse the adverse effects of those with the least.

But before we can properly evaluate each of these foods, we need to understand a number of important factors to make an informed choice. We have to qualify each food before we can make an informed choice. First we'll review a few of the tests that are available to measure them. We'll look at their power as well as their limitations. An understanding of other criteria, like the distance our food travels, the case for the local farmer, the importance of eating organically, and other key issues, will guide us in the ultimate selection of our foods.

EVALUATING FOOD: GLYCEMIC INDEX AND GLYCEMIC LOAD

All carbohydrates are converted into blood sugar when we eat them, not just the simple ones. The time it takes them to do so is an important consideration in our evaluation of a food—a factor we need to understand to assist us in regulating our blood sugar. In general, those carbohydrates containing the largest amount of fiber require a longer period of time to be digested than those containing the least. The GI (Glycemic Index) measures the time it takes to break down a food's carbohydrate and convert it to blood sugar. Several good foods, such as carrots and watermelon, have relatively high GI scores. A GI of 70 or more is high, 56 to 69 is medium, and 55 or less is low.

But measuring how fast these foods are broken down and enter our bloodstream is not the same thing as measuring the amount of glucose found in a normal serving size. For example, while a given food may contain carbohydrates that can be broken down to glucose quickly, it may contain a relatively small amount of glucose. Although the food may spike your blood sugar, that surge may not last very long. So, the amount of insulin required to usher it out of your bloodstream and into your fat cells may be miniscule. Carrots and watermelon are examples of this.

Keep in mind that GI levels for all foods are based on eating a portion of exactly 50 grams of carbohydrate. One carrot weighs approximately 75 grams, with only 6 grams coming from carbohydrate. You would need to eat 8 to 9 medium-sized carrots, or 1.3 pounds (highly unrealistic) to obtain the amount required for a GI ranking. Although they have a high GI (131), their Glycemic Load, or GL, is quite low (10). Given its high GI ranking, you may have heard that it's best to avoid them. Yet, as we can see, basing that decision on the GI level would be short-sighted. Since only a small percentage of their weight takes the form of carbohydrate, their important nutrient value makes them a healthy option. That's why the Glycemic *Load* is based on *typical serving sizes* in our diet. A GL of 20 or more is high, a GL of 11 to 19 inclusive is medium, and a GL of 10 or less is low.

By the same token, a low ranking on the GL index doesn't necessarily mean that a food is healthy. For example, the fat found in certain desserts can allow them to enter your bloodstream *slowly*. Recall that fat slows the absorption of carbohydrates, but that doesn't mean that these sugary foods are good for you. *Combining* foods groups can greatly alter their GL ranking. As you've already learned, fats, acids, and protein, eaten in conjunction with a high GL food can collectively slow their absorption. That's why sourdough bread is your best bread choice for blood sugar moderation when dining out, unless you're certain your whole-grain bread is 100 percent whole grain. It's not that sourdough bread is a healthy food. It's just not as *unhealthy* as other breads. On the other hand, coconut bread, absent from most menus, is the healthiest option.

The manner in which some foods are processed can also make a difference in the rate they enter your bloodstream. Foods stripped of their fiber, like instant oatmeal, designed to cook quickly, are just as rapidly absorbed as other high GL foods. However, the same food eaten in its more natural state, like steel-cut oatmeal, retains its fiber. It's a good low GL food.

If all this sounds complicated, please know that it's not. While both the GI and GL are good tools to assist you in making a sound determination of whether to include a particular food in your diet, they don't tell the whole story. Because different foods, such as rice, can have significantly different GIs based on the different varieties and the manner in which they are processed or prepared. A 50-gram serving of sticky rice found in most Chinese restaurants can have a GL of almost 100; but parboiled long grain converted rice made on your stovetop contains a measly 44.

The amount of amylase enzymes in the starch has a great deal to do with how easily it's digested. The higher the amylase, the more difficult it is to break it down. This makes those starchy foods with a higher degree of amylase a healthier choice, from a GI perspective. Amylase is one of two components of starch. Most starch consists of about 20 percent amylase; while the other 80 percent consists of amylopectin. White rice spikes your insulin and breaks down faster than other rice because it contains a higher percentage of amylopectin than amylase. So, while both the GI and GL have great value in helping us select the right foods, there are other important considerations: how the food was grown (remember, you are what you eat-*ate*), prepared (less is generally best), combined (with a small amount of healthy fat and protein), and stored.

EVALUATING FOOD: THE ORAC AND TAC SCORES

In 1992, Dr. Guohua Cao of the National Institute of Aging developed the first test to measure the Oxygen Radical Absorption Capacity of Food. Three years later he joined the Jean Mayer USDA Human Nutrition Research Center on Aging and teamed up with Dr. Ronald Prior and succeeded in partially automating the original test. The test measures the ability of a given food's antioxidants to minimize free radical damage. In 1997, a private corporation named Brunswick Laboratories, working in conjunction with Prior, developed and patented an improved means of measuring the capacity of antioxidants to fight free radicals. According to Brunswick Laboratories, the original research was performed using an aqueous buffer solution, so only water-soluble antioxidant activity could be measured. Fat-soluble antioxidant activity was simply not tested. So foods high in *fat-soluble* antioxidants never received the important credit they deserved.

As more information and larger databases became available, scientists were able to develop still another rating, based on more detailed considerations, using better probes. This permitted researchers to measure activity of antioxidants in lipids as well.

In 2004, the results of an important study conducted by Wu and colleagues refined the ORAC scoring method (*Journal of Agriculture and Food Chemistry*,

2004, pp. 4026–4037). They created an entirely new technique that substantially improved the value of the original design. After carefully analyzing over 100 foods for their hydrophilic (water-based H-Orac), and lipophilic (fat, L-Orac), and TP (total phenolic) capacity researchers, a TAC score (Total Antioxidant Capacity—TAC) measured its total antioxidant activity, not just its ability to punish free radicals. It is an important method of comparing the ability of a given food to absorb free radical activity *and* guard against damage on a cellular level. The total antioxidant action of lipid-based sources scored far higher in the revised ORAC than those measured from water-based sources alone. In simpler terms, the higher the ORAC value, the lower the level of oxidative stress.

According to the company, ORAC scores are now being touted by many food makers like bragging rights; with hopes of convincing the public that their food is healthier than another food based on its higher score. Before we can make an informed choice, there are a number of other factors that must be considered. While there *is* merit to the test, which will be used as one of our evaluation criteria, there are also some serious shortcomings in the way some have chosen to interpret them. It's important to understand both the value and shortcomings of this tool.

First, having a good deal of power to defeat free radicals doesn't necessarily make one food a better choice than another. For example, a food with a high score may be nutrient dense in one antioxidant, while a food with a lower score may have a better dispersion of many nutrients that collectively provide us with far more value as a food. The test also doesn't measure a food's ability to defeat *all* free radicals—only peroxyl and hydroxyl radicals, according to the company. That means a food with a high ORAC score may defeat some free radicals and not others.

In addition, the scores are often based on unrealistic serving sizes. Comparing the activity in one whole cup of blueberries (the average serving size that *few of us* would eat in one sitting) to the activity in one black plum (an average serving size that *many of us* would easily eat in one sitting) is unfair and misleading if not properly understood. ***Foods are also scored without regard to their water weight.*** That means you might compare a score of one water-dense food to another that's dried. You're comparing the activity found in a great deal of dried food without water, to a much smaller amount of wet food.

Brunswick discourages makers from using ORAC as a means to compare their foods to rivals. But many disregard these warnings, instead marketing their scores against other foods with lesser ones on their packaging. A number of dried food makers (providing everything from gogi and noni, to raisins), invite such a comparison. Raisins, for example, have no more health value than grapes. After all, they began life as a grape. But if ORAC values are compared based on wet weight per gram, raisins would shine given the absence of water in a raisin. It also takes far more dried raisins to fill up a one-cup serving size than it does to fill it with grapes. Of course, a cup of raisins is more nutritionally dense and contains more antioxidants than a cup of wet grapes. It took an army of raisins to fill the same cup requiring a lower number of grapes. Does this mean that raisins are more healthful than grapes? If you looked at their ORAC value, one would think so. But in reality, despite its ORAC score, the opposite is true. All dried fruits, such as raisins and prunes, have no vitamin C, according to the Food Standards Agency, while their water-laden younger selves do. They also have none of the important vitamin D, and contain a lot more sugar "per serving size" than their formerly hydrated selves.

Given the significant reduction in their water content, the dried version of the fruit is far more calorie dense than its natural plumped up predecessor. And makers that play that game need to let consumers know it works both ways. That cup of raisins is also loaded with calories (more than 400!) compared to that same one cup of grapes (with approximately 60 calories per serving).

And pay particular attention to the manufacturer's stated average serving size. They may be as ridiculously low as some ORAC's are high. Still, other makers use weight to indicate their average serving size. Be aware of food companies that tout high ORAC values based on weight, rather than realistic serving sizes. Don't buy into claims based on bent information designed to boost the legitimacy of manufactured or processed foods.

To get a better handle on the value of a given food, I decided to measure their reported activity based on more realistic serving sizes. I call this TRAC (Total Realistic Antioxidant Capacity) in order to permit realistic scoring for the purposes of our discussion. Certain TRAC scores were not based on serving sizes as listed on the USDA Database for Standard Reference[9] as the TAC scores were. While most serving sizes found in the database are pretty realistic, several are not, which can make quite a difference in their scoring. So, I added my own.

In the future, I hope that our government will require manufacturers to not only list realistic serving sizes, but also to determine them on the basis of other important factors such as age, weight, height, amount of physical activity, ethnicity, nationality, genetics, and other variables.

Another weakness with ORAC scores is that they only show antioxidant activity and free radical absorbance capacity (in vivo) *outside* our bodies. Inside of us it's entirely possible that a food with a high ORAC score may have little or no value at all. That activity and capacity, and our ability to absorb this value, may be limited. The food may still be of value, but in this case, not because of a high ORAC score. Even if a nutrient was shown to be bio-available, it doesn't mean it's useful. Your body only uses what it needs to meet its requirements. Water-soluble vitamins such as vitamin C, taken in excess of what we require, aren't retained; instead, they're eliminated. An unrealistic serving size can provide a distorted view of a given food's true radical scavenging ability. The TRAC puts that in perspective.

In the case of berries, that's one third of a cup, rather than an entire cup. Even that will vary based on the serving size that's right for you. The TRAC score for one cup of cultivated blueberries is a whopping 9019, and one cup of whole cranberries is 8983, while one black plum is 4844. While all three foods have extraordinary power potential regardless of their TRAC or TAC score, their TAC ranking suggests that a single serving of either one of these berries trumps that of a black plum.

But when viewed in light of its TRAC score, the reverse is true. The black plum's TRAC of 4844 (based on a serving size of one black plum) is actually much higher than the 3006 TRAC score of blueberries (based on approximately one- third of a cup, or one-third the TACS 9019) and the TRAC score of cranberries of 2994 (approximately one-third of its TACS 8983). *The plum's TRAC is almost 40 percent greater than the cultivated berry.*

As we'll soon see, the method of growing a given food is another important factor in our understanding its potential as an antioxidant. Let's look at another example of how misleading it can be, to use one measure alone, to select our food.

If the TRAC score of cranberries is 2994 (almost equal to the 3006 TRAC score of blueberries) does that mean that one, from an antioxidant perspective, is as healthful to eat as the other? Not necessarily. Few of us would eat one third of a cup

... THE METHOD OF GROWING A GIVEN FOOD IS ANOTHER IMPORTANT FACTOR IN OUR UNDERSTANDING ITS POTENTIAL AS AN ANTIOXIDANT.

of cranberries that weren't already *pre-sweetened*. But no sugar is added to blue-berries. And while plums may be a better choice than both, they rank 18th of 42 foods tested by the Environmental Working Group for contamination from pesticides (the lower the ranking the worse). So, whether it's a TAC score or a TRAC score, use it wisely (certainly not as a definitive indicator of the value of a given food). It's only one of several important criteria that may be useful in evaluating a food.

And there's another consideration worth noting ...

While the total free radical activity of carbohydrates is important, the *type* of free radical protection they provide may be even more important. For example, while avocados didn't distinguish themselves on the original ORAC scores, their lipophilic antioxidant score (one of the components in calculating their total antioxidant capacity) was off the chart in the follow-up study. While their TAC score was high and respectable, avocados delivered *several hundred times* the amount of antioxidants from important monounsaturated fat than nearly every other fruit tested (and 250 percent more the raspberry, which ranked second).

The more cultivated or processed a food is in general, the lower its nutritional content. However, some vegetables, such as tomatoes, had a far *lower* antioxidant capacity served raw than when lightly cooked. It appears that antioxidant activity is far higher when tomato cell membranes are broken down by heat.

Seasonality, time of harvest, distance traveled, cooking, and storage methods are among other important influences that need to be considered when evaluating the potential of food. And while we often don't have access to all this information, we can make better decisions in general by being well informed.

The list of foods that has been suggested in this book are those that have proven themselves in other ways, beyond a whopping ORAC score. Collectively, this information provides the means to identify those foods capable of making the greatest contribution to our health. But identifying wonderful foods isn't enough. If eating *whole foods* has superior health benefit when compared to eating isolated nutrients, than eating whole foods alone also falls short of the mark. *In other words, a thoughtful meal, rather than a single food, is the key to good health.*

The medley and power of the right Super-Nutrients, *eaten collectively,* is powerful; more powerful than a single food, and the very foundation of our Synergy of Super-Nutrient Program.

EVALUATING FOOD: THE CASE FOR BUYING LOCAL—SUPPORT THE AMERICAN FARMER

There has never been a better time to go back to our traditional means of raising and purchasing food. At the time of this writing, food prices are skyrocketing (thanks to the rising costs of transporting them). The price for corn today, an important part of animal feed and ingredients affecting a broad array of foods, continues to spiral upward. And its scarcity, due to the ethanol craze, further exacerbates the problem.

The manner in which our food is grown and purchased is a key factor in determining their value in our selection process. Remember, we are what we eat-*ate*. There's good reason to buy fruits and vegetables that are grown as closely to home as possible. *Sadly, the average fruit or vegetable travels some 1,500 miles from the farm where they were grown, to the shelf at your local grocer.* According to a study from Iowa State University's Leopold Center for Sustained Agriculture ("How far do your fruit and vegetables travel?" *Leopold Letter,* Vol. 14, No. 1. Spring, 2002), broccoli travels an average of 1,836 miles from the farm to your dinner table. Hard to believe, given the fact that, for most Americans, broccoli is grown only twenty miles away from our homes. A green bean can be grown about 40 feet away from your dinner table. But the average American buys beans at their local grocery store that has traveled 1,700 miles to get there. Other locally grown fruits and vegetables travel similar distances. If the average American only drove ten to fifteen miles to a farmer's market, the positive impact on our environment and our economy would be startling. Even mail-order purchases made from growers based closer to home would markedly improve our lives.

Our consumption of fossil fuel has also gone through the roof in the past few decades. In 1997, in the United States alone there were 1,797,000 registered combination trucks that used 20,294 billion gallons of fuel. By 2006, 49.8 billion gallons of fuel were consumed annually by commercial trucks, more than double the consumption less than a decade earlier. According to the Air Transport Association, approximately 30 percent is gasoline and 70 percent, or 35 billion gallons, is diesel fuel. Every gallon of gasoline produces almost 20 pounds of CO_2 emissions; and more than 22 pounds of CO_2 is produced for every gallon of diesel fuel we burn. At our present level of consumption, that amounts to 770 billion pounds of CO_2 annually.

A staggering amount of other pollutants are generated to produce these fuels. According to the U.S. Environmental Protection Agency, the most important of the greenhouse gases released through fuel burning and other human activities are CO_2, methane, nitrous oxide, hydrofluorocarbons, per-fluorocarbons, and sulfur hexafluoride. Of these, CO_2 is by far the largest component of gas released by diesel fuel trucks, comprising over 99 percent of the emissions by weight.

There are over forty other known toxins in diesel exhaust, including cancer-causing arsenic, formaldehyde, nickel, benzene, acetaldehyde, polycyclic aromatic hydrocarbons, and butadienes. The sulfur dioxide emitted is the primary component found in acid rain, and the release of nitrogen oxide contributes to ozone depletion. Other absorbable compounds include sulfate, metals, and nitrates. According to the EPA, "Fine particles in the air are a serious public health problem. They pose a significant health risk because they can pass through the nose and throat and lodge themselves in the lungs. These fine particles can cause lung damage and premature death. They can also aggravate respiratory conditions such as asthma and bronchitis."

In addition to the obvious health risk, the economic impact is pretty dramatic. A one-penny increase in the price of diesel fuel costs the trucking industry an additional $350 million dollars annually according to the American Trucking Association (ATA). At the present time, wars are being waged, due in large part to our dependence on foreign reserves of fossil fuel.

In 1998, the United States signed and agreed to the terms of the Kyoto Global Warming Accord. The treaty called on the world's largest industrialized nations to collectively reduce greenhouse gases by 5.2 percent from the levels of accumulated gases emitted in the decade before. This meant that the United States, the world's single largest offender, was required to reduce its level of greenhouse gas emissions by 7 percent. For the treaty to be in effect, it had to be ratified by the industrialized nations responsible for 55 percent of these emissions. But only three years after signing this important agreement, the Bush Administration announced that they opposed the Kyoto Accord on the grounds that it put an unfair burden on our nation's economy. One hundred and forty countries ratified the agreement—but the U.S. refused to do so.

An unfair burden? Can eating locally grown produce closer to home, and utilizing biofuel and other alternative sources of energy, be as painful as death, disease, war and the eventual (potential) destruction of our planet? Eating foods grown in closer proximity to where you live would go a long way toward reversing the most destructive eco-trend in the history of mankind.

You can help save the planet by buying locally, and be around longer to enjoy it. That's how important it is to select the most efficient fuel to power your journey. The right sources of energy will increase the number and quality of each stage of our trajectory.

EATING FOODS GROWN IN CLOSER PROXIMITY TO WHERE YOU LIVE WOULD GO A LONG WAY TOWARD REVERSING THE MOST DESTRUCTIVE ECO-TREND IN THE HISTORY OF MANKIND.

Today's food system is inefficient. It wastes valuable resources, adds toxic pollutants that endanger our lives, and requires hazardous fuel emissions that threaten the survival of our planet. It's also taken what little profit was left out of family farming.

The following is an excerpt from the book *Hungry for Profit* (Monthly Review Press, 2000) that puts this plight into historical perspective: "The farmer's share of the food dollar (after paying for input costs) has steadily declined from about 40 percent in 1910 to less than 10 percent in 1990. The enormous power exerted by the largest agribusiness/food corporations allows them essentially to control the cost of their raw materials purchased from farmers, while at the same time, keeping prices of food to the general public at high enough levels to ensure large profits. It is no accident that the food industry is the second most profitable one in the United States, following pharmaceuticals ... In the extreme situation, such as poultry growers under contract to Tyson or Purdue, or hog producers under contract to Murphy Family Farms, independent farmers are reduced to the position of laborers, but without the rights of workers to collectively bargain." Even a free-market economy needs to be socially responsible—and that responsibility belongs to us.

All too often we opt for convenience over conventional wisdom. It's important that we understand the enormous global consequences of our simple behaviors. Doing so may allow us to take greater responsibility for ourselves and the world we live in. While many foods may not be available locally, others are, and still others can be purchased closer to home. While farmers' markets may not be conveniently available, we can request that our local grocer stock more locally-available produce.

If farmers have no incentive to produce, their children will find a different way to make a living. This means still less control and a continuation of the trend toward the diminishing integrity of our food supply. Big businesses' message to our farmers is clear—grow bigger, and do so faster, or vanish. Work for less, and yield more. This is the same fate that's befallen our health care system. Doctors must sign on with large PPOs to survive. They must turn more patients in less time or lose their affiliation with insurers.

Basic health care and our food supply have been compromised for profit. We need to give incentives to our farmers and our family physicians to think small. Paying both groups more money to keep us healthy is ultimately cheaper than paying the irresponsible hands that currently feed them. Keeping us from breaking is far less expensive than fixing us. Paying doctors each month for keeping us well would significantly improve our health care system. It also adds years to our lives, which puts money in our pockets. Supporting our local farmers would do so as well. Returning to a system where integrity is rewarded would be a good step in the right direction. A system is needed where those with the knowledge, training, and experience to do their jobs are fairly compensated for doing so, and where responsibility goes hand-in-hand with accountability. The *quality* of the goods and services provided should take precedent over the quantity. It's time the provider, not the marketer, keeps a bigger piece of the profit for getting it right.

RELYING ON ETHANOL HAS ONLY SERVED TO INCREASE CORN PRICES IN THE LAST TWELVE MONTHS, WHICH HAS IN TURN INCREASED THE COST OF THE GRAIN WE FEED OUR CATTLE, AND ALL CORN-RELATED PRODUCTS.

While subsidizing farmers and legislating artificial demand sounds good on the surface, I believe it's misguided, ultimately destroying the livelihood and way of life of those it's designed to protect. These policies are often little more than large bones thrown to constituents by politicians who have no more than their own political interests at heart. Quick fixes are designed to capture the support of powerful lobby groups to win elections, with little concern for the long-term impact on the lives of those most affected. To a poor farmer, such programs may appear to be a blessing. But in the end, they do little more than exacerbate the problem by failing to address the real issues. Relying on ethanol has only served to increase corn prices in the last twelve months, which has in turn increased the cost of the grain we feed our cattle, and all corn-related products. At the same time, the cost of a gallon of gasoline has skyrocketed. The effect of this on the poor in this country, and on those in developing third world nations, is tragic.[10]

Land use formerly reserved for the production of other important crops has shifted to corn. According to the USDA (Agricultural Baseline Projections: U.S. Crops, 2008–2017):

"Strong expansion of corn-based ethanol production in the projections affects virtually every aspect of the field crops sector, ranging from domestic demand and exports to prices and the allocation of acreage among crops ... Soybean planting declined to less than 70 million acres after 2008, reflecting more favorable returns to corn production ... Cotton stocks declined in the first several years of the projections as some acreage shifts to corn." According to the United States Department of Agriculture (*Technology Review*, Published by MIT, February 2007), this year the country is going to use 18 to 20 percent of its total corn crop for the production of ethanol, projected to grow by at least 25 percent a year going forward.

What about the importance of crop rotation? According to a report from Iowa State University Professor and Extension Grain Economist Robert Wisner (*Impacts of Iowa's Rapid Expansion in Corn-based Ethanol Production on Crop Acreage Needs, Grain Prices, Basis Behavior and Distillers Grain Supplies*, Iowa State University, October 2006): "Agronomic research at Iowa State University indicates that when rotations are shifted from a corn/soybean rotation to corn following corn, a yield reduction of 10 to 12 percent should be expected. If so, that might require even more acreage." Government mandates for continued increases in ethanol production, coupled with huge tax credits, will continue to prop up artificial demand for ethanol in the foreseeable future. According to the International Monetary Fund (*Finance and Development*, March 2008), "Ambitious mandates about biofuel use in the United States and the European Union imply that diverting crops toward biofuel production will continue for at least another five years, when new technology in the form of second-generation biofuel feedstocks—made of inedible vegetable matter that does not compete for the land and the water resources used for major food crops—become commercially viable."

In the United States, the 2007 Energy Bill almost quintuples the biofuel's target to 35 billion gallons by 2022, and the European Union has mandated that 10 percent of transportation fuels must use biofuels by 2020. This means that upward pressures on prices of some of the major food crops will continue for some time. Economies are now growing increasingly dependent on this growth, in production and facilities that appear to be spinning out of control.

Is this what our government calls sustainable agriculture? Has it made a dent in our dependence on foreign oil or lowered the price at the pump? Have we been told the truth about ethanol? Several ethanol manufacturing facilities have been found to release volatile organic compounds (VOCs), which include known carcinogens such as acetic acid and formaldehyde. And they're smelling up the towns. While we're told that the use of ethanol reduces tailpipe emissions from our automobiles, we later discover that it *increases* our automobile's output of VOCs into the air. Is this truly in the best interest of the American farmer?

Well, for those farm families needing to feed their children, of course it is. But in the end, it's the kind of policy, like so many that came before it, that manipulates the farmer, ushering in false support that hastens their demise. In the end, synthetic materials that are truly sustainable will take the place of ethanol, leaving some farming families and local governments holding the bag, (until the next round of artificial supports).[11]

If technology is required to meet our growing need for food, why is there more hunger in our world today? According to the United States Department of Agriculture (USDA, Food Assistance and Nutrition Report, 2004) the number of Americans living in households that suffered from food insecurity rose from 33.2 million in 2000 to 36.2 million in 2003, an increase of 9 percent. The number of hungry children in such households rose from 12.9 million to 13.3 million during that time. The number of people who lived in households that directly suffered from hunger rose from 8.5 million in 2000 to 9.6 million in 2003, a 13 percent increase. In this land of plenty and in others, where technology to produce higher priced food for export took priority over basic foods required to sustain local populations, hunger has skyrocketed.

The following is an excerpt from a GreenPeace Study of agricultural practices in Argentina, a country that was convinced ("Record Harvest Record Hunger: Starving in GE Argentina," 2002) that the introduction of genetically engineered products would help feed the world. But the facts support the opposite conclusion: "Argentina has adopted GE crops more enthusiastically than any country other than the United States. Since their introduction in 1996, the area under soya cultivation has more than doubled. But during the same period food insecurity has greatly increased. Half the population—18 million out of 37 million—are now on the bread-line. Set aside exported growth and models of globalization. The reality in Argentina is that hundreds of thousands of children are malnourished or at risk of being. Millions of people go to bed hungry."

According to this research, Argentina was sold a bill of goods: the promise of greater yields through genetically engineered foods. But the only increase in yield was due to deforestation and cannibalization of more acreage out of the hides of small- and medium-sized farms. Farms that formerly produced food at reasonable prices consumed by the local people have all but vanished. In its place stands raped industrialized land depleted of nutrients, and higher priced food for export to those that could afford it. Argentina's bountiful agricultural resources were stolen from the poor to be shipped to the rich.

Expensive pesticides and lack of respect for sustainable agricultural practices, without regard for the local poor, resulted in record exports for the country and record hunger for its people. According to that same study, "In spite of record-breaking harvests nearly half of Argentineans are living in poverty. As of May 2002, 18 million people, almost 50 percent out of a population of approximately 37 million, cannot afford to meet their basic needs."

IN SPITE OF RECORD-BREAKING HARVESTS NEARLY HALF OF ARGENTINEANS ARE LIVING IN POVERTY. AS OF MAY 2002, 18 MILLION PEOPLE, ALMOST 50 PERCENT OUT OF A POPULATION OF APPROXIMATELY 37 MILLION, CANNOT AFFORD TO MEET THEIR BASIC NEEDS.

We fatten, inoculate, radiate, vibrate, and eradicate. The way we treat our livestock reflects our disregard for the world around us and ourselves. The trend today is that things must be done faster and be more conveniently available. However, as you've learned, there are consequences when we do so—consequences we pay for dearly.

There's just never enough time. But if we took the time, in the end we'd have more time. Today, according to Eric Schlosser in his book *Fast Food Nation: The Dark Side of the All-American Meal* (2001), **Americans spend more money on fast food than on higher education.** But now let's journey even closer to home. For the moment, let's put concerns about the environment, economy, society, and morality aside and focus on just *you*. What kind of bang are you really getting for the buck? Nutritionally, most of the foods you buy at the grocery store bear little resemblance to those you can buy closer to home.

Buying closer to home means eating foods which have had far less transit time. Less transit time means that the foods you purchase are allowed to keep producing the nutrients you need *longer*. When a fruit or vegetable is harvested before its time, so it can travel 1,500 miles to reach your dinner table, it lacks the nutrients it would have contained if it were allowed to ripen on the vine. Harvesting before maturity short-circuits its potential to achieve vivid color. Among other things, it will fall far short of its ability to deliver important phytochemicals. And phytochemicals, one of the two groups we've classified as Super-Nutrients, are a significant recently discovered component of healthful eating. More on these shortly ...

While some fruits such as tomatoes can continue to ripen after harvest, Arias and colleagues (*Journal of Agriculture and Food Chemistry*, May, 2000;48(5):1697–702) found that they lost more than 33 percent of their lycopene content when they're prematurely picked. While many growers are genetically modifying food so they can delay ripening, in the case of tomatoes, this further depletes its lycopene. Now truck it 1,500 miles, handle it, and let it sit under a grocery store's light for another week or two; beyond lycopene, significant vitamin and mineral loss occurs.

Many fruits can't ripen after they're picked. These include oranges, tangerines, apples, strawberries, pineapple, cherries, grapes, tangerines, and watermelon. Picking a fruit or vegetable before it ripens means it lacks the level of nutrients contained in its counterparts that were allowed to more fully complete their cycle of life. As Henry Brockman pointed out in his article "Organic Matters" (October, 2001), you can eat certain vegetables until the cows come home, but if enough time has transpired since they were harvested, their nutrient value may be quite shallow. "Leeks, for example, lose over *50 percent* of their total carotene in only three days. A study by Mary Eheart and Dianne Odland showed that even under optimal storage temperatures, green beans lose *60 percent of their vitamin C in the first three days* after harvest and lose another third by the end of the fourth day. By the end of the week, it won't matter if you eat a whole bushel of beans—you'll have to look elsewhere to get your U.S. recommended daily requirement of vitamin C."

Researchers L. A. Howard et al. (*Journal of Food Science, Food Chemistry*, Volume 83, Issue 1, October 2003, Pages 33–41) found that after green beans were refrigerated for 16 days immediately following their harvest, they had lost *90 percent* of their original ascorbic acid content. Broccoli, after only 5 days of refrigeration post harvest, lost about 50 percent of its ascorbic acid. Given an average of 1,500 miles to complete the journey, few of us will be fortunate enough to get store-bought broccoli from the farm to our table in less than two to three weeks. Is it any wonder why nutritional supplements have become a $5 billion dollar industry?

... GREEN BEANS WERE REFRIGERATED FOR 16 DAYS IMMEDIATELY FOLLOWING THEIR HARVEST, THEY HAD LOST 90 PERCENT OF THEIR ORIGINAL ASCORBIC ACID CONTENT.

The USDA's comparative analysis of fruits and vegetable nutrient content as reported in 1950 versus 1999, found that the amount of riboflavin declined almost 38 percent, while ascorbic acid declined 15 percent, and iron, calcium, and phosphorous declined between 9 and 16 percent. Similar studies done in Canada and the UK support the same conclusion. Many of the same foods we are eating today are considerably less nutritious than they were fifty years ago. Now consider the effect of light, handling, transportation, mishandling, cutting, chopping, heating time, cooking method, genetic manipulation, early harvesting, and how long we keep what we purchase in storage. Unless you wish to remain *Misinformed About Food,* you will need to make a concerted effort in today's world to get the nutrition required to truly sustain your life.

Buy your food as locally as possible. If you can't find what you're looking for at your farmers market or local food co-op and don't wish to grow it, order it from a reliable source in closer proximity to your home. Pester your grocer and favorite local restaurant to purchase or serve more locally grown foods. Avoid vegetables and fruits that don't ripen after harvest and appear unripe on the grocer's counter. Eat your vegetables raw or lightly steamed. High heat reduces the value of certain vitamins and minerals in some foods. Avoid purchasing large quantities of fruits and vegetables that will require longer storage than necessary. If you must shop at your supermarket, find out what day of the week the items you want are typically delivered.

A couple of Web sites that will help you in your new quest to eat locally grown are www.localharvest.org and www.foodroutes.org. As you'll see, it's not all that difficult to find good food grown closer to home. The Web site www. farmtoschool.org also explores a very exciting and fairly new initiative, bringing fresh, locally grown produce from the field to the school.

For those of you that feel growing your own herbs and veggies in your own greenhouse is too much work, wait until you see what's on the horizon.

Electrolux's VEGE may be introduced in the not too distant future. It makes "growing your own" more convenient and fashionable than you ever imagined. Roughly the size of a freezer, it's rumored to hold up to 40 plants, giving them just the right amount of light and nutrients.

You can taste the difference. Choose to eat fresh, crisp, textured, locally grown foods brimming with flavor and chock full of important vitamins and minerals. In contrast, voyaged veggies, characterized by bland flavor and sallow color, often lack natural sugar which is quickly converted to starch after harvest. Typically sprayed with chlorine for sanitation, they're regassed with ethylene to promote continued ripening in transit. Many fruits are also waxed, fumigated, disinfected, artificially colored, and overly handled.

Proponents of processed foods would argue that you can't buy coconuts locally. This may be true for most of us. But why do we import the majority of coconuts from the Philippines, when they're grown much closer to home, in Florida and Northern California? Buying "closer to home" means just that—minimizing transportation time, cost, processing, refrigeration, pollutants, global warming, storage, and handling. Choose to maximize your food's nutrients, texture, and flavor—and minimize the impact of our present delivery system on our environment, economy, and our health. By doing so, you'll support your local farmers, putting them in a better position to support you.

EVALUATING FOOD: THE CASE FOR "ORGANICS"

Most of us are willing to pay a reasonable premium to eat wholesome products. But these days the premium we pay to purchase foods organically grown can amount to as much as 50 percent more than the same food manufactured conventionally.

The very word "organic" conjures up thoughts of happy chickens waving good-bye to hen houses, roaming the land for insects, playing poker at night with happy grass-fed cows, all treated with warmth and hospitality by local farmers who just want what's best for us. Hearty vegetables are grown from rich soil laden with organic mulch, ripening to maturity in nature's sunshine and permeating our nostrils with the raw pungent but healthful odor of fresh dung. Wholesome foods, grown by wholesome farmers willing to pull insects out of the ground rather than subjecting us to food tainted with dangerous pesticides. Sure, they have to work a little harder, and understandably, the labor they use to protect us will cost us more.

We show our appreciation by putting our money where our mouths are. By stepping up to the plate and rewarding natural food stores for providing us with organically grown produce. The premium is a small price to pay for supporting their almost spiritual approach to safeguarding our health. But it's time to debunk yet another myth. Big business is rarely sleeping at the switch. This is precisely their kind of story. Organics *are* where the action is. The profit potential is enormous. In this great land of ours, an enterprising bad guy can quickly become a good guy by just buying him out. It's a simple process that often repeats itself.

So if in this business, at first you don't succeed, there are always options. One is to *morph*, by buying one of the well-respected organic guys. The way Dean Foods® bought Stoneybrook Farms. Now, you're invited to return to a time where life was simpler—with county fairs, uncomplicated living, and wholesome food. Just the word "Stonyfield" conjures up thoughts of a lush green pasture nestled in idyllic surroundings—a world so sublime that the cows are free to roam and graze at whatever pace they choose; a land where unadulterated products are churned by the hands of local farmers.

But it's just an illusion. Stonyfield's major thrust of old-world organic farming appears to be a shell of what it was. As Raymond Powers points out in "Sounding Circle the Organic Myth" (October 2006), Stonyfield's "main facility is a state-of-the-art industrial plant just off the airport strip in Londonderry, NH, where it handles milk from other farms." This is a far cry from 1983 when current Chairman, CEO, and early save-the-planet advocate Gary Hirschberg, joined forces with natural foods advocate Samuel Kayman to found Stonyfield Farms.® Kayman's motivation was to sell small amounts of plain full-fat organic yogurt to feed his six kids and educate the world to the importance of supporting the local farmer. What was Hirshberg's motive? I believe it was to find a way to benefit mankind and continue his devotion to the environment and reusable resources. Another one of those "better for you than" beliefs marketed to a public that simply wanted to make the best decisions they could to improve their health.

However, the organic apple did appear to have fallen far from the tree. It isn't that these aren't great men, because they are. It's clear that both did everything they could, given the reality of growth, to cling to their vision. But often, the realities of growth and lofty ideals are incompatible with your needs. After all, Kayman has returned to his roots. And Hirschberg, who is now running an industrialized food giant, appears to be doing his best to try to be as true to his aspirations as big business will allow him to. It's called compromise. Kayman chose not to; Hirschberg appears to be trying hard, but seems to be slowly sinking in the quicksand of corporate America.

As Samuel Fromatz wrote in the introduction to his article "Organic Inc. Natural Foods and How They Grow" (Harvest Books, March, 2008): "I was particularly interested in people who sought to manifest their values in their businesses ... The intersection of idealism and business was not an easy place to stand, since one usually trumped the other." Fromatz earlier wrote (while focusing on start-up businesses in publications such as *Inc.* and Fortune's *Small Business*): "While buying organic may be better than the alternative, it's not as noble as the cottage industry that grew out of barrels of barley at your corner health food store. What began as a benevolent grass roots movement has morphed into a government-regulated agribusiness exceeding $15 billion dollars in annual sales."

The term "organically grown" tells us that these foods were grown without the use of synthetic pesticides and synthetic fertilizers. So what? Arsenic is organic. While far more hazardous in its inorganic form, you sure wouldn't want it in your sourdough bread. Critics of organic farming argue that growing foods with natural pesticides (such as oil, pyrethrum, neem, rotenone, sulfur, and copper compounds) does not make them less of a danger than those grown with synthetic pesticides. After all, sludge and oil are organic substances. But you wouldn't want them in your baby food. In fact, the two most heavily used pesticides on earth—oil and copper—are organic. Are they dangerous?

Let's begin our discussion by defining what we mean by "dangerous." Dangerous to what? If we're talking about the danger to our health in the short term, the data is in and it's clear. In general, there is less danger from pesticides used in organic farming than those used in conventional methods of farming. In general? Less dangerous?

Scientists obtained test data from three independent U.S. sources: the Marketplace Surveillance Program of the California Department of Pesticide Regulation, the Pesticide Data Program of the U.S. Department of Agriculture, and private tests conducted by the Consumers Union. They focused on foods sold with claims of reduced pesticide use or use of integrated pest management (IPM), foods claimed to have no detectable residues (the former and the latter classified as organically grown), and foods with no market claims at all (that were believed to have been grown conventionally).

Collectively, the three data sets provide an enormous amount of information on residues in conventionally grown samples of twenty major crops. The data also include 1,291 samples of organically grown foods and 240 samples with IPM claims of no detectable residue (NDR). Enough information to support statistical analysis and comparison of residue patterns across the three market categories.

Researchers Brian P. Baker and colleagues (*Food Additives and Contaminants*, 19:5, May 2002, pp. 427–446) conclude: "Our analysis shows convincingly that organically grown foods have fewer and generally lower pesticide residues than conventionally grown foods. This pattern was consistent across all three independent data sets. Organic foods typically contain pesticide residues only one third as often as conventionally grown foods do. Foods marketed with an IPM or NDR claim to fall in between organic and conventional foods in both the frequency of residues and residue levels. Organic samples are also far less likely to contain multiple residues than conventional or IPM/NDR foods are. While the risks to health associated with dietary pesticide residues are still uncertain and subject to debate, risk is relative, and lower exposure undoubtedly translates into lower risk. Consumers who wish to minimize their dietary pesticide exposure can do so with confidence by buying organically grown foods."

> *ORGANIC FOODS TYPICALLY CONTAIN PESTICIDE RESIDUES ONLY ONE THIRD AS OFTEN AS CONVENTIONALLY GROWN FOODS DO.*

The researchers found that organically farmed produce utilized one third the amount of pesticides required by commercially grown foods. In another study from the University of Washington (*Environmental Health Perspectives*, 2003 March; 111(3): 377–382) that focused on pesticide breakdown products (metabolites), results showed that children who ate organic diets had concentrations of pesticide metabolites six times lower than those who ate conventional diets.

There appears to be *significantly* lower risk of pesticide contamination in organically grown foods. But here's the rub. *Significantly les*s is not what most of us bargained for. It's also not the reason many of us are willing to pay through the nose for organic food. The myth that organic farming means we can expect to eat produce that's pesticide free is just that, a myth. The amount of pesticides will vary depending on which were selected by the farmer. They will range anywhere from the same level to one third the amount found in conventionally grown produce.

But a lower *amount* of a pesticide doesn't necessarily mean it's *less of a danger*. Toxic pesticides are permitted for use in organic gardening by the U.S. Department of Agriculture, because they break down more rapidly than certain synthetic pesticides, and must come from mineral and botanical bearing sources. *Persistent* pesticides are those that don't break down rapidly. Instead, they build up over time in humans and wildlife. Copper sulfate, banned in Europe due to the danger it posed to the health of humans and the environment, is an example of a pesticide approved by the USDA that's both highly toxic *and* persistent. It's been implicated in cancers of the liver and kidney and is highly toxic to fish.[12]

The Extension Toxology Network (a Pesticide Information Project of Cornell University, Michigan State University, Oregon State University, and University of California at Davis) profiles copper sulfate as "a fungicide used to control bacterial and fungal diseases of fruit, vegetable, nut, and field crops. Some of the diseases that are controlled by this fungicide include mildew, leaf spots, blight, and apple scab. It's used in combination with lime and water as a protective fungicide, referred to as *Bordeaux* mixture, for leaf application and seed treatment. It's also used as an algaecide, an herbicide in irrigation and municipal water treatment systems, and as a molluscide, a material used to repel and kill slugs and snails."

While proponents will argue that it takes at least 1 gram of copper sulfate orally ingested to produce these onerous effects, the long-term impact of this persistent pesticide is cumulative. You can liken these arguments to those that support the use of microwaves, because *allowable limits* are established by the government (Performance Standards for Microwave and Radio Frequency Emitting Products, Title 21 Code of Federal Regulations, Part 1030.10) without taking into consideration the *total* amount of microwaves we're bombarded with each day. Some, even as close to home as your next door neighbor's. Or, perhaps from a TV or an FM radio station's broadcast antenna. Like mercury, copper is retained in body tissue. It's also rapidly absorbed through skin and eye contact. While that won't typically cause allergic reactions and burning, it *will* cause fluid buildup in the eyelid and may result in the deterioration of

LIKE MERCURY, COPPER IS RETAINED IN BODY TISSUE. IT'S ALSO RAPIDLY ABSORBED THROUGH SKIN AND EYE CONTACT.

your cornea. After only 3 to 15 years of exposure to copper sulfate solution in the Bordeaux mixture, some vineyard sprayers reported liver disease. So, while there appears to be *less* danger of toxic exposure in organically grown foods, you may still be exposed to potentially deadly pesticides that accumulate in your body.

We remain unprotected from serious and persistent toxins in organic food, and the FDA appears unable to insure otherwise. It's important to note that **organic farming requires significantly *higher* doses of insecticide than is normally found in conventional farming**. It follows that the more we farm organically, the more pesticides will be required to sustain this movement. Laurie Pickett Pottoroff of the Colorado State University Extension ("Some Pesticides Permitted in Organic Gardening," 1999) points out that there are several allowable pesticides in organic gardening that have a good deal of downside risk, like nicotine, for example. "Nicotine is extracted from tobacco or related nicotiana species and is one of the oldest botanical insecticides in use today. It's also one of the most toxic to warm-blooded animals and it's readily absorbed through the skin," says Potornoff. "It breaks down quickly, however, so it is legally acceptable to use on organically grown crops ... Rotenone is a resinous compound produced by the roots of two members of the leguminosae family. It's commonly used to control various leaf-feeding caterpillars, beetles, aphids, and thrips on a wide variety of vegetables and small fruits. A slow-acting chemical, rotenone requires several days to kill most susceptible insects, but insect feeding stops shortly after exposure," Pottoroff explains. "Rotenone is moderately toxic to most mammals but extremely toxic to fish."

While certain organically grown foods have been shown to give us less exposure to pesticides than their conventionally grown counterparts, less exposure, again, may not mean less danger. If an organic farmer applies copper pesticides, you may have no more protection from the crop than its commercially grown counterpart. If the organic product you purchased was shipped 1,500 miles, picked prematurely, and gassed into maturity as it was being trucked and stored, you may have paid much more, for much less.

Research *does* continue to support the fact that foods grown organically are denser than their conventionally grown counterparts. One such study ("Organic Food Is More Nutritious Than Conventional Food," *Journal of Applied Nutrition*, 1993, 45:35–39) clearly supports this. Organically and conventionally grown apples, potatoes, pears, wheat, and sweet corn were purchased in the western suburbs of Chicago over two years, and analyzed for mineral content. The organically grown food was found to be on average

THE ORGANIC FOOD AVERAGED 29 PERCENT LOWER IN MERCURY THAN THE CONVENTIONALLY RAISED FOOD.

63 percent higher in calcium, 73 percent higher in iron, 118 percent higher in magnesium, 178 percent higher in molybdenum, 91 percent higher in phosphorus, 125 percent higher in potassium, and 60 percent higher in zinc. The organic food averaged 29 percent lower in mercury than the conventionally raised food.

This is consistent with other studies. But again, this doesn't mean that organic foods are necessarily brimming with nutrients. They're just generally less depleted than conventionally grown foods.

In terms of the atmosphere, most organic farming creates the same problems as conventionally grown foods if they're transported long distances, and picked before they're mature, gassed, and stored. Organics are big business. Today, they enjoy well in excess of $20 billion dollars a year in annual sales. The majority of organic farming is no longer done by small family farms. Most of those companies with wholesome names that you've come to trust have been purchased by the bigger guys. And they're nobody's fool.

Whether it's cooking oil, cattle, fish, poultry, or even milk and cheese, they essentially play the same game. If the market for industrialized dairy products is only growing a few percentage points a year, and their wholesome organic counterparts businesses are growing by 20 percent or more, it doesn't take long for the marketing geniuses to step up to the plate. True, double-digit growth in a small business is chopped liver next to single-digit sales growth in a far larger one. A small percentage of a larger pie can be quite meaningful.

But smart marketers follow the trends of where consumer dollars are being spent; they ride them like a horse—in the direction they're going. If tyrants can convince nations to harm others to help themselves, imagine what big business can do with a little help from the FDA. All they need to do is convince them to take a weak-kneed step forward for mankind, and let industry write the rules—then legislate it (wrapped in coddle talk). As we've seen, the FDA is no stranger to weak-kneed steps. And all big business had to do was find someone who embodied all things good, like Hirschberg for example; compensate him well, and pay dearly for his company. Groupe Danone, the same company that fooled you into believing that high-calorie sugary yogurt with little if any active friendly bacteria, actually made you healthy, did just that.

Once the FDA paved the way for the big boys to enter the game, the rest was a cakewalk. Up until that time, most of us thought we knew the meaning of the word "organic." But then the FDA stepped in and *redefined* that word. That enabled "the boys" to legislate and actually *certify* it. Prior to this time, there was no such thing as certification. A new era was born with the simple stroke of a pen. You see, you can't certify something and a get a special seal of approval, until you can convince the government to *legislate* a standard definition for it. More often than not, the force that's behind this legislation consists of special interest groups, whose interests may have little to do with yours. In fact, they often undermine what's best for you by legalizing what's not. It's nothing new really.

A special report entitled "PAYBACKS: How the White House and Congress Are Neglecting Our Health Care Because of Their Corporate Contributors," (August 18, 2004) co-authored by a number of public watchdog groups[13] explains how the Bush Administration and Congress helped pay back campaign contributors with ridiculous giveaways, forgiving regulation, and tax breaks that damaged our health care. According to the report, since 1999 pharmaceutical makers alone have contributed $46,964,230 to members of Congress.

So if you think the FDA's new standard announced on December 20, 2000, was created with the sole purpose of benefiting humanity, think again. Remember when the government defined "saturated fat" and ushered in margarine and other unstable polyunsaturated fats? Today, while the product may be different, the game's essentially the same. It's not that there isn't value in certification. In fact, quite the opposite is true. Only that all too often the requirements are too lax, and consumers trust in the fact that they aren't.

Just as troubling is the FDA's failure to legally define the term *natural* for any products other than meat and poultry. According to the Consumers Union, "Unless otherwise specified, there is no organization independently certifying this claim. The producer or manufacturer decides whether to use the claim and is not free from its own self-interest." And Consumer Reports Eco-Labels Center defines natural as: "Claims used on products that are not independently verified. They are often placed on the product by the manufacturer."

Today, what organic says is not necessarily what organic does. Thanks to the FDA, the word "organic" is so loosely defined that it only vaguely resembles what we thought it did. If the big industrial food guy's products were becoming increasingly less attractive, all they needed to do was to give their industries and products a face lift. Take a wholesome brand name and *buy it*. Then stock their stable with a respected pioneer of the naturalist movement and buy him to support you. Overnight, you've gained enough respect and marketing muscle to go from the local food store to the world's mass market. According to Phil Howard, assistant professor at Michigan State University's Department of Community, Agriculture, Recreation and Resource Studies, 25 of the largest conventional food corporations have done just that.

As the big have gotten bigger, the small guys either saw their margins diminish, or sold out. The tree trunks gobble up the water, one way or another, from the grass roots. What does all this mean for you, a person simply trying to make the right purchasing decisions? Well, according to Stonyfield: "In Groupe Danone, we've found a partner that provides cost-saving efficiencies and growth opportunities, while allowing us to manage ourselves autonomously and remain true to our mission." Saving efficiencies? What mission?

The company, established in 1983, was a nonprofit venture of the Rural Education Center originally founded by Samuel Kayman in 1971. Now, Stonyfield buys strawberries from China and apple puree from Turkey. California's strawberry production, once by far the world's largest, is in danger of being surpassed by China. In "China's Strawberry Industry: An Emerging Competitor for California?" authors Carter, Chalfant, and Goodhue et al. (*ARE Update*, Volume 9, Number 1 September 1, 2005) point out that frozen strawberry imports from China are increasing while those from California are decreasing: "China is becoming an important player in the world strawberry market. Although its yields per acre are much lower than California's, its costs per acre are much lower as well. China's production and exports are growing rapidly. For some countries, frozen strawberry imports from China are increasing while frozen imports from California are decreasing."

But wasn't Stonyfield's *mission* all about supporting the local farmer? Or is this what the company means when it says its partnership with Groupe Danone provides significant cost efficiencies? Ask New England dairy producer Rob Howe about cost efficiencies.

Howe, one of the first New England dairy producers that provided organic milk made a respectable wage by selling pure, high-quality milk to a small co-op known as the "Organic Cow of Vermont" (OCV). But when Horizon, the leading organic milk company bought out OCV, Howe received a letter from the company telling him they were going to pay him less money. Horizon, now owned by conventional milk giant Dean Foods, was certainly within their rights to do so. After all, they're marketing a commodity in a highly competitive world. But people are paying large premiums to buy organic milk. Many might believe there must some correlation between lower wages for the local maker, and a lower quality product. After all, we all have to make a living.

In addition to sourcing ingredients thousands of miles from home (adding to global warming by doing so) and hurting the local farmer in the process, Stonyfield Farms and other organic giants feed their cows a diet primarily consisting of grain. Feeding cows who produce organic milk a grain-based diet is in itself a contradiction—and so is selling organics to a mass-market retailer who must transport it often hundreds and even thousands of miles away. We know what that does to the environment. Yet, Hirshberg has stated that he feels Wal-Mart would be the best partner he could possibly have.

> *FEEDING COWS WHO PRODUCE ORGANIC MILK A GRAIN-BASED DIET IS IN ITSELF A CONTRADICTION ...*

Grazing in a beautiful green pasture on a diet of tall, rich blades of grass is not common. But isn't that what Horizon's label suggests? Happy cows grazing in a valley of lush green grass. Grazing is costly. The activity itself is a calorie burner, not a protein builder. Feed-lots may provide a lousy life for a cow, but they're far more cost effective in beefing up the beef. Recently, Horizon, Organic Valley, and Humbolt Creamery joined forces to co-author a recommendation written to the secretary of the USDA, imploring him to keep the percentage of free access to pasture land *vague*. They also refused to support an initiative that would have specified a maximum percentage of grain permissible in the diet of their milk cows. To qualify as organic, one of the FDA requirements is that cows must be allowed to "have access" to pasture land. We all know what that means. I have *access* to millions of dollars whenever I'm at the bank and the vault door swings open. Once again, the government's interpretation of the word "access" is deliberately vague and deliberately non-deliberate. Dean Foods' and Aurora Organics' insistence that their dairy animals have "access" to pasture land provides us with little peace of mind.

Dean Foods actually owns a couple of their own farms under their Horizon name. Horizon, like many other wholesomely-named companies you once thought you knew, is owned and cleverly hidden from public scrutiny by Dean Foods®, under the name "Whitewave," their organic milk holding company.

Cornucopia Institute (a Wisconsin-based farm policy group) who supports family farms) visited Deans/Whitewaves/Horizons farms in Idaho. Their report paints a very different and quite grim picture of a horribly crowded industrialized feed lot. It would appear that organic farming is being as carefully crafted, woven, spun, and marketed to us now in the same deliberate way as so many other "natural" food products we've examined.

The following photos from their site tell the story:

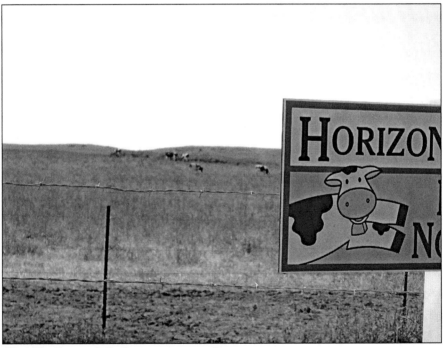

Photo: The Cornucopia Institute, www.cornucopia.org

**At the Horizon Idaho farm, 50 of the 3500 heifers
are out on grass in the midday sun.**

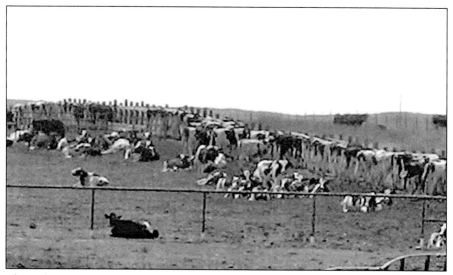

Photo: The Cornucopia Institute, www.cornucopia.org

The heifer dry-lot facility.

Based on their investigation of many such dairies, the only cows that appear happy here were the ones in the photo above.

On Cornucopia's Web site (www.cornucopia.org), Dean Foods, the largest commercial and organic milk producer in the world, is profiled as follows: "They operate two corporate-owned farms, in Maryland and Idaho. Their Idaho facility, milking 4000–5000 cows, was originally a conventional factory-dairy that they converted to organic production. It has, according to widespread industry reports, very little access to pasture. Unlike the majority of all organic dairy farmers in the United States, who concentrate on the health and longevity of their cows, caring for them from birth, the Dean/ Horizon Idaho farm sells off all their calves. Later, presumably to save money on organic feed and management, they buy one-year-old conventional animals on the open market. These replacements likely have received conventional milk replacer (made with blood—considered to be a "mad cow" risk), antibiotics, other prohibited pharmaceuticals, and genetically engineered feed. Many practices on a farm of this nature put ethical family-scale organic farmers at a competitive disadvantage."

Cornucopia posts ethical rankings of most of the major organic producers on their Web site. On a scale of 1 to 5 of ethical rankings among the major producers (one being the lowest), Horizon scored a lowly rating of 1. In fact, Cornucopia's Web site advises us that they "recently filed formal complaints with the USDA against three industrial dairies, including allegations that these mega-farms in the arid West were violating the law by confining their cattle to feedlots and sheds rather than grazing as the organic regulations require. The dairy farms in question include the one owned by Dean Foods in Idaho and California shipping milk for distribution under the Horizon label. Because of inaction by the USDA, the Institute is now preparing to seek court intervention in order to compel the agency to investigate the alleged improprieties."

So, where does all of this leave the consumer? The only ones we can trust to watch out for us, is us. You know by now that the FDA isn't likely to do so, nor are the major food and drug companies. Maybe it's time you make the time to do so, so you can have more time. Shouldn't staying alive become everyone's principle objective?

Yes, organically grown fruits and vegetables *have* been shown to contain more nutrients and fewer hazards than their conventionally grown counterparts. Organic, for those that can afford it, remains a better choice. Locally grown foods, or foods grown as close to home as possible, grown naturally, organically, and responsibly are nutritionally superior when compared to either of these other approaches. Taking time to determine the best way to do so may provide you with many additional years of health and vitality. Purchase what you can from farmers whose methods you're free to question at your local farmers' market. You may wish to call the principal at your local school and tell them about the farm to school program (www.farmtoschool.org). This program connects schools with local farmers. Their goal is to develop healthy, locally-based food programs in school cafeterias, improving student nutrition and providing important education on health.

Eat ORGLOC (*org*anic and *loc*al). You'll quickly feel the difference eating organic and locally grown products. Help make raising your children a different kind of love story. Provide healthy habits that your children's children may choose to emulate. Walk the talk. Stop feeding them to death. Feed them to life. In the process, you'll also help support the family farm, a vanishing legacy of free enterprise in our country and throughout the free world. And, if at all possible, grow your own food!

EVALUATING FOOD: COLOR COUNTS, THE POWER OF SUPER-PHYTOS

Another factor we need to consider in evaluating the potential of a food is its ability to optimize immunity. In this regard, the color of a fruit or vegetable is almost a *tell*. **In general, the more vivid the color of a fruit or vegetable, the more healthful your choice of food.** Purple cabbage is a better choice than green. Not that there is anything wrong with the color green, nor with green cabbage. But given the choice, green cabbage, in contrast to the green color in kale, is a more sallow looking shade of that color. Romaine lettuce is far more colorful than iceberg lettuce and so on. And browns, beige, and white choices are often the worst (like most potatoes). But, as we've consistently found, not always!

Color is due to the type and density of what are known as phytochemicals or phytonutrients. These names are often used interchangeably (even by the FDA), though technically, using the term *phytonutrient* is a misnomer. A chemical is, by definition, not a nutrient. Nutrients are substances required to *sustain* life. Recall that *essential* nutrients must be obtained from food since our bodies can't produce them.

Phytochemicals are also incredibly protective mechanisms designed by nature to safeguard its plant's fruits, vegetables, teas, grains, legumes, and nuts. There are too many classifications and subclassifications to list for the purpose of this writing. However, what follows is a brief description of a few of the most popular and broad classifications of phytochemical Super-Nutrients, and some of their subclassifications:

CAROTENOIDS

There are nearly 700 of them. Not only plants, but animals and insects can thank these phytos for their vivid color. Egg yolk's bright yellow color is due to a high density of these phytochemicals that nature provided them with, to protect *their* important unsaturated fatty acids. A subclassification of carotenoids known as the "terpenes" help give oranges, tomatoes, parsley, grapefruit, and even spinach, as well as other fruits and vegetable, their bright colors.

FLAVONOIDS (POLYPHENOLS) INCLUDING ISOFLAVONES (PHYTOESTROGENS)

Over 1500 of this important phenol subclass of phytochemicals has been identified. They've been shown to reduce inflammation, fight free radicals and microbes, and to even protect us against tumors, microbes, and certain allergies. Long ago they were all lumped together as simply, vitamin P. But our knowledge and the proof of their power continues to grow. Among their many virtues, flavonoids help prevent estrogen-induced cancer. They're able to do so by blocking the enzymes that produce estrogen itself. They also appear to enhance the effectiveness of vitamin C. A partial listing of some of their well-known subclassifications is as follows:

Flavones (containing the citrus bio-flavonoid apigenin found in parsley, peppermint, perilla, chamomile, and more), and flavonols (found in onion, tomato, kale, broccoli, cacao, lettuce, tomato, apple, grape, berries, tea, and red wine to name a few). Quercetin is found in grapefruit and rutin (research has shown it fortifies our capillaries and is often recommended for those suffering from hemophilia) is found in buckwheat. And lastly flavanones (hesperidin—plentiful in citrus fruits; and silybin found in milk thistle are the primary flavonolignan that's extracted from the seed of milk thistle).

LIGNANS

Foods that break down into the *lignans* we ingest include legumes, whole grains such as barley and rye, fruits such as berries, and vegetables like kale and broccoli. Flax has the highest concentration and is healthy, as long as your intake is accompanied by sulphur-based protein. If taken without this protein (like that found in cottage cheese), the converse is true and it will act to punish your immune system.

LIMONOIDS

Found in citrus fruit peels, they *appear* to be effective in protecting lung tissue and in reducing oral cancer. Though impressive, most studies to date were performed in-vivo or using lab animals. Purdue University scientists recently discovered that adding lemon to green tea increased catechin levels five-fold. Though limonoids appear to hold great promise, more research in human subjects is called for.

ISOTHIOCYANATES AND INDOLES

Isothiocyanates combat carcinogens by neutralizing them, reducing their growth by inhibiting the production of enzymes they require to metabolize (*Drug Metabolism Review:* 2000 Aug-Nov; 32(3-4):395-411; Inhibition of carcinogenesis by isothiocyanates). Studies have shown that isothiocyanates help prevent lung cancer and esophageal cancer. Isothiocyanates can also lower the risk of other cancers, including gastrointestinal cancer and bladder cancer. Tang et al. ("Dietary Isothiocyanates Inhibit the Growth of Human Bladder Carcinoma Cells," *Journal of Nutrition*, August, 2004) showed that isothiocyanates literally abolished cell progression activity in low micromolar concentrations. Isothiocyanates can be found in cruciferous vegetables such as broccoli, cauliflower, kale, turnips, collards, brussels sprouts, cabbage, radish, turnip, and watercress. Glucosinolates are precursors of isothiocyanates found in cruciferous vegetables like broccoli and cabbage, and appear to protect us against many forms of cancer.

PHENOLS AND CYCLIC COMPOUNDS

Phenols protect plants from oxidative damage and perform the same function for humans. Blue, blue-red, and violet colorations seen in berries, grapes, and purple eggplant are due to their phenolic content. Bilberries, for example, are high in phenolic anthocyanidins and are red in color. The outstanding phytonutrient feature of phenols is their ability to block specific enzymes that cause inflammation. They also modify the prostaglandin pathways and thereby protect platelets from clumping.

SAPONINS

These are soap-like phytochemical surfactants, designed by nature to help certain plants and animals avoid the taste buds of predators found in many herbs. These incredibly complex compounds are continually shown to act as powerful anti-inflammatory agents that stimulate our immunity, while fighting microbial growth and bacteria.

SULFIDES AND THIOLS

Phytonutrients of this sulfur-containing class are present in garlic and cruciferous vegetables like cabbage and turnips and are members of the mustard family. A subcategory known as "terpenes" (yes, the derivative of the word turpentine), they are the major compounds found in the essential oils of many plants and flowers. Also found in many grains, green foods, and soy products, they make up one of the largest and most intently studied classes of phytonutrients. Included in this group are the carotenoids, such as famed beta-carotein. The terpene family functions as antioxidants, protecting fatty acids from assault by free radical oxygen species including those from superoxide.

All of the above, and many more not listed, evolved to protect living things in a number of remarkable ways. Some protect plants from animals. Others protect our foods from damaging sun as they grow. Still others fight bacteria, or work to strengthen one another. An impressive and mushrooming body of research supports their powerful contribution to our health, handily proving their power to protect and defend us. While vitamins can be phytochemicals by virtue of the antiquated definition of a nutrient, not all phytochemicals can be nutrients. I've used the term "Super-Nutrients" to include those nutrients classically defined (both essential and non-essential, including vitamins and mineral supplements), as well as phytochemicals. All have the potential to heal and protect us. In my opinion, the current definition of nutrients is far too limiting. And all *Super-Nutrients* are derived from foods that can be bought organically.

While our understanding of phytochemicals is growing and their powerful contribution to our health is a relatively recent discovery, they're of enormous value.

Many non-nutrient antioxidants are phytochemicals, such as the anthocyanins found in cranberries and the lycopene found in tomatoes. The Synergy of Super-Nutrients Program considers how we can maximize our potential using both phytochemicals and classically defined nutrients. By the time you've completed Chapter 6, you'll receive and understand the most powerful program of its kind. A program that, if used properly, will change your life.

Antioxidants are found in certain foods that neutralize free radicals. These include the nutrient antioxidants; vitamins A, C, and E; and the minerals copper, zinc, and selenium. Other dietary food compounds such as the phytochemicals found in plants and zoo-chemicals, from animal products, are believed to offer even *greater antioxidant protection* than many vitamins or minerals. These are traditionally referred to as non-nutrient antioxidants and include phytochemicals such as lycopene in tomatoes; quercetin found in apples, beans, and onions; anthocyanins found in cranberries; and the catechins found in cocoa, wine, green tea, and lentils.

Flavonoids (one of many families of phytochemicals), such as the catechins, are believed to be responsible for the low rates of heart disease in Japan and elsewhere. Lutein, found in dark green vegetables such as kale and spinach, is credited with lowering the incidence of eye degeneration and blindness in the elderly, based on information reported by the Australian government's Better Health Channel. Foods containing lycopene (particularly tomato-based foods) show this Super-Nutrient's amazing ability to significantly lower the risk of prostate cancer in men. Vividly colored fruits and vegetables provide powerful protection when properly combined. The best approach is to eat *as many different colored foods as you can in a given meal,* every day, to the extent that's possible. Principally those which have been carefully identified and qualified to be listed in The SOS program found in Chapter 6.

The National Cancer Institute's (NCI) "5 a Day" program, also known as "Sample the Spectrum," advises people to color their daily diets with fruits and vegetables that are bright orange, deep red, dark green, blue, purple, and yellow. "We're trying to make people understand that fruits and vegetables in their more colorful form have the most nutritional bang for the buck," says Linda Nebeling, chief of health promotion at the NCI (*Washington Post,* 2001). Data shows that *in combination with each other*, the ability of each respective phytochemical is greatly enhanced. While the Spectrum program is a good start, it doesn't qualify *which* colored foods are best, and provides only one pillar of the foundation we need to maximize our health from food. While eating different colors of the spectrum is helpful, learning to eat the *most powerful foods* in combination with each other, along with important supplementation, will add "years to your life and life to your years."

EVALUATING FOOD: FIRST, A WORD ABOUT TOP 10 FOOD LISTS

We all want quick and simple fixes, but achieving optimum health is not done by limiting your intake to two handfuls of "super-food" that made the cut from a top 10 list! Such lists are a disservice to those that use them. We have our own list, of course; but it's far from short, and it's based on real criteria, from solid research that's stood the test of time. It respects and indeed emphasizes the *real* power of a broad spectrum of synergistic Super-Nutrients.

Is one food better than another because it has more vitamin C, as some researchers suggest? What if it's not absorbable, or only found in foods that are among the most pesticide laden? Perhaps it's been shown to be effective on animals but not humans, females and not males, or younger folks but not older. What if a food was not selected for a top 10 list because it ranked poorly in vitamin C, but contained a broad array of amazing compounds which when packed into one food, work *together* to protect your DNA?

What's the best way to *prepare* this super-food? The way we chose to do so may completely alter its characteristics and value. It's simply *not* possible to receive the right kind of protection we need from a narrow list of foods. As you'll soon see, it's important for us to understand the food choices we make, and enjoy as many of their unique characteristics as we possibly can to enrich our lives. Even for a chapter such as this, primarily focused on carbohydrates, providing a top 10 list is of little value. *Many* foods have a unique ability to protect us. Their nutrients or chemicals combine in special ways that empower them to empower you.

A BRIEF INTRODUCTION TO THE SYNERGY OF SUPER-NUTRIENTS (SOS) PROGRAM

Many researchers have contributed to the collective body of information used to develop this program. More often than not, their focus has been in one particular area. The Synergy of Super-Nutrients Program, from the vantage point of our food, is a compendium of powerful information that pulls it all together.

The SOS program:

- Identifies the world's most powerful foods using a number of important criteria. Even the criteria themselves are interrogated. We've already begun by identifying the finest sources of protein and fats in chapters 1 and 2.
- Combines the right amount of each food group to properly balance our hormones—an area of understanding that Dr. Barry Sears, Dr. Robert C. Atkins, and others have underscored.
- Identifies the value of important phytochemicals in those foods, and how to use them together to maximize their effectiveness.
- Sets the record straight on supplements, what you need, and how they work together to collectively empower each other.
- Identifies and utilizes the power of phyochemicals—the new frontier. Identifying the foods boasting the most powerful combination of phytochemicals, and illustrating the best way to increase their healthful value.
- Takes the best of all the well researched work in this area, eliminating the need for guesswork to select and combine the best foods.
- Identifies the most formidable supplements that work together to protect us, bolster our immunity, and permit us to grow older by minimizing and even reversing many of the characteristic signs of aging.

Based on what you've already learned, along with what you're about to, you'll be armed with a broader base of knowledge than most of the experts. And by the time you've read Chapter 6, you'll have a true blueprint for a better quality of life that you can put to work now; a powerful plan for change based on a vast body of cutting edge research. A simple program with the power to change your life! Lester Packer and others have shown the power of this synergy with certain supplements. Sears has shown that other protection occurs by regulating our hormones when we properly balance them at mealtime.

We've already identified a number of poor food choices; what remains are the good ones, and the truly great ones. The more vivid they are in color, the higher they are in fiber. The lower their GL and the less contaminated they are, the greater their ability to heal and protect us. Now let's learn about the finest carbohydrates on earth, based on all the criteria we've indentified.

The most healthful selections are SOS foods purchased pesticide-free and organically grown whenever possible. But don't find *too* much comfort in this. Allowable levels of pesticides that may be used by growers have been based on experiments with animals. For decades, the allowable guidelines have been calculated using what's known as the "Inter-species Rule of Ten." This calculation set by the government requires that growers evaluate the speed in which a food breaks down into glucose after entry, relative to serving size. But it leaves it up to *them* to determine serving size.

Consuming as many of these carbohydrate foods each day along with the other amazing food groups in this book, and pairing off at least one color with another from a different subset, will start you on the road to supercharge your immunity.

Now that we've explained some of the basic criteria to assist us in the selection process, the following will help explain each measurement used to qualify the special foods that will follow in a quick, "at a glance" list for the foods we will detail shortly.

CARBOHYDRATE RATING AND VALUE INFORMATION:

Old ORAC (Oxygen Radical Absorbance Capacity) score. A score that measures a food's lipophilic (fat-based) constituents.

New ORAC TAC (Total Antioxidant Capacity) score. A more recent test that scores the combined lipophilic (fat-based) and hydrophilic (water-based) constituents.

TRAC (Total Realistic Antioxidant Capacity). Provided where the new ORAC TAC score is based on an impractical serving size.

GI—Glycemic index. 70 or more is high; 56 to 69 is medium; 55 or less is low.

GL—Glycemic load. 20 or more is high; 11 to 19 is medium; 10 or less is low.

EWG (Environmental Working Group)—Conventionally grown food's pesticide content ranking: 14 or less is high, 28 or more is low

THE POWER OF HIGH FIBER CARBOHYDRATES. AN IMPORTANT CLASS OF SUPER-NUTRIENTS

The following section reveals the *most* important carbohydrate foods that I recommend you eat as often as possible. Doing so will optimize your drip system and bathe your cells with a constant flow of these bio-miraculous compounds.

While space won't permit a detailed profile of every important fruit and vegetable, one or more of particular interest have been selected that represent each color category. Other important foods within that category have also been indicated. Eating the featured foods in each group daily, along with profiled members of the other color groups, provides you with an antioxidant soup containing nutrients that build upon each other. Adding to your regime one or more of the "other" important members that are indicated, and varying these choices often, is the best way to take advantage of the full range of nutrients provided by nature.

BLACK AND BLUE AND PURPLE FOODS

This pigment found in certain plants, fruits, and vegetables contains a large family of polyphenolic compounds known as "flavonoids." Over 4,000 flavonoids have been identified at the time of this writing. The simple path we should all take toward understanding them has once again been made all the more difficult by the language used to name them. The flavonoid family encompasses important sub-groups. These include flavenols, flavanols, flavenones, flavanones, flavones, and isoflavones (words should be used to facilitate our understanding of what they are chosen to describe, not confuse them).

Chief protectors among these flavonoids are *blue anthocyanins*, a powerful class of antioxidants that function as natural sunscreens. These phytochemicals protect plants from cellular damage by absorbing blue-green light. They also serve to insulate them from radical damage formed by UV light. **All phytochemicals evolved as bio-protective mechanisms**, permitting plants to better cope in the world around them. Different sub-classifications evolved for different reasons. While anthocyanins developed to protect the seed, pulp, and DNA of the plant from the ravages of the sun, other biochemical defenses evolved to protect plants against oxidation, bacteria, predators, environmental toxins, viruses, fungi, and other potentially threatening situations. This amazing antioxidant protection found in certain fruits, vegetables, and beverages is conserved in certain foods, and actually passed on to other organisms that eat them, like us.

This means that we can influence the character and the quality of our protective mechanisms by simply eating theirs.

BLACK RASPBERRIES

Old ORAC: 1220
(Serving size: 3.5 ounces)
New ORAC TAC: 6058 (Total Antioxidant Capacity)
(Serving size: 1 cup)
TRAC: 2019
(Serving size: 1/3 cup)
GI: 40
GL: 5
EWG Ranking: 17

Note: Only red raspberries were tested in the new ORAC [Wu] study. But research by Leslie W. Ada and colleagues ("Antioxidant Activity and Phenolic Content of Oregon Cane-berries," *J. Agric. Food Chem*, 2002) measured the values of each color. Their research showed that *black* raspberries had a far higher ORAC, anthocyanin, and phenolic content than even super-healthy red raspberries.

Black raspberries contain almost 20 percent of the RDA dietary fiber per total weight (8 grams per cup) and top the list of foods ranked for important phenolic compound content. These include compounds from phytonutrients such as ellagic acid, quercetin, gallic acid, kaempferol, anthocyanins, and salicylic acid. This powerful group of polyphenols has been the subject of a rapidly growing body of research that underscores their huge contribution to your health. Research has shown their ellagic acid has powerful anti-mutagenic, anti-carcinogenic, anti-bacterial, and anti-viral properties. Just as noteworthy, black raspberries contain five times more of this important antioxidant than any other berry!

Dr. Danielle Nixon and colleagues at Hollings Cancer Institute of South Carolina found that raspberries prevent the development of cancer cells (just one cup a day). In one study, the ellagitannins in raspberries gave cultured infected human cervical cells the ability to stop mutatgenis by preventing the degradation of P53 cells. According to the Rockefeller Foundation, "P53 protein is a tumor suppressor encoded by a gene whose disruption is associated with approximately 50 to 55 percent of human cancers. The p53 protein acts as a checkpoint in the cell cycle, either preventing or initiating programmed cell death. Since cancer is the unchecked proliferation of cells, p53's role is critical."

Other research has shown that raspberries protect cells from DNA damage. They bind with the carcinogens themselves interfering with their ability to latch onto DNA's bacteria (encapsulating them), which prevents them from causing cell mutation.

"Raspberries contain vitamin C and anthocyanines," says Jules Beekwilder, "but these can also be found in other products. However, approximately 50 percent of the antioxidant effect of raspberries is caused by ellagitannins. These you find in small doses in strawberries and practically nowhere else."

While there are lots of good reasons to tout black raspberries, signaling out one particular photochemical misses the point. The real power appears to be in the way the *medley* of fruits and important phenols and other antioxidants react among themselves. In turn, that determines how their "molecular soup" chemically reacts with the other material present in your body.

Does raspberry's high content of salicylic acid provide the same benefit against heart disease as aspirin? The Washington Red Raspberry Commission ("Photochemicals in Red Raspberries," 2004) thinks it might. According to them, "Salicylic acid is found in red raspberries and is suspected of having the same protective effect against heart disease as aspirin."

Its presence in combination with other factors and foods containing salicylic acid has the power to significantly reduce internal inflammations. Some believe it provides the heart with the same type of protection found in baby aspirin. After all, aspirin is actually the synthesized form of salicylic acid. In fact, it's actually a buffered descendent. Salicylic acid, in its purest form extracted from the willow bark tree, was found to be too hard on the stomach. According to *A History of Aspirin* by Mary Bellis, writing for the Inventors series featured on About.com, a French chemist Charles Gerghardt found a way to neutralize salicylic acid, in 1853, by buffering it. Almost five decades later, Gerghardt's original formula was discovered by a young scientist named Felix Hoffman. He administered it to his own father who was suffering with painful arthritis.

And the rest is history. He convinced Bayer, his employer, to market the new miracle formula as a powder when their patent was issued in 1889. In 1915, Bayer aspirin was produced in tablet form.

According to Bellis, "Aspirin® and Heroin® were once trademarks belonging to Bayer. After Germany lost World War I, Bayer was forced to give up both trademarks as part of the Treaty of Versailles in 1919." As a point of interest, for over ten years Bayer mistakenly marketed *heroin* as a non-addictive cough syrup for kids and a cure for heroin addiction. They eventually discovered that the liver converts heroin to morphine.

ACCORDING TO BELLIS, ASPIRIN® AND HEROIN® WERE ONCE TRADEMARKS BELONGING TO BAYER.

Some contend that a small non-buffered dose of salicylic acid, when combined with other sources of this antioxidant, may very well protect the heart and reduce inflammation. Scottish researchers hypothesized just that. Their research comparing 37 vegetarians to non-vegetarians found marketed increases in the vegetarian's blood serum level of salicylic acid levels. So it's entirely possible that this increase in those consuming large amounts of fruits and vegetables may help explain why diets high in these foods are associated with a reduced risk of heart disease and colon cancer.

Many other fruits and vegetables that contain high levels of salicylic acid, including almonds, green peppers, tomatoes, and more, when eaten regularly, may indeed provide enough of this polyphenol to protect our hearts. We just don't know yet.

Raspberries also contain large amounts of kaempferol, a natural flavonoid that's been shown to reduce the risk of heart disease when consumed in tea and broccoli. While a good indicator that the kaempferol in raspberries is just as effective, the data would be even more compelling if it were based on the kaempferol found in raspberries themselves, rather than in combination with other flavonoids.

Eaten with foods such as our recommended nuts and seeds, in a mixture of other colored berries and pure plain yogurt (such as Athena brand) and topped with powerful and delicious cinnamon, your meal is a rhapsody of healthful nutrients that work to empower each other.

Research on animals ("Inhibition of the mutagenicity of bay-region diol epoxides of polycyclic aromatic hydrocarbons by naturally occurring plant phenols: Exceptional activity of ellagic acid, *"Biochemistry,* September, *1982)* suggests that ellagic acid appears to deactivate metabolites of such cancer-causing compounds as polycyclic hydrocarbons (PAHs). We get these by eating char-grilled meat. We also inhale these from breathing in contaminated air with toxins from the incomplete burning of gasoline and certain fossil fuels, garbage, or other organic substances such as tobacco.

RASPBERRIES' ANTHOCYANINS ALSO CONTAIN ANTIOXIDANT PROPERTIES FOUND TO PREVENT AN OVERGROWTH OF CERTAIN BACTERIA AND FUNGI IN THE BODY ...

While human toxicology studies intentionally exposing humans to hazards for the purpose of research is not possible, a study could be constructed comparing a subject's level of polycyclic aromatic hydrocarbons who ate sufficient amounts of ellagic acid, to those that don't and have chosen to live in polluted areas. Raspberries' anthocyanins also contain antioxidant properties found to prevent an overgrowth of certain bacteria and fungi in the body, such as yeast. Fungal infections contribute to both irritable bowel syndrome and vaginal infections.

We can't yet say, with certainty, that eating raspberries will help prevent cancer, or heart disease, or halt the growth of virulent microbes in humans. Though, in at least one human study and in several animal studies, it had a major impact on one or more of these disorders. We can conclude that black raspberries are one of the most biologically active foods known to man, full of important nutrients that appear to hold great promise in our fight against cancer and heart disease. The powerful nutrients in black raspberries have been incredibly effective in animal studies where they've been shown to reduce cancer growth and promote cancer cell apoptosis (programmed cell death). Hopefully, more research in human populations is on the horizon.

Beware of claims by some makers touting supplements of ellagic acid. According to the research, it's the *ellagitannins* that are broken down from ellagic acid that we need. If you can't eat of cup of red raspberries a day, approximately 80 milligrams of red raspberry seed powder would be equal to one cup of whole raspberries a day. The finest source is organic, freeze-dried powder. Resource information is available at: www.RKInformedLiving.com.

Other equally important black foods ...

BLACK BEANS

Old ORAC: 503 (baked beans tested)

Serving size: 3.5 ounces

New ORAC TAC: 4181

Serving size: 8.1 ounces

TRAC: Same as above

GI: 30 GL: 7

EWG Ranking: Not tested/ranked.

Their wonderfully high content of water-soluble dietary fiber will slowly feed your blood sugar. Black beans absorb a good deal of water and slow down the absorption of its own carbohydrate content. Nutritional heavy weights and rich in anthocyanin, they trump all other beans in important antioxidant activity. An amazingly nutrient dense food, black beans have a concentrated tapestry of anthocyanins. The deepest, darkest hues pack a phytochemical powerful punch. Researchers Choung et al. found ("Anthocyanin profile of Korean cultivated kidney bean [Phaseolus vulgaris L.]" *Journal of Agriculture and Food Chemistry,* 2003 Nov. 19;51(24):7040–3) that the darker the bean's seed coat, the higher their level of antioxidant activity. Chemical analysis based on the same gram weight revealed that they were followed (in descending order) in bio-available activity by red beans, brown, yellow, and white.

Eating only a few portions a week will significantly lower your risk of heart disease. Hannia Campos and a team of researchers from Harvard University's Department of Nutrition (*Journal of Nutrition*, 2005) interviewed 2,118 healthy individuals in Costa Rica and compared them with an equal number of people who had suffered nonfatal heart attacks. They discovered that those who ate one third of a cup per day, regardless of other risk factors such as smoking and obesity, were 38 percent less likely to have suffered a heart attack than were those who ate beans less than once a month. An important source of folate, regular consumption of black beans can help lower homocysteine levels in your blood. Just one third of a cup provides more than 20 percent of the daily value of folate.

An excellent source of iron (best absorbed when eaten in combination with animal protein according to a study published in the *American Journal of Clinical Nutrition*, 21, 1175–1183), black beans are particularly important to pregnant women and growing children. They also provide more than 30 percent of our daily value for magnesium (the fourth most abundant mineral in our body), which relaxes blood vessels, improves blood flow, reduces heart attack risk, and is often prescribed to improve the flow of the blood to the heart.

EATING ONLY ONE THIRD OF A CUP OF BLACK BEANS PROVIDES ALMOST 60 PERCENT OF THE DAILY VALUE FOR THIS HELPFUL TRACE MINERAL.

Are you allergic to sulfites? Black beans are loaded with an important and rare trace mineral known as "molybdenum," a metal that's antagonistic to copper and tungsten. Several enzymes can't be created in our bodies without the co-factoring activity of this important inorganic substance. One of those enzymes is sulfite oxide, whose presence is required to detoxify sulfites. These preservatives are found in almost all wine, the majority of beers, most canned, bottled, and frozen juices, dried fruit mixes, cookies, pizza crust, pretzels, potato chips, pickles, olives, gelatins, all clear hard candy, cornstarch, dried fruits and vegetables, jams, jellies, frozen shrimp, lobster, crab, soy products, and more. If you have adverse reactions to any of these products, it may be due to insufficient molybdenum reserves needed to create sulfite oxide, required to detoxify them. Eating only one third of a cup of black beans provides almost 60 percent of the daily value for this helpful trace mineral. Fortunately, other food sources can contribute to your daily requirement, including dark green leafy vegetables, eggs, and grains.

Bacteria cause beans' complex sugars to ferment in the large intestine. Soaking beans the night before in water and apple cider vinegar (the sugars are water-soluble), cooking them with garlic, or taking a commercial product such as Beano™ prior to eating them, helps reduce or eliminate flatulence.

Other great black foods include: black plums, black currants, blackberries, black mulberries, Beluga caviar, and black lentils.

BLUE AND PURPLE

The original ORAC testing was performed on cultivated blueberries. Testing was subsequently performed again in 2004 on the wild lowbush variety. For comparison purposes with other foods tested on those same dates, I've listed the results on each below:

BLUEBERRY (CULTIVATED)

Old ORAC: 2400
(Serving size: 3.5 ounces)
New ORAC: TAC: 9,019 (Total Antioxidant Capacity)
Serving size: 1 cup, cultivated

LOWBUSH BLUEBERRIES

New ORAC: TAC: 13,427- Lowbush-Not cultivated
TRAC: Low Busch 4471
TRAC: Serving size= 1/3 cup
GI: 53
GL: 6.5 Serving size 1/2 cup
EWG: 31

According to the U.S. Highbush Blueberry Council, North America is the world's leading blueberry producer, accounting for nearly 90 percent of the world production at the present time. The North American harvest runs from mid-April through early October, with peak harvest in July. I consider blueberries to legitimately be the second highest ORAC carbohydrate food (given the shortcomings of the old ORAC scale) based on the measures taken in the second ORAC study. They were only exceeded by prunes at 5770, and raisins at 2830. But both of these are dried versions of other fruits (plums and grapes respectively), and don't lend themselves to accurate comparisons with whole, wet fruits that aren't dried. While black plums lagged right behind blueberries in ORAC and TAC rankings, they do, in actuality, rank higher (#1), based on density and a realistic serving size.

In the new and more accurate ORAC scale published in 2004, wild lowbush blueberries blew all other fruits that were tested out of the water, showing once again that the manner in which a food is grown, processed, or cultivated directly affects its nutrient value. Conventionally grown blueberries ran a distant but respectable second place on the scoreboard of fruits tested with a TAC of 9019. All of this, as well as a low GI, low GL, and a low EWG pesticide ranking of 31 characterize blueberries as a truly amazing food.

Scientists at the U.S. Department of Agriculture's Human Nutrition Research Center on Aging proclaimed blueberries to be one of the world's most healthful foods on earth, while acknowledging that certain flavonoids in blueberries may actually reverse aging of nerve cells (a 2006 study by Galli and colleagues of the Human Nutrition Research Center on Aging at Tufts University confirmed this). Dietary supplementation with antioxidant-rich blueberries was shown to decrease the level of oxidative stress in certain regions of the brain, while ameliorating age-related deficits in neuronal and behavioral function. Short-term supplementation with blueberries was also shown to enhance the brain's ability to generate a mediated neuroprotective response.

Previous studies by Tufts/USDA researchers had already shown that rats, which corresponded in age to that of a 75-year-old human being, showed marked improvement in coordination after regularly consuming a supplement that was the equivalent of one cup of blueberries a day. In an interview in 2002, *Newsweek* (June 17, 2002) quoted Tufts neuroscientist James Joseph as stating: "When it comes to brain protection, there's nothing quite like blueberries." Studies show that regular consumption of blueberries is beneficial in fighting everything from diabetes to cancer, macular degeneration to heart diseases, stroke, urinary infections, circulatory problems, and stubborn body weight (with just over 40 calories for a half cup, it's an incredibly dense food as well).

While red wine is touted as protective due to its rich antioxidant content of anthocyanins, a study by Sánchez-Moreno et al., published in the *Journal of Agriculture and Food Chemistry* (August 2003 13;51(17):4889–96), found that blueberries delivered a whopping 38 percent more of this important phytonutrient.

Mary Ann Lila Smith PhD, a cancer researcher at the University of Illinois, found that proanthocyanidin (a related group of flavonoids that are also free radical scavengers) in wild blueberries (and to a lesser extent in cultivated blueberries) suppresses an enzyme that encourages the growth of cancer cells (*Journal of Food Science, 2000*, "Bioactive properties of wild blueberry fruits," 65:352–356).

Regular feeding of blueberries to animals was shown to significantly lower the damage caused by stroke. All berries contain tannins, which are a substance proven to help in the prevention of bladder infections. They do so by preventing potentially damaging bacteria from attaching to organs and cells.

REGULAR FEEDING OF BLUEBERRIES TO ANIMALS WAS SHOWN TO SIGNIFICANTLY LOWER THE DAMAGE CAUSED BY STROKE.

While the effectiveness of cultivated blueberries on our health appears to be nothing short of amazing, the *lowbush wild* variety (tested in the 2004 ORAC study) blows all other fruits tested away, with a TAC score that was off the chart.

What is a "lowbush blueberry"? Again, the facts differ from what various trade groups and certain commercial operators would have us to believe. In most languages, the term "wild" would imply that something has been left alone to develop naturally without the assistance of mankind. But the FDA's language often defies logic. So, it should come as no surprise to you that we actually have no legal, regulatory definition for the term "wild," like so many other important terms we've discussed.

This leaves the door wide open for commercial growers to "farm" and market what they label and promote as "wild" blueberries. In fact, these are often plants grown from the *seedlings* of native, forest-grown, truly wild blueberries. However, there is nothing wrong with them. Maine, the largest grower of "harvested" wild blueberries, has now surpassed Michigan as the largest U.S. producer, harvesting some 60,000 acres of this farmed crop. Eastern Canada is also a large producer of this produce as well.

Although some lowbush producers seemed pleased to tell us the "improved cultivated, highbred" highbush variety found in most stores are not truly wild, both lowbush and highbush varieties may be found in their natural habitat. The highbush blueberry is the most common grocery store blueberry available for purchase. It's not as rich in important antioxidants as its lowbush cousin (both of these fruits are grown from different plants).

In 2001, researchers Kalt et al. published the results of their work in the *Journal of Agriculture and Food Chemistry* (2001, 49 (10), 4761–4767) that compared the breadth and value of antioxidants between both highbush and lowbush blueberry species. Their conclusion: "Regardless of the method, lowbush blueberries were consistently higher in anthocyanins, total phenolics, and antioxidant capacity, compared with highbush blueberries." Always buy them organic locally grown, of course, and never canned. The World's Healthiest Foods reports a study in the *Journal of Food Chemistry* that found that anthocyanins were nearly *undetectable* in canned foods and suggests this may be due to their unique chemical structure that causes them to become unstable at a neutral pH. However, organic freeze-dried powder (that includes pulp) and frozen (freezing stops the nutrient loss) are as good or better than what we call fresh (stored and trucked after harvest). Hand-picked and quickly eaten blueberries remain your healthiest option. Please see our web site for recommended resources on this and other foods in this book.

PURPLE CABBAGE

Old ORAC: 105 (white cabbage tested)
(Serving size: 1/2 cup)
New ORAC: TAC: 2359 (Total Antioxidant Capacity)—Red (purple)
(Serving size: 75 grams or approximately 1/3 of a cup)
TRAC: same

GI: 10 GL: 2 Serving size: 1 cup (70 grams)

EWG Ranking: 36

Research has focused on the green and so-called red cabbage variety. But, most cabbage labeled as red is actually purple in hue, which will be the focus of this discussion. Purple cabbage has much denser clusters of important anthocyanins than the green variety. Cornell University scientists compared the phytochemical content in 100 grams of red cabbage to that of the green variety (also known as white). They found that red cabbage contained 190 milligrams per 100 grams of polyphenols and an incredible 23 versus 0.01 milligrams of anythocyanin. Research published in the *LWT—Food and Science Technology*, 2006 (the official journal of the Swiss Society of the Food Science and Technology and the International Union of Food Science and Technology) based on a study conducted by Cornell's Ho Jin Heo and Chang Yong Lee (*Food Science and Technology*, "Phenolic phytochemicals in cabbage inhibit amyloid protein-induced neurotoxicity," Volume 39, Issue 4, May 2006, Pages 331–337) found that that the total amount of active antioxidants found in red cabbage was six to eight times greater than that found in white cabbage. They also found that regular consumption of red cabbage may help protect us against degenerative diseases of the brain. And that it's capable of substantially reducing plaque in the brain, which may cause Alzheimer's disease.

According to Heo and Lee, "The phenolics from red cabbage significantly blocked a beta-induced toxicity in a dose-dependent manner (greater than 600 micrograms per millilitre), while white cabbage showed lower activity. Additional consumption of vegetables such as red cabbage may help increase the chemo-preventive effects in neurodegenerative diseases such as Alzheimer's."[14] Once again studies appear to support the fact that the anthocyanins found in red cabbage evolved to protect it against oxidation and heavy metal contamination (respectively), which appears to be of similar value to us when incorporated into our own line of defense.

Several studies have isolated compounds that evolved to protect cabbage against a variety of fungal infections. Lab studies reveal that sulforaphanes in cabbage are truly effective in preventing various types of cancer from developing in animals. By stimulating the production of beneficial enzymes that prevent tumor growth, sulphoraphanes have been shown to decrease the development of tumors in the breast by as much as 40 percent!

An important source of indoles, the indole-3-carbinol (known as I3C) found in cabbage has been shown to favorably alter estrogen levels. This may explain their potential role in reducing cancer rates, particularly cancers of the breast in women. In animal studies, I3C has been shown to interfere with the binding activity of aflatoxins to DNA, a precursor to tumerogenesis.

In addition, cabbage's glucosinolates are metabolized by your body into powerful anticarcinogens known as "isothiocyanates." *Plants contain substances that evolved to contain sulfur to protect them.* This sulfur is derived from glucosinolates. They impart the bitter or sharp taste to cabbage and other cruciferous vegetables that you're familiar with.

Other key foods in this color category include bilberries, black currants, black mulberries, black horseradish, boysenberries, elderberries, purple asparagus, purple Belgium endive, purple figs, purple grapes, and purple peppers. Although purple-fleshed potatoes are also part of this food group, they are not a recommended food. Nor are eggplant, raisins, and prunes (the latter two due to their high sugar content).

RED IS RIGHT

This group of antioxidants improves and protects vision, reduces the risk of prostate and other cancers, guards against urinary infection, helps neutralize environmental carcinogens, and reduces the risk of stroke and heart disease. This color family is the key contributor of antioxidant beta-carotene and lycopene, as well as ellagiac acid and anthocyanins. Characteristically high in vitamin C, certain members of this group contain other important, harder-to-find antioxidants, such as resveratrol; a powerful, incredibly protective antibiotic produced by certain plants in response to attack by pathogens. Nature provides plants with the ability to produce this and other agents, known as phytoalexins, that are toxic to these invading fungi and bacteria. Also found in the skin of red grapes, it's one of the components of red wine that provides you with important protection as well. Certain family members such as cranberries contain proanthocyanidins (PACs) that prevent E. coli and other bacteria from adhering to the wall of the urinary tract. This appears to reduce urinary tract infections by interfering with the ability of many threatening forms of bacteria as they adhere to the bladder cells, which form the epithelial. Their anti-adhesion property may also inhibit the bacteria associated with gum disease and stomach ulcers.

The family members of the red-pigmented color group contain strong biodense nutrients that can help protect against prostate cancer and heart disease. Beta-carotene may also reduce the risk of other cancers and heart disease and is an important contributor to ocular health.

POMEGRANATES

No or new ORAC, GI or EWG testing data available

GL: 10

Serving size: 1 Pomegranate

EWG Ranking: Not ranked

Caution: Well-tolerated in most humans, it's possible for dogs to damage their nervous system by consuming the fruit.

The pomegranate bush or small tree produces one of the oldest and most fascinating foods known to man. Its beautiful ornamental fruit, often used for decorative centerpieces, contains juicy, red, glistening seeds called "arils." These ruby-like kernels are tucked into paper thin sacks or membranes. Their slender skins are easily discarded, exposing a tiny treasure chest of arils bursting with enzymes, antioxidants, and other hard-to-find nutrients. The mysterious healing properties of pomegranates have only just begun to unravel. One of the first cultivated foods in the history of mankind, some scholars suggest it was actually a pomegranate, not an apple, that Eve plucked from the Garden of Eden. The confusion is understandable. Its name itself is derived from the Latin syllables pomum ("apple") and granatus ("seeded").

Dating back to nearly 2000 BC, this mysterious fruit is mentioned no less than nineteen times in the Bible. Cultivated before the time of Moses, Jewish tradition holds that a pomegranate has 613 seeds, which correspond to each of the 613 commandments (referred to mitzvoth) in the Torah. The Persians believed that the seed of this fruit made their warriors invincible on the battlefield.

JEWISH TRADITION HOLDS THAT A POMEGRANATE HAS 613 SEEDS, WHICH CORRESPOND TO EACH OF THE 613 COMMANDMENTS.

According to the Pomegranate Council, pomegranate trees do well in a hot, dry climate with little or no care. The pomegranate bush (considered by some to be a small tree) is arguably one of the most beautiful plants on earth. With its early roots throughout the Mediterranean, Iran, and the Himalayas, the pomegranate's global habitat has expanded. Today, they're found in the South Pacific Rim, parts of Africa, as well in the more arid parts of California and Arizona. In fact, the largest commercial production in the world is now based in California's San Joaquin Valley.

Only now are we rediscovering the incredible healing power of this ancient fruit; knowledge that had been seemingly lost in time. While the recommendations made in this book are principally confined to solid foods, pomegranates and orange juice (for quite the opposite reason) are exceptions. Juice has a great deal of sugar—natural sugar and often added sugar. You've learned by now that sugar is pretty bad stuff. So is cancer—and cancer loves sugar. But pomegranates are just plain difficult to eat and are quite tart. Fortunately, sweet cultivars continue to be developed that are not as sour as the original fruit. But for those of you who are determined to eat them as nature intended, the Pomegranate Council offers this advice: "Cut off the crown, then cut the pomegranate in half, then place the section in a bowl of water, then roll out the arils (juice sacs) with your fingers, discard everything else, strain out the water, then eat the succulent arils whole, seeds and all." By the way, the French were so taken by the scattering of the pomegranate seeds themselves, and the size and shape of the fruit, that they named their hand thrown explosives "grenades"(the French name for pomegranates) in honor of this fruit.

If you have the fortitude to do all of this, I believe you'll be rewarded. But for those of us that don't, just drink *a little*. No more than one ounce of pomegranate juice (PJ) at night occasionally (no more than a couple of times weekly), along with one ounce of pure unsweetened organic cranberry juice. Add four ounces of spring water with lemon (always rinse your mouth with water after eating lemon before bedtime) and one teaspoon (eventually graduating to a tablespoon) or more of psyllium husk (which we'll discuss in more detail shortly), depending on your tolerance for this amazing source of fiber. The small amount of sugar (a good portion will be absorbed by the psyllium) is more than offset by the treasure of nutrients you'll discover in this simple drink. (Note: too much psyllium or excessive ancillary consumption of any fiber is not recommended).

My favorite variation of this drink:

1 ounce of R.W. Knudsen Blueberry Pomegranate juice
(about 33 calories)

1 ounce of pure unsweetened organic cranberry juice

4   ounces of spring water with lemon

1   teaspoon of psyllium husks (you can gradually increase this
    to an amount that is right for you)

Always top with husks or you'll be bottom fishing for them. Please make sure you drink this before you brush your teeth, not after, because again, the citric acid in lemon can corrode tooth enamel.

The benefits of a small amount of pomegranate juice are staggering. The nitric oxide in pomegranates may be a natural way to enhance penile erection. Research, such as the work of Aviram et al. *(2001, Atherosclerosis 158; 195–198,* "Pomegranate juice consumption inhibits serum angiotensim-converting enzyme activity and reduces systolic blood pressure") and others, has consistently shown that pomegranates as well as the consumption of pomegranate juice relaxes blood vessel, improving the flow of blood to the heart and other important organs.

> THE NITRIC OXIDE IN POMEGRANATES MAY BE A NATURAL WAY TO ENHANCE PENILE ERECTION.

Pomegranate juice also enhances the biological action of other nutrients and cofactors while stopping the body's destruction of nitric oxide. Researchers L. J. Ignarro and colleagues at the David Geffen School of Medicines Department of Molecular and Medical Pharmacology (*Nitric Oxide*, September 2006, Volume 15, Issue 2, Pages 93–102): "Pomegranate juice protects nitric oxide against oxidative destruction and enhances the biological actions of nitric oxide." Researchers found pomegranate juice to be a potent inhibitor of super oxide anion-mediated disappearance of nitric oxide, which is significantly more potent than blueberry juice, grape juice, red wine, or even ascorbic acid.

Johns Hopkins cardiologist Charles J. Lowenstein, MD, and his team reported that results showed this fruit's amazing ability to inhibit inflammation in endothelial cells that line blood vessels (*Cell*, 2003).

Many researchers have begun to tout pomegranate juice's ability (particularly its high content of punicalagins) to protect us against several cancers such as cancer of the prostate. A broader body of research is required on large human populations before we definitively conclude this. But it is fair to say that the research that has been done is quite encouraging.

In a recent study by scientists at UCLA based on a subset of forty-eight male prostate cancer victims (*Clinical Cancer Research,* July, 2006 Vol. 12, 4018–4026,

"Phase II Study of Pomegranate Juice for Men with Rising Prostate-Specific Antigen following Surgery or Radiation for Prostate Cancer"), all had rising PSA levels after surgery. Prostate Specific Antigen (PSA) is a protein enzyme produced by the cells within the prostate gland and secreted into seminal fluid, according to the Northern Institute of Urology. It's an important biomarker that alerts physicians to the probability and early detection of prostate cancer. Researchers wanted to test the effectiveness of regular PJ consumption on what's known as "doubling time," or the time it normally takes for PSA levels to double. The subjects were required to drink 8 ounces of PJ daily for two years.

The results were astonishing. 80 percent of the subjects experienced a whopping 350 percent jump or more in PSA doubling time, from a mean baseline of 15 months to 54 months! This suggested PJ's ability to substantially impede a rapid progression of residual cancer. They also discovered that when they injected prostate cancer cells in vitro from the blood of these men after this treatment, cell apoptosis skyrocketed, and cell growth plummeted. Here too more expansive studies are warranted. But sufficient evidence supports the value of this important carbohydrate.

Enjoy the tremendous benefits of this ancient fruit, a fruit so beautiful that a pair of decorative silver pomegranates adorn and protect the two upper wooden handles of the Torah, arguably the most important book of teachings in the history of Judaism. A fruit so powerful that it has been shown to actually reduce anti-inflammatory LDL oxidation, arteriolosclerosis, heart disease, and perhaps even cancer, while promoting nitric oxide production and penile erection. The latter just may have something to do with why Eve chose it over an apple in the Garden of Eden.

WATERMELON

Old ORAC: 100
Serving size: 3.5 ounces
New ORAC: TAC: 216 (Total Antioxidant Capacity)
Serving size: 1 cup diced
TRAC: same as above
GI: 72 GL: 3
EWG Ranking: 31

One of the most fascinating foods I've studied, watermelon, is *both* a fruit by definition, as well as a vegetable. From a botanical perspective, it's the ripened ovary of a seed plant, making it technically a fruit. But it's also a cucurbitaceae plant family of gourds, classified as citrullus lantus (Maynard, 2001), and planted from a seed like a pepper, pumpkin, cucumber, or tomato, raised and harvested like other vegetables. More than 1200 different varieties are grown throughout the world to provide us with one of nature's ultimate miracle foods. The amazing watermelon is as close to a perfect food as we get—high in fiber, low in calories, with over 40 percent *more* lycopene than a tomato, according to USDA researchers. And its phytochemical citrulline gets converted to arginine, which helps to relax constricted vessels, promoting greater blood flow (men out there, listen up!). According to Dr. Bhimu Patil, director of Texas A&M's Fruit and Vegetable Improvement Center in College Station (Texas A &M Ag news and Public Affairs, June 30, 2008; "Watermelon May Have Viagra-Effect: Secrets of Phyto-nutrients Are Being Unraveled"), "The citrulline-arginine relationship helps heart health, the immune system, and may prove to be very helpful for those who suffer from obesity and type 2 diabetes. Arginine boosts nitric oxide, which relaxes blood vessels, the same basic effect that Viagra has, to treat erectile dysfunction and maybe even prevent it," he added.

A watermelon steak (sliced with olive oil and lightly grilled) handily trumps cooked tomatoes' bio-available lycopene (the now infamous and much touted antioxidant). Research has shown that watermelon has a whopping 40 percent more of this purported anticarcinogen and important cardiovascular nutrient. So, why haven't we heard about this before? Processors of powdered lycopene and lycopene supplements have found it far easier to extract lycopene from a tomato than from the juice or rind of watermelon. Extracting it this way is the cheapest and most preferred way for processors.

Most supplements touting lycopene are of minimal value as a bio-available source of this important chemical compound, particularly if they're synthetic. I was unable to find any significant research that shows that isolated lycopene, unheated, affords the type of protection provided by consuming the whole food. In order for us to properly absorb, metabolize, and maximize the potential of lycopene from food, a fruit or vegetable must release it. And the most efficient way to do so is by heating it. In a discussion appearing in *The Journal of Clinical Nutrition* (2000), Dr. Lenore Arab tells us why: "You have to break down the cell wall and the chromoplast; without that, lycopense is in a crystalline structure. Then, before it can be absorbed, it has to be in a lipid form. So actually it has to be extracted from the food matrix."

Heating does just that. And cooking oil dissolves it and helps shuttle it into the bloodstream by facilitating absorption, according to Harvard Health University researchers. If it's not broken down properly and absorbed, the lycopene in tomatoes is of minimal value. But cooked tomatoes rock. And watermelon rocks even harder. Heat breaks down this tightly bound substance releasing wonderful flavor, particularly when char-grilled. It's been shown to have a good deal of bio-available lycopene even when eaten cold (unlike tomatoes).

MOST SUPPLEMENTS TOUTING LYCOPENE ARE OF MINIMAL VALUE AS A BIO-AVAILABLE SOURCE OF THIS IMPORTANT CHEMICAL COMPOUND, PARTICULARLY IF THEY'RE SYNTHETIC.

Watermelon has gotten a bit of a bad rap since the advent of the GI index, but the punishment never fit the crime. While watermelon has a GI of 72 and the sugar from this carbohydrate can theoretically enter your bloodstream fast, it won't. Watermelon is 93 percent water, which actually makes it among the lowest carbohydrate counts of any fruit or vegetable. If you brush it with EVOO, the GI is even lower. While we know a GL under 10 is low, watermelon's GL is an *incredibly* low 4 grams for a 120-gram serving.

Mounting evidence further suggests that oral health may rapidly improve from regular exposure to moderate amounts of lycopene. In a study, even leukoplakic lesions of the mouth, the most common form of oral precancerous sores, disappeared from regular yet minimal exposure (only 8 milligrams a day) to watermelon's powerful lycopene (*Journal of Oral Oncology*, July 2004). This was accomplished in only three months. To put this feat in perspective, only a cup and a half of watermelon contains approximately 10 to 12 milligrams of lycopene.

Researchers further found that blood plasma concentrations of lycopene were just as high for those consuming watermelon juice (which was not heated), when compared to those that drank tomato juice that was heated. According to chemist Alison J. Edward, and nutritionist Beverly A Clevidence, of The USDA's Agriculture Research Services (ARS) Phytonutrients Laboratory (note the word "phytonutrients" used by this government agency) who conducted the study (*Agricultural Research*, June, 2002; "Watermelon Packs a Powerful Lycopene Punch"), it didn't matter if the subjects received 40 milligrams or 20 milligrams. The blood plasma concentration of lycopene remained the same. So, not only is there *substantially more* lycopene in watermelon than tomatoes, but it's far more bio-available. Watermelon is also a terrific source of vitamin C and A, as well as important B vitamins, such as B6 and thiamin.

As with all fruits and vegetables, it's important to purchase them whole and not sliced. Watermelon is no exception. It loses lycopene and other nutrients when cut and refrigerated. According to a study by the U.S. Department of Agriculture (*Journal of Agricultural Food and Chemistry*, August, 2006), storing watermelon at room temperature actually increases lycopene content 11 to 40 percent and its beta-carotene a whopping 50 to 139 percent, compared to eating it on the vine. "What we found was very surprising," said study author Penelope Perkins-Veazie, a plant physiologist at the USDA Agricultural Research Services' South Central Agricultural Research Laboratory in Lane, Oklahoma. "The amount of lycopene in watermelons went up about an average of 20 percent when we left them out uncut at room temperature, while beta-carotene actually doubled," she said.

> AS WITH ALL FRUITS AND VEGETABLES, IT'S IMPORTANT TO PURCHASE THEM WHOLE AND NOT SLICED. WATERMELON IS NO EXCEPTION.

So buy your watermelon whole and store it at room temperature for several days. Just slice, brush with EVOO, and lightly grill. It could save your life.

TOMATOES

Old ORAC: 195
Serving size: 3.5 ounces = 0.435 of a cup
New ORAC: TAC: (Total Antioxidant Capacity) = 552 (cooked)
Serving size: 1/2 cup
TRAC: same as above
GI: So low that no test data was available other than negligible
GL: 2
EWG Ranking: 29

Cooked tomatoes may be one of the healthiest foods you can eat. Even though lightly cooked watermelon tops them for bio-available lycopene, tomatoes are a close runner-up. There may be an even better choice in the end, in a way, based on the availability of a number of such a wide variety of tomato-based foods.

I frequently eat both watermelon steak and lightly cooked tomato and garlic, both topped with EVOO. Tomatoes are easy to cook along with other carbohydrate foods that collectively enhance its power. According to Dr. Edward Giovannuci of the Harvard School of Public Safety (*Journal of the National*

Cancer Institute, Vol. 94, No. 5, March 6, 2002; "A prospective Study of Tomato Products, Lycopene, and Prostate Cancer Risk"), men can enjoy a *35 percent decreased risk of prostate cancer* by simply eating two or more servings of tomato products per week. Organic ketchup is also an easy addition to any diet.

But there's a lot more nutrient value in the tomato than lycopene. Though watermelons contain large amounts of vitamin C (one cup contains almost 15 milligrams), a single cup of tomatoes has more than twice that amount (almost 35 milligrams). The *tamarillo* red variety (also known as the tree tomato) boasts even more. You can purchase these oval-shaped tomatoes year round at many food stores. Somewhat bitter, they are best enjoyed cooked, as they should be. Quite perishable, tomatoes quickly soften after they're picked from vines where they were permitted to ripen and mature. There is nothing quite like vine-ripened tomatoes. Many of us still enjoy this wonderful food the way nature intended us to, by growing our own, or purchasing them from local farm stands.

But for the rest of us, tomatoes are bought in grocery stores after traveling over 1,500 miles. They're picked before they're ripe to avoid bruising in transit. Then they're gassed with ethylene spray to help them mature off the vine. They can now hitchhike across the country, artificially ripening as they go. By the time they hit your grocery counter, they've been primped, gassed, trucked, stored, and refrigerated. All of this is done to assist them in appearing firm, ripe, and ready for your consumption.

Today, the average American eats almost two pounds of tomatoes or tomato-based products per week. Though encouraging, consider that it's a little more than double the one pound a week we consume of high fructose corn syrup. A growing body of evidence suggests that regular consumption of real tomato-based products is far more effective than getting your lycopene from a supplement. Coupled with the need for heat and oil to maximize availability and absorption, supplements containing lycopene are a far less effective way to boost immunity to cancer and other disease. Research indicates the role of other nutrients found in tomatoes that may be activated by lycopene, which enhances its ability to protect against prostate cancer.

In 2007, the *Journal of Cancer Research* published the results of a study led by University of Illinois' Professor of Food Science and Human Nutrition, John W. Erdman, Jr., in support of these findings. A powder made from whole tomatoes and another made from whole broccoli were fed to tumor-induced rats. Researchers sought to compare the effectiveness of whole food extracts on prostate tumor progression versus supplementation of the isolated yet active form found in supplements, and to measure the effectiveness of tomatoes in conjunction with another important carbohydrate.

The *combined* whole food powders of broccoli *and* tomato resulted in an amazing 52 percent reduction in tumor weight when measured after just 22 weeks. The broccoli powder alone shrunk tumors by 42 percent, and the tomato powder by 34 percent. But the isolated active lycopene supplement only shrank tumors by 7 percent and 18 percent respectively, depending on the two dosages that were given. Researchers concluded that the whole food powders made from tomato or broccoli were far more effective than supplements of lycopene alone. It's another example of combining foods *synergistically* to increase their immune boosting capacity.

> THE COMBINED WHOLE FOOD POWDERS OF BROCCOLI AND TOMATO RESULTED IN AN AMAZING 52 PERCENT REDUCTION IN TUMOR WEIGHT WHEN MEASURED AFTER JUST 22 WEEKS.

Of course, *both* whole foods contain many other important bioactive compounds. Tomatoes, for example, contain other proven cancer-fighting nutrients such as quercetin, folate, and other carotenoids, as well as vitamins K, E, and C, and fiber. Broccoli also contains important potentially bio-available plant compounds found in cruciferous plants known as glucosinolates. Two of these, sulphoraphane and indole-3-carbinol, can be hydrolyzed into metabolites with known anticarcinogenic activity. Broccoli is also loaded with other important nutrients such as potassium, folate, vitamins A, C, and E, and harder-to-find vitamins K and selenium. Selenium activates an antioxidant enzyme called glutathione peroxidase. Discovered in 1957 by Gordon C. Mills, its main biological role is to protect the organism from oxidative stress.

Dr. Giovannucci also found that men who regularly ate ten or more servings of tomatoes (or tomato-based foods) per week *reduced their risk of prostate cancer by an amazing 45 percent!* (*Journal of the National Cancer Institute*, March 6, 2002 Vol. 94, No. 5, 391–398). While red tomatoes contain lycopene (and vine ripened contain far more than those picked green, then gassed to maturity, trucked, stored, and shelf ripened), research shows that cooking tomatoes more than *doubles* its bio-availability. The *heat* breaks down the cell wall of the tomato.

Cooking with a small amount of fat or oil more than *triples* our ability to absorb this important cancer fighting carotenoid, as previously discussed.

Researchers Unlu et al. (Carotene absorption from salads and salsa is enhanced by the addition of avocado or avocado oil, *(Journal of Nutrition,* 135, 431–436) have shown that those eating salads with this healthy fat received *seven times* more alpha-carotene, *fifteen times* more beta-carotene and *five times* more lutein, than those who ate salad without it. This supported work done in earlier smaller studies conducted by Brown et al. (*American Journal of Clinical Nutrition;* 80, 396–403; Carotenoid bioavailability is higher from salads ingested with full fat than with fat reduced salad dressings as measured with electrochemical detection) which showed that subjects eating salads with fat free dressing received minimal amounts of lycopene and carotenes in their blood. It's as true with tomatoes as it is with all fruits and vegetables. Healthful fat significantly enhances our ability to *absorb* their important nutrients.

Research suggests it may also protect us against certain cancers and heart disease. Combining powerful Super-Nutrients such as those found in cooked tomatoes and broccoli enhances their ability to combat tumerogenesis. Clearly, the whole tomato (the entire fruit, not the whole *plant*—the leaves and stems are actually poisonous) and tomato-based products are an important part of our "self-defense." As is our next super-food, the cranberry.

CRANBERRIES

Old ORAC: 1750
Serving Size: 3.5 ounces = 0.433 of a cup
New ORAC: TAC: (Total Antioxidant Capacity) = 8983
Serving size: 1 cup
New TRAC: 2698
Serving size: 1/3 cup
GI: 64
GL: 19 EWG Ranking: Not tested/listed

One of only three fruits native to North America (the other two are blueberries and Concord grapes), Native American Indians discovered the importance of this fruit long before the Pilgrims arrived at Plymouth Rock. According to the Wisconsin State Cranberry Growers Association, these inventive people developed unique applications for this natural resource that went well beyond their role as a staple in their diet. From brewed cranberry poultices used to draw the poisons out of animal wounds, to a unique source of red dye for their blankets and rugs, the Indians were onto something long before the rest of us. But it was the Pilgrim's name for these berries that ended up sticking over time. "Crane berries," the name they gave them due to the plant's resemblance to the head, neck, and beak of a crane, was eventually replaced with the abridged version we know today as the "cranberry."

Cranberries have a proven anti-adhesion ability that can prevent urinary tract infections by stopping harmful bacteria from clinging to cell walls. In 1994, a Harvard study (*Nutrition Review*, May 1994;52(5):168—70, "Cranberry juice reduces bacteriuria and pyuria in elderly women") of elderly women showed that those who drank just over a glass a day (300 mL) enjoyed a 58 percent reduction in these infections. Several compounds in cranberry juice acidify your urine. This includes hippuric acid, an antibacterial agent not normally found in human beings that reduces the ability of dangerous bacteria to adhere to the walls of the urinary tract. E. Coli, which is responsible for more than 80 percent of urinary tract infections, simply can't hang on and are carried away in the urine before they can create infection.

> CRANBERRIES HAVE A PROVEN ANTI-ADHESION ABILITY THAT CAN PREVENT URINARY TRACT INFECTIONS BY STOPPING HARMFUL BACTERIA FROM CLINGING TO CELL WALLS.

Researcher and oral surgeon Dr. Hyun Koo and his colleagues at New York University's Rochester Medical Center (*FEMS Microbiology Letters*, 2006;257(1):50–6, "Inhibitory effects of cranberry polyphenols on formation and acidogenicity of Streptococcus mutans biofilms") found that cranberry juice had a similar anti-adherence effect in the mouth, disarming the ability of pathogens to stick to tooth enamel. They also found that cranberry juice interfered with the enzymes known as "glucosyltransferases" required by certain bacteria to form a sticky bio-film providing the foundation for the building blocks of plaque. Once this film is in place, bacteria actually have a roof over their heads, a safe but sticky haven where they can hang out while they produce acid as they catch and process sugar.

Not surprisingly, pure cranberry juice can significantly reduce tooth decay, and Koo hopes to create natural toothpaste to isolate these compounds. While many of us have heard of the effect of cranberry juice on bacteria in the urinary tract, we've also been told that other tannin-rich foods such as grape juice, dark chocolate, and green tea are capable of bestowing these same virtues. Though red wine was not part of this study, its grape content is purportedly responsible for producing this antibacterial effect.

Additional research shows that other unique compounds found in cranberry juice, such as quinic acid (usually eliminated from the body within twelve hours), produces a slightly acidic effect in the urine, which appears to prevent the formation of kidney stones. Most of the oncological studies, particularly in the area of ovarian cancer, were performed on cancer cells *in vitro*. But the powerful action of phenolic compounds in cranberry juice and its ability to protect us in many other important areas is less than clear. Most of this protection is conferred with a daily dose of just 8 ounces of cranberry juice per day. If you decide to do so, drink two glasses filled evenly with 4 ounces of organic cranberry juice and 4 ounces of water. Adding a dash of psyllium fiber and a squirt of fresh lemon will slow the rate its fructose is absorbed in your liver.

There are other equally delicious and important red carbohydrates. Beets contain more iron than spinach and are loaded with boron, a mineral that plays an important role in the production of human sex hormones. But studies that support its ability to elevate estrogen are inconclusive and evidence actually contradicts their ability to do so. There are also better sources of iron from carbohydrates, such as pumpkin seeds and black beans. It's important to note that the best source of available iron is found in the hemme form found in animal protein. Vegetable sources contain the less available non-hemme variety. That's why vegetarian diets often require moderate supplementation of iron.

As much as I enjoy the flavor of beets, their high sugar content should be reason enough for any diabetic to avoid them. While further research may support their alleged power to protect the body against calcium and magnesium loss, enhance cognitive functioning, bolster the immune system, and normalize the metabolism of cells, most of the current research is based on small study groups, or animals, or is anecdotal. Their high content of betaine, which is responsible for their vivid color, has also been shown to protect the body against certain cancers.

My grandfather Harry drank borsht, a drink containing beets and many other powerful nutrients to relieve his indigestion and constipation. I loved Grampa Harry and his borsht, and believe beets have redeeming health value that's yet to be explored.

But given the research available at the time of this writing, the most compelling reason to eat beets is their high fiber content (a small beet has approximately 1.6 grams of soluble fiber)—and because they taste great.

As far as Grampa Harry, he passed away still complaining about gas and indigestion. The bottle of borsht was not far away, which may not be the best testimonial for the borsht industry. But I think it would have been worse for Grampa Harry had it not been for the borsht. Harry was a very bright guy.

Other important red fruits and vegetables include: blood oranges, cherries (an important source of dietary melatonin, quercetin, and other anti-inflammatory enzymes), currants, guava (a good source enzyme that clobbers free radical "singlet oxygen," a highly destructive free radical that reacts destructively when combined in the normal metabolic process with polyunsaturated fat), kidney beans (for heart health, fiber, its ability to stabilize blood sugar, and more), papayas (avoid if you have an allergy to latex; they contain substances called chitinases that precipitate latex-fruit allergy syndrome), pink grapefruit (contains important tumor inhibiting limonoids, an enzyme that reduces the likelihood of tumor formation by increasing the production of the powerful detoxifying glutathione-S-Transferase), radichio, radishes, red apples (prostate health from their flavonoids, respiratory health, and more), red beans, red grapes, red mulberries (a great source of both resveratrol, a cancer preventing compound, as well as anthocyanins), red onions (loaded with important antioxidants such as quercetin and other anti-inflammatory sulpher-based compounds), red pears, red peppers, red-skinned potatoes (if you must), and strawberries (the conventionally grown are heavily laden with pesticides, according to the EWG).

THE GREENER THE GREATER

ASPARAGUS

Old ORAC: Not measured/listed
New ORAC: TAC (Total Antioxidant Capacity) = 2021
Serving size: 1/2 cup
TRAC: same
GI: 15
GL: 3
EWG Ranking: 39

If you want a healthy low-calorie food that actually has the ability to protect your DNA, that contains lots of hard-to-find B9 (100 grams contains a mere 24 calories but a whopping 1/3 or 149 milligrams of the B9 required daily), *asparagus* is it! B9 is particularly important for pregnant women. A deficiency of B9 can cause the crippling spinal birth defect known as spina bifida. A good source of free radical scavenger quercetin, asparagus packs a healthful wallop, including its ability to relieve your kidneys and tissues of excess water. But if you're consuming it to help detoxify your gastrointestinal tract, be sure you don't hang out with your significant others. Asparagus contain a potent, smelly, sulfur compound that can make you gasp for fresh air when it's eliminated in your urine.

Other green vegetables include amaranth greens, known as "Chinese spinach." Avoid them if you have a kidney disorder, gout, or arthritis. Its high oxalates inhibit the absorption of zinc and calcium. The same doesn't appear to be the case for grain amaranth. According to researchers Gelinas et al. of McGill University's Department of Plant Science (*Journal of Agriculture and Food Chemistry*, 55 (12), 4789–4794, 2007), the insoluble form contains extremely high concentrations of calcium and magnesium that offset the absorbability of the oxalates.

AVOCADO
Old Orac: 782
Serving Size: 3.5 oz
New Orac: TAC: 3344
Serving Size: 1 fruit
TRAC: (Total Realistic Antioxidant Capacity):
Serving size: 1/2 avocado
GI: 0
GL: 1
EWG: 44

You've already learned a lot about one of our favorite foods. While their total antioxidant capacity is topped by some other foods, it's the *type* of activity you want to focus on here. They topple all other fruits and vegetables for lipid soluble antioxidant activity. Those that are conventionally grown are tied for first place with onions, as foods containing the lowest amount of contamination from pesticides. Always seek to buy organically grown foods. They'll be far more nutrient dense than the trucked, conventionally grown variety.

KIWI

Old Orac: 610
Serving size: 3.5 ounces
New Orac: TAC: 698
Serving size: 1 fruit
TRAC: (Total Realistic Antioxidant Capacity):
Same as above.
GI: 53
GL: 8
EWG Ranking: 38

Native to Northern China's Yangtze River, Yang Tao (known today as kiwifruit) was first eaten by Asia's great Kahn warriors more than 700 years ago. They're one of the most nutrient dense fruits on earth. The kiwi packs almost twice as much vitamin C as a same-size orange and topples bananas as the best fruit source of potassium. Sodium-free and teeming with a wide range of nutrients, the kiwi provides heart protecting, insulin regulating, soluble fiber, as well as important insoluble fiber that may help reduce the risk of certain diseases while maintaining regularity.

Research shows that the kiwifruit offers significant protection against asthma and other respiratory diseases, while reducing the incidence of macular degeneration. Kiwifruit also ranks higher than all other fruits in *lutein*, a unique carotenoid pigment that's been linked to the prevention of cancer in the prostate and lung. Several studies have shown regular consumption of lutein is associated with a 20 percent to 50 percent lower risk of cataract disease. Moderate consumption also decreases the incidence of blood clots associated with heart disease. The protection it provides the immune system may enhance cell-mediated immune responses that allow the cell to resist tumor formation. Emerging studies suggest a potential contribution of lutein toward the prevention of heart disease and even stroke. Motahashi et al. ("A study of kiwifruit extracts," *Journal of Ethnopharmacology*, Vol. 81, No. 3:357–64. 2002) found kiwifruit to contain abundant amounts of valuable anti-cancer bioactive materials that are also pro-oxidant in high concentration and

THE KIWI PACKS ALMOST TWICE AS MUCH VITAMIN C AS A SAME-SIZE ORANGE AND TOPPLES BANANAS AS THE BEST FRUIT SOURCE OF POTASSIUM.

antioxidant at lower concentrations, and nutrients that activate tumor-specific antimicrobial activity.

A study published in *Thorax* of 18,000 children between the ages of 6 to 7 years old ("Consumption of fresh fruit rich in vitamin C and wheezing symptoms in children," April, 2000: 5(4):283-8) compared those eating 5–7 servings of kiwi to those eating less than 1 serving per week. Researchers found a 32 percent reduced incidence of shortness of breath, a 27 percent reduction in nighttime coughing, a 28 percent reduction in runny nose, and 25 percent reduction in chronic coughing. *Asthmatics showed marked improvement after eating only a couple of servings of this fruit a week.* Another study (*Plasma*, August 2004) 15 (5), 287–297 Effects of kiwifruit consumption on platelet aggregation and plasma lipids in healthy human volunteers) found that subjects enjoyed a *15 percent reduction in triglyceride*s and an 18 percent reduction in blood clot potential for those eating two to four kiwis for 28 days when compared to those who ate none.

Kiwi contains the protein-dissolving enzyme actinidin, making it a high-quality natural meat tenderizer. Rub the flesh over meat, or mash it and spread it over the side facing up. There's no need to peel a kiwi to eat it. If you can handle eating the skin, by all means do so. The seeds and skin are also an important source of nutrients and fiber. Another alternative is to simply wash the skin and drop it in your masticating blender, skin and all.

Avoid eating if you have an allergy to latex. Avoid consumption for children under the age of five. In one study done at the University of Southampton (Ref: 04/101, July 2004), 75 percent of children in this age group, but only one fifth of adults tested, experienced allergic reactions to this otherwise healthful fruit.

BROCCOLI

Old Orac: 890

Serving size: 100 grams or approximately 3.5 Ounces

New Orac: TAC: 982

Serving size: 1/2 cup cooked

TRAC: (Total Realistic Antioxidant Capacity):

Same as above.

GI: 15

GL: 8

EWG Ranking: 35

Broccoli is also a valuable source of indoles. These aromatic organic compounds inactivate dangerous estrogens that precipitate tumor pro-genesis. Sulforaphane and diindolylmethane (another compound from brassica vegetables) have recently been shown to work synergistically to inhibit cancer growth.

In 1999, the *Journal of Nutrition and Science Care* published the results of research from scientists at the Tokyo Graduate School of Agriculture showing that isothiocyanates can block the growth of melanoma skin cancer cells. Diindolylmethane, one of the stable indoles found in broccoli and other cruciferous vegetables, also promotes proper estrogen metabolism in women as well as in men by reducing harmful estrogen metabolites, while simultaneously increasing healthy estrogen metabolites.

Recently, broccoli has even been shown to protect your eye health. According to Dr. Paul Talalay, food scientist at Johns Hopkins University, these enzymes neutralize potential cancer-causing substances before they have a chance to damage the DNA of healthy cells. Talalay fed rats hearty servings of the vegetable for a few days and then exposed them to a potent carcinogen known to trigger a form of breast cancer in the animals. Broccoli-munching rats were half as likely to develop tumors as animals eating standard food, according to results published in the April 1994 proceedings of the National Academy of Science: "Even those rats that did develop cancer ended up with fewer and smaller tumors, which is an important advantage in itself," said Talalay.

As a nutritional powerhouse, broccoli is loaded with important beta-carotene and its florets contain *eight times* as much of this important nutrient as the stalk. Just one cup contains 200 percent of the RDA for vitamin C. How you cook mature broccoli greatly affects the density of its nutrients; either steam "lightly" or sauté in EVOO on low heat. *The best* way to cook broccoli and other vegetables is by lightly steaming them, since boiling them often results in a leaching of their nutrients into the water. A study published in the *Journal of the Science of Food and Agriculture* (October, 2003 Volume 83, Issue 14, Pg 1511–1516, "Phenolic compound contents in edible parts of broccoli inflorescences after domestic cooking") investigated the effects of various methods of cooking broccoli. Of all the methods of preparation, steaming caused the least loss of nutrients. Microwaving broccoli resulted in a loss of 97 percent, 74 percent, and 87 percent of its three major antioxidant compounds—flavonoids, sinapics, and caffeoyl-quinic derivatives respectively.

In comparison, steaming broccoli resulted in a loss of only 11 percent, 0 percent, and 8 percent respectively. Co-author Dr. Cristina Garcia-Viguera noted that "most of the bioactive compounds are water-soluble; during heating, they leach in a high percentage into the cooking water. Because of this, it is recommended to cook vegetables in the minimum amount of water (as in steaming) in order to retain their nutritional benefits."

I was even more intrigued by the health value of broccoli *sprouts*. Fascinating research conducted by the Johns Hopkins School of Medicine and Johns Hopkins University in Baltimore by Paul Talalay and colleagues was published in 2001 by the American Association for Cancer Research (*Cancer Epidemiology Biomarkers & Prevention*, 10:501–508, May 2001). What they found was startling. Young broccoli sprouts, sprouts that were only three days old, had a *twenty to fifty times* greater concentration of protective glucosinolates than those found in mature plants. In fact, the amount of protection decreased as the plants continued to develop. Research has shown that broccoli sprouts and their component glucosinolates and isothiocyanates induce phase 2 enzymes, which protect against chemically induced tumors. According to the scientists, on a fresh gram basis, broccoli sprouts contain *fifty times* more glucoraphanin, the glucosinolate precursor of sulforaphane, the most potent natural phase 2 enzyme-inducer known to man.

I WAS EVEN MORE INTRIGUED BY THE HEALTH VALUE OF BROCCOLI SPROUTS.

While sprouts are not a substitute for eating mature broccoli florets, they're a powerful way to alternatively receive an amazing amount of broccoli's protective anticarcinogenic bang. In fact, it's possible to obtain the exact variety of special seeds used by researchers in the study (because all seeds were not found to have the same benefit). If you wish to do so, contact the Caudill Seed Company at (800) 695-2241, according to the Brassica Protection Products Corporation. The company packages these sprouts under the brand name of BroccoSprouts™. They've obtained an exclusive worldwide license from Johns Hopkins University (who owns the patent) to market the sprouts. By design, they contain particularly high levels of glucosinolates. I plan on ordering the seed and growing the sprouts at home. Talalay's son, who now runs the company, does what he can to eat four ounces a week of his product. Maybe you should too?

BRUSSELS SPROUTS

Old Orac: 980

Serving size: 3.5 ounces

New Orac: TAC: Not listed/tested

GI: (Approx.) 15

GL: 3-raw; 5-cooked

EWG Ranking: Not tested

The mere mention of its very name may send shivers down your spine. But it's right up there with cabbage and kale as one of my favorite green family foods. My wife's terrific yet simple recipe brings out its most flavorful characteristics, even for those of you who would rather starve than eat them. For those who are allergic to onions, as I am, Kelly's brussels sprouts creation is the next best thing to mimicking the flavor of a well-done onion. Most would agree that simply boiling them falls gastronomically short, to be kind. But leading chefs have discovered what Kelly has—that adding a few choice ingredients can wake up the incredible intrinsic flavor of a brussels sprout. A surprising culinary touch that will put many a chef's creation over the top, this, as well as few other simple recipes we enjoy, are included in Chapter 7.

THE MERE MENTION OF ITS VERY NAME MAY SEND SHIVERS DOWN YOUR SPINE.

Unlike french fries, brussels sprouts do hail from their namesake, Brussels, Belgium, where they were first cultivated from wild cabbage. While their exact origin is vague, they became a popular food in northern Europe in the sixteenth century. They're classified among 3,200 species of the Brassicaceae family and are also known as being members of the Crucifier family. The word *Crucifier* itself originates in an even older name, cruciferae, which means "cross bearing." The flowers of Crucifiers contain four petals that actually fashion a cross. Despite all these species, only two of them, the B. oleracea and B. campestris, are the source of edible crops. Brussels sprouts are members of the former.

While they appear to be no more than a miniature version of cabbage, there's considerable disparity among their nutrients. In fact, *brussels sprouts have a whopping two to three times more important glucosinolates than red cabbage.* Sulforaphane, one of most potent glucosinolate phytonutrients, helps guard against active substances that are potentially carcinogenic. It does so by super-charging detoxification enzymes. When exposed to sulphurane, precancerous cellular material (created in response to environmental pollutants) and other molecules are literally derailed. Rather than spiraling into more hazardous carcinogens that molecularly divide, they become water-soluble. Through a process known as glucuronidation, sulforaphane from brussels sprouts facilitates the binding of certain hazardous material from radical cells to a substance known as "glucorinic acid." Once engaged, the process permits the easy removal of these toxic molecules from your body.

In an important animal study published in *Carcinogenis, the Worlds Healthiest Foods* (The George Mateljan Foundation), and reported by www.whfoods. com, drinking water supplemented with juice from brussels sprouts offered amazing protection against the development of both liver and colon cancer in subjects. For those of us who enjoy grilling or char-broiling meat, the power of brussels sprouts may provide important protection that just might save your life. Animals exposed to heterocyclic amine carcinogens, a by-product of barbecuing certain foods high in protein, showed a startling 41 percent to 52 percent reduction in the development of precancerous cells in the colon, and a 27 percent to 67 percent in the liver after regular consumption of its juice.

Eating brussels sprouts fights cancer in still another important way. Not only by detoxifying carcinogens, but by releasing important *singrin*, a powerful, sulfur-based compound derivative. When singrin comes in contact with an enzyme known as "myronsinase," allyl isothicynate (a highly reactive compound) is released which actually inhibits cell division, known as "mitosis." Its powerful two-prong assault on carcinogens makes this food an important ally in the prevention of several types of cancer. It also offers humans powerful protection against DNA destruction.

KALE

Old Orac: 1770
Serving size: 3.5 ounces
New Orac: TAC: Not tested
GI: Negligible. Not listed/tested.
GL: 3-raw, 4-cooked
EWG: Not tested

Contrary to popular belief, calcium from high oxalate spinach is poorly absorbed. But it's well absorbed from low oxalate kale. Kale's kaempferol, a potent flavinol, has been shown to prevent the dangerous oxidation of LDL and other harmful lipids. Not many foods have such bragging rights. And that's just the tip of the iceberg.

According to the long running and highly respected Nurse's Study, other vegetables such as broccoli sprouts, also containing important kaempferol, inhibit the development of certain cancer cells. Researchers found a remarkable 40 percent decrease in rates of ovarian cancer in women who regularly ate diets high in kaempferol-laden foods when compared to those that did not (*Science Daily*, "Flavonoid-rich Diet Helps Women Decrease Risk Of Ovarian Cancer," November, 2007).

In 2004, Huyng Hung reported in the *Journal of Cellular Physiology* ("Inhibition of estrogen receptor alpha expression and function in MCF-7 cells by kaempferol") that "breast cancer cells with kaempferol resulted in a time- and dose-dependent decrease in cell number."

Kale also helps protect your eyes against macular degeneration; not surprising, because kale contains a good dose of zeazanthin and lutein; carotenoids that appear to protect our eyes from oxidative damage caused by exposure to sunlight.

I love steamed kale with olive oil, minced garlic, sea salt, and pepper. Over 2,000 years old, this easily grown ancestor of wild cabbage is still waiting to be discovered by most Americans.

WATERCRESS

Old Orac: Not tested/listed

New Orac: TAC: Not tested/listed

GI: 0

GL: 0

EWG Rank: Not tested/ranked.

The ancient Romans and Anglos ate watercress to prevent baldness; the Greeks did so to boost their intellect; the Cretes believed it to be an aphrodisiac, and the Anglo-Saxons ate it to purify their blood. Famed statesman Francis Bacon believed it to be capable of restoring a woman's vim and vigor and youthful bloom, while herbalist John Gerard identified it as an early cure for scurvy.

In addition to its bounty of important flavonoids, one cup of raw watercress provides 106 percent of the daily value of vitamin K. This important nutrient is required for the synthesis of certain protein necessary for the coagulation, as well as anti-coagulation, of our blood. But with or without the help of watercress, a deficiency is rare.

This same 1 cup of watercress delivers an incredible 1961 mcg of lutein and zeaxanthin, carotenoids that have been found to significantly reduce the risk of wet age-related macular degeneration. This disease is the most common disorder responsible for the loss of vision in the elderly. Not surprisingly these carotenoids exist in the human body in their highest concentration in the back of the eye. There, in a specialized area of the retina called the macula, they help filter out damaging blue light; the concentration of these important carotenoids is so dense that it forms a dark yellow spot known as the macular pigment. Research has shown that a significant loss of these two natural pigments is closely associated with risk for this disease. These carotenoids protect the retina from leaky blood vessels due to the deteriorating effects of light.

... RESEARCH SHOWED THAT SMOKERS WHO REGULARLY CHEWED WATERCRESS (2 OUNCES A DAY AT INTERVALS OVER SEVERAL DAYS) WERE ABLE TO INHIBIT OXIDATION OF THE LUNG CANCER CARCINOGEN NNK.

In a 1995 study led by Hecht and his colleagues on behalf of the American Association for Cancer Research, and published in Cancer Epidemiology Biomarkers & Prevention (Vol 4, 1995), research showed that smokers who regularly chewed watercress (2 ounces a day at intervals over several days) were able to inhibit oxidation of the lung cancer carcinogen NNK. This amazing protective action came from the release of powerful phenethyl isothiocyanate (PEITC) simply by chewing it!

Further research has supported the ability of phenethyl isothiocyanate (PEITC) to induce cell apoptosis in a variety of cancer cells, including those found in the prostate (*Journal of Biological Chemistry*, 277:42, October 2002). Thankfully, a number of additional studies, many that involved large populations of subjects, have corroborated the important protection provided by dietary carotenoids.[15]

Subjects fed diets with the highest levels of lutein and zeaxanthin had a far lower risk for Age-Related Macular Degeneration (AMD) when compared to those receiving the least (5.8 milligrams a day versus only 1.2 milligrams a day). Finally, at the University of Ulster, lead researcher Ian Rowland and associates showed that eating one bowl of watercress a day provided incredible protection to the DNA in human red blood cells. A true power-food, regular consumption of this green vegetable provides tremendous health benefits supported by abundant research. But the USDA carotenoid database doesn't even list watercress in its ranking.

From a culinary perspective, watercress provides unique flavor to soups, salads, and sauces; it cleanses the pallet between courses and its mustard oil appears to stimulate circulation of your blood. Could it be that the Anglo-Saxons from ancient times were correct in their belief that watercress gave blood a boost of vitality through cleansing it? Research seems to support what the ancients knew dating back to 456 BC when Xerxes, a Persian emperor, ordered that his soldiers be given watercress to keep them healthy on long marches.

Watercress contains almost magical properties that protect us. The mysterious means by which its "compounds interact" is only beginning to unfold. It appears to have taken us thousands of years only to substantiate the claims of our ancestors.

ARTICHOKES

Old Orac: Not tested/listed
New Orac: TAC: 7904
Serving size: 1 cup (hearts)
TRAC: (Total Realistic Antioxidant Capacity): 3952
Serving size: 1/2 cup
GI: 15
GL: 3
EWG Ranking: Not tested /listed.

It's about time artichokes got their due. I enjoy artichokes, which many liken to eating crawfish; the struggle to get to the meat is worth the effort. However, it appears the majority of nutrients are in the leaves that protect it. According to ORAC researchers, the artichoke blew away all other fresh vegetables in important H-ORAC (hydrophilic [or water-based] antioxidant capacity). But the sodium in a typical artichoke is a whopping 152 milligrams. Contrast that with a serving of beans from the garden at 5 milligrams; that's about 10 to 15 percent of the daily intake we require, and I believe even less is best.

For those on a low-sodium diet, I suggest you avoid artichokes, or, simply drain them if they're canned. They're often packed in brine. From a health perspective, they're worth the effort. An excessive amount of sodium in the average American diet is one of the most damaging aspects of our food supply. Make sure you buy standard artichokes such as the globe variety that are fresh. Marinated artichokes that are jarred often contain excessive oils that are typically unhealthful. Several studies have shown artichoke leaf extract's unique ability to protect the liver. This is not surprising, because artichokes are actually the immature portion of the thistle plant. As one of the foremost foods for promoting bile flow, it enjoys unique protective status. The consumption of its leaf boosts your liver's ability to eliminate harmful toxins from your body. Ancient people used artichoke leaves as a digestive aid and recent research confirms their wisdom. A German study of 553 patients with digestive disorders (*Zeitschrift fur Allgemeinmed*, 1996; 72:1–19; "Antidyspeptic and lipid-lowering effect of artichoke leaf extract") found that 85 percent experienced significant relief. Another important study lead by Holtmann et al. had similar results. Two-hundred and forty-seven subjects with functional dyspepsia participated in the investigation (*Aliment Pharmacol Ther*, 2003;11–12:1099–105; "Efficacy of artichoke leaf extract in the treatment of patients with functional dyspepsia"). In the end, the researchers concluded that "the artichoke leaf extract tested was significantly superior to a placebo in the treatment of patients with functional dyspepsia."

Artichokes offer value to diabetics as one of the foods that actually *helps lower blood sugar* (as does garlic, onions, gooseberries, cabbage, and even vinegar) with a high content of insulin, (naturally occurring) it helps balance your blood sugar requiring less work for your pancreas.

The Jerusalem artichoke, also known as a "sunchoke," has also been helpful in balancing blood sugar, but you may be surprised to know that it's *not* an artichoke. It's actually a member of the sunflower family. It hails from Cape Cod, not Jerusalem, where it was first discovered by an explorer named Samuel de Champlain, and grown by native American Indians long before he arrived. Higher in calories and glycemic load, Jerusalem artichokes have their own share of important nutrients, but they can't hold a candle to the value of the genuine article.

THE JERUSALEM ARTICHOKE, ALSO KNOWN AS A "SUNCHOKE," HAS ALSO BEEN HELPFUL IN BALANCING BLOOD SUGAR, BUT YOU MAY BE SURPRISED TO KNOW THAT IT'S NOT AN ARTICHOKE.

Other green vegetables include arugula, bok choy, broccoli rabe, celery (high in glycation precursor galactose sugar), chinese cabbage, chard, chives, collard greens (very nutritious), cucumbers, endive, and garden cress (an easy-to-maintain perennial with great health benefit that can grow two feet tall). Garden cress can be used as a border ornamental and is an important part of India's Ayurvedic medicine that originated some 4,000 years ago. Other green foods include green apples (great if you can grow your own and avoid the pesticides; Granny Smith is your best bet), green beans, green cabbage, green grapes, and green onions (avoid green onions or take the time to wash them thoroughly; they've been associated with too many outbreaks of Hepatitis A).

Our list of green vegetables continues with green pears, leeks, lettuce, lima beans, limes, mustard greens, okra, and parsley. Parsley, another guardian of our DNA, is *loaded* with important flavonoids such as polyphenol luteolin. A team of researchers led by Ju Wei et al. (Lovelace Respiratory Research Institute, Albuquerque, NM) found that luteolin made colorectal cells and lung cancer cells more sensitive to normal cell death, and further suggested that treatment with luteolin may provide an effective method for the prevention of lung cancer (*Molecular Biology*, May 2007).

Other key green vegetables that warrant primary consideration include peas, spinach,[16] collards, mustard greens, romaine lettuce (loaded with nutrients and healthier than you might think), Swiss chard (teaming with important nutrients such as vitamin K, shown to activate osteocalcin, which supports calcium molecules and mineralization in the bone, as well as vitamin A, C, and others), and turnip greens (one of the healthiest of the healthy green vegetables).

Turnip greens are a great source of copper; those suffering from rheumatoid arthritis may benefit from its consumption. Copper is required for healthy connective tissue. Turnip greens are the leaves of the turnip plant. They're a great source of vitamin K, C, A, and more.

So what about green olives? After all, if the right kind of EVOO is so good for us, should we be chowing down on its source, the olives themselves? And aren't black olives even healthier than green? What you're about to learn may surprise you.

The first of more than 35 varieties of olives were grown in Crete as early as 3000 BC and were found in Egyptian tombs dating back to 2000 BC. That's the same time historians believe the Mount of Olives was originally planted. At the foot of the mount in Jerusalem's Kidrom Valley lies the Garden of Gethsemane. According to the New Testament, it's where Christ was betrayed by Judas, and where he and his disciples prayed together after the Last Supper. It's also believed to be the resting place of the Blessed Virgin Mary. Though botanists have found exact age dating hard to determine, some believe that eight of the trees winding down the road to Jericho were standing in the Garden at the time of Christ. Tree ring analysis was successful on a well-known olive tree on the Island of Brioni Istria in Croatia. Still producing abundant olives that continue to be used to make the highest grade oil, the tree is certified to be over 1,600 years old. The olive branch has symbolized peace and healing, and was the first sign of vegetation carried in the beak of a dove to Noah after the Deluge (Jeremiah 11:16). Cited in Homer's *Odyssey*, several were even found in the tomb of Tutankhamen. While the trees themselves may be ancient, twisted, and mangled looking, they're actually an evergreen; and the fruit is a member of the drupe family (along with coconuts, coffee beans, mangos, and pistachios).

It wasn't until 1769 that olive trees found their way to the United States, when a Franciscan missionary planted the first such tree in San Diego. Today, all olives grown in California are known as missionary olives.

Unfortunately, you can't eat green olives off the tree. They're inedible and incredibly bitter due to their high content of valuable phenolic compounds, such as their unique glycoside, oleuropein, and their powerful metabolite hydroxytyrosol (one of the most powerful of all the antioxidants). Both of these phytochemical compounds, along with the organic compound oleocanthal, collectively produce the bitter taste we find in EVOO. Good EVOO, that is. While much is lost in the pressing process (oleuropein is water-soluble, not fat-soluble, so healthy fats are lost in the oil) many of its descendent fats survive; enough to still produce that wonderfully pungent yet bitter flavor.

> UNFORTUNATELY, YOU CAN'T EAT GREEN OLIVES OFF THE TREE. THEY'RE INEDIBLE AND INCREDIBLY BITTER ...

When was the last time you tasted a bitter table olive? And why would you? They wash all of those precious bitter tasting phenols right out of them. That's right. While olives produced for oil go right to the mill, where they're pressed and separated from the bitter fruit, a very different fate awaits table olives.

While methods vary, here's a typical journey:

First, workers beat the dickens out of trees with sticks to remove them. Then they're washed, often with a great deal of pressure, and soaked in saltwater for long periods of time (from one to six months) to remove important but bitter polyphenols.

Black table mission olives are not fermented and are carefully picked to preserve their flesh. They *start out green*, as all olives do, get power washed, are soaked in saltwater, and treated with lye or chemicals if canned. Lye speeds the process along, breaks down their cell structure, and makes them uniformly mushy.

Green olives are typically firmer. They're often allowed to ferment before they're packed in brine. Some are just soaked in oil for a few months.

While some varieties of olive are naturally dark (not black as molasses like lye-soaked table olives), they turn that color when their harvest is postponed. But remember that good fats degrade from heat, light, and time. So, *darker olives typically have less healthy monounsaturated fat*, and fewer important nutrients than the greener variety. Though, the latter eventually catch up. Most are stuffed with pimentos, garlic, or one of any number of other ingredients to enhance their flavor through the use of high speed machines.

This leads the pretty table olive as a shell of the first pressed oil that's so eagerly sought after. In fact, all this brining results in a food that's off the chart with sodium. About 68 milligrams of sodium in an average-sized large olive! In my opinion their fat, relative to their nutrient and sodium content, makes most a poor choice. Stick with the right EVOO, a mission worth the effort.

The last in alphabetical order of the greens is zucchini. There's not much I can say about them. While they're a reasonably good source of potassium and carotenoids, vitamin C, A, and more, there are better sources. In fact, they're really not even a vegetable, but the swollen ovaries of the zucchini flower. Botanists don't usually regard vegetables as coming from any part of a flower (which would also, technically, knock tomatoes and peppers off the veggie list). Nutritionally, they simply don't provide much value.

YELLOW AND ORANGE FOOD

This color class contains over 600 kinds of carotenoids, that can protect you against several types of cancer and even optical degeneration, while boosting your heart health and immunity. Each of these foods provides one or more important nutrients and antioxidants. A few of them are particularly noteworthy.

My favorite member of this family, containing vision-protective lutein, is the yellow bell pepper. Though there's also plenty of lutein in corn, I'm not a big fan of this starch. It's high on the glycemic scale and I'd prefer to live without it.

Cantaloupe hails from the Italian commune of Cantalupo in Sabina near the city of Tivoli where it was first cultivated somewhere around the year 1700 AD. Most of what we know today and buy at the grocery store are actually muskmelons, *not* cantaloupes. True cantaloupes are a different species and are rarely found in the United States. Both are a terrific source of both vitamins A and C and other important carotenoids.

Lemons, another important member of this family, contain flavonol glycosides. Several studies have suggested that intake of this class of these polyphenolic compounds can stop cancerous cell division and lower your risk for heart disease. But some studies contradict each other, due in large part to confounding variables. To determine validity, Greek scientists (*British Journal of Cancer*, *89*:1255–1259, 2003) applied results of these studies against dietary information gathered in a large case-controlled study. Eight hundred and twenty subjects were women with breast cancer while another 1,548 women were in the control group. The researchers found a significant reciprocal correlation between flavone intake and breast cancer.

This conclusion was again supported with research conducted by Fink et al. (Department of Epidemiology, School of Public Health, University of North Carolina, Chapel Hill, NC) when he and colleagues investigated the impact on breast cancer from flavonoid consumption on a U.S. sample population base (*American Journal of Epidemiology*, March 2007 ;165(5):514–23,"Dietary Flavonoid Intake and Breast Cancer Risk among Woman on Long Island"). In this study, 1,434 women and 1,400 control subjects completed food frequency questionnaires regarding their average intake for the prior twelve months. The results showed that a substantial decrease in breast cancer risk was associated with flavonoid intake, which was most pronounced in postmenopausal women.

Citrus compounds called limonoids stopped neuroblastoma cells in the lab, according to research by Texas Agricultural Experiment Station scientists. Dr. Ed Harris, a biochemist and lead researcher, worked in conjunction with Dr. Bhimu Patil, a plant physiologist at the Texas A&M University-Kingsville Citrus Center in Weslaco. In a 2004 interview in *Science Daily*, Patil called citrus fruit "a vast reservoir of anti-carcinogens." In their study, limonoid extract stopped neuroblastoma cells in the lab. Lemon's kaempferol was shown to work in conjunction with other molecules to inhibit tumor growth.

While all this research shows great promise, it doesn't mean that eating lemons or drinking lemon juice will produce these same results. Isolating enough limonoids is no small task, according to Patil, because they're "present in very small concentrations." But the research is clearly promising. I predict that lemons and other citrus fruits, and in particular their compounds and pectin, will prove to be effective in the treatment and prevention of disease. Because acid helps slow the breakdown of carbohydrate into glucose, I routinely squirt a little lemon in my red wine, my water, and my "good night sweep" drink before bedtime. But due to lemon's corrosive effect on tooth enamel, again, remember to always rinse or brush your teeth following its use.

Other yellow citrus fruits include grapefruit. I prefer the ruby red over the yellow. I'm including them both here because they are such close cousins in the family of healthful carbohydrates. They're among the few foods that have been proven to actually lower pro-inflammatory LDL, as well as triglyceride levels. While yellow grapefruit was very effective, the red variety had almost *twice* the power to lower inflammatory lipids. The study was headed by Dr. Shela Gorinstein of the Hebrew University School of Pharmacy's Department of Medicinal Chemistry and Natural Products, in cooperation with Prof. Abraham Caspi, head of the Cardiology Institute at Rehovot's Kaplan Medical Center and published in an online edition of the American Chemical Society's *Journal of Agricultural and Food Chemistry.*

All participants in the study group had recently undergone coronary bypass surgery and suffered from highly elevated levels of lipids in their bloodstream (hyperlipidemia). These include LDL as well as triglycerides and other pro-inflammatories that lay the groundwork for internal inflammation. After only thirty days of eating one grapefruit per day, subjects eating the yellow variety saw their LDL drop an average of 10.7 percent. Those that ate the same amount of red grapefruit enjoyed almost twice this reduction, a significant 20.3 percent drop in pro-inflammatory LDL. The red group also enjoyed a 17 percent reduction in triglycerides, with a 5.6 percent reduction in the yellow group. There was no change in the control group.

As exciting as these results are, further studies are warranted with larger groups for even longer periods of time. But as yellow foods go, grapefruit produces a great deal of bang for the buck. I don't recommend it for everyone. Grapefruit has much greater potential than other fruits for interactions with medications and drugs. If you take any form of medication or recreational drug, ask your pharmacist if there are known interactions they suggest you avoid. For more information on this, please go to a grapefruit-drug interactions Web site at www.powernetdesign.com/grapefruit.

And, in a recent meta-analysis (*Drug Safety*; 2005;28(8):677-94. Undesirable effects of citrus juice on the pharmacokinetics of drugs: focus on recent studies) researchers Saito et al. found significant evidence to warrant that we avoid the consumption of "all" citrus juices while taking medications.

YELLOW ONIONS

Old Orac: 450
Serving size: 1 cup
New Orac: TAC: 1281 (yellow)
Serving size: 1/2 cup
TRAC: (Total Realistic Antioxidant Capacity): 641
Serving size: 1/4 cup
GI: Negligible. Not listed/tested GL: Negligible. Not listed/tested.
EWG Ranking: 45—the lowest!

The ancient Egyptians literally worshipped the onion. Its concentric circle within a circle symbolized eternal life. There were even carved onions in gold revered on altars of the gods and buried with their pharaohs. One pharaoh was all over this vegetable as much in death as he was in life. Ramses IV, a veritable onion head, simply couldn't get enough. He was buried with onions in each eyeball socket and onion skin in each nostril.

THE ANCIENT EGYPTIANS LITERALLY WORSHIPPED THE ONION. ITS CONCENTRIC CIRCLE WITHIN A CIRCLE SYMBOLIZED ETERNAL LIFE.

If the exact origin of the onion is sketchy, its old age is unquestionable. At least 5,000 years old, they appear to have existed in most or all parts of the world at the same time. The Bible refers to both garlic and onions in the diet of the Israelites in Numbers 11:15: "We remember the fish which we used to eat freely in Egypt, the cucumbers and the melons and the leeks and the onions and the garlic."

Onions are a member of the Allium family, which includes garlic, leeks, scallions, shallots, and chives. Their pungent odor and their ability to produce tears in our eyes are due to their powerful immune protecting sulfoxide, an amino acid that forms sulfonic acid. Enzymes are immediately released when the cells of an onion are cut or sliced. These combine with sulfonic acid to form another sulfur compound, a gas called "lachrymator," that combines with fluids in the eye to produce irritation in the nerve endings of your eyes. Tears are immediately produced to protect them.

Soaking an onion in water for a couple of minutes before slicing will help dilute its sulphur content. Then throw it in the freezer for a mere five to ten minutes; this will slow the action of the enzymes. Cut or slice near a flame on your stove top (not too close, of course) or a burning candle (always keep a candle on a glass surface for safety), which will help burn away the irritating vapor. Finally, breathe through your nose (not your mouth) as you slice. Nature gives all of its creatures various means of protection. The gas released by the enzymatic action of an onion cell is only one of their many incredible natural defenses. Even their saponins can be toxic to fish–but not to you.

Remember, in addition to the nutritive soup from its vitamins, minerals, and other phytonutrients, and the manner in which they interact, when you eat an onion you're eating all of its own natural protective compounds. To the extent they are available, active, and absorbable, you're dousing yourself with their powerfully protective phytochemical soup. A large body of research suggests exactly that.

Considered a rich source of the flavonoid and powerful antioxidant quercetin, studies show that the properties of the onion's constituents rapidly assimilate into blood plasma after they're eaten. Studies show that the more pungent the variety, the greater the level of important flavonoids. Western variety *yellow* onions contain *eleven times* the amount of these important molecules than either the white or red variety, and several times the amount of powerful quercetin. In fact, white onions were shown to have only small amounts of quercetin.

But don't throw your red onions into the pharaoh's crypt just yet. Research conducted by Anna Maria Nuutila and colleagues of VTT Biotechnology in Finland (*Food Chemistry*, Volume 81, Issue 4, June 2003, Pages 485–493; "Comparison of antioxidant activities of onion and garlic extracts by inhibition of lipid peroxidation and radical scavenging activity") found that red onions had more radical scavenging ability than yellow, and significantly more than garlic. They also found that the **skin of the onion that we generally peel and discard had the greatest amount of antioxidant activity.** Eating raw onions is actually healthier than cooking them, if you can tolerate it. If not, steam or lightly sauté them in a skillet with EVOO, though keep in mind that some of the phytonutrients will be damaged from the heat.

A large body of published and respected research shows the almost magical ability of regular onion consumption to improve bone health and substantially reduce the risk of cancers of the esophagus, prostate, mouth, kidney, colon, larynx, and more. In a case controlled study of a large population in northern Italy, by Galeone et al. (*American Journal of Clinical Nutrition,* November

2006, Vol. 84, No. 5, 1027–1032, "Onion and garlic use and human cancer"), research showed more than an 80 percent decrease in risk for abnormal tissue growth in esophageal, pharynx, and certain other oral cancers for those that ate up to 14 servings a week, which amounts to more than a *70 percent decrease* in risk for prostate and ovarian cancer. Even the risk of renal cell carcinoma (only surgery seems to effectively eradicate this cancer at the time of this writing) plummeted by a whopping 38 percent, and breast cancer by 25 percent.

SUFFICIENT EVIDENCE EXISTS WHICH DEMONSTRATES THAT THE REGULAR CONSUMPTION OF RED AND YELLOW ONIONS CAN QUITE LITERALLY SAVE LIVES.

Amazing studies like this are so prolific that space doesn't permit us to include them. But sufficient evidence exists which clearly shows that the regular consumption of red and yellow onions can quite literally save lives. Numbers like this are hard to ignore and make eating more onions well worth the effort.

CARROTS

Old ORAC: 200
Serving size: 3.5 ounces
New ORAC: 741
Serving size: 1 raw carrot
TRAC: Same
GI: 47 GL: 4
EWG: 13

Pity the foolish veggie that even thinks it can topple the beta-carotene content found in this important food. But carrots have gotten a bad rap by more than one of the experts in the last couple of decades. The first shoe dropped when carrots were wrongfully maligned for spiking glucose, allegedly breaking down rapidly after consumption and racing into the bloodstream. One of the early victims of the often misleading glycemic index (which used a baseline measurement of foods that were far from normal realistic serving sizes as we've previously discussed), the poor carrot became a co-conspirator to everything from diabetes to obesity in one failed swoop of the GI branding iron.

Thankfully, it would later be vindicated by the glycemic load that measured the *speed* in which a normal serving size entered the bloodstream. Dr. Andrew

Weil correctly pointed out the fallacy of categorizing the carrot as a high glycemic food. In the end, an apology of sorts to the beleaguered vegetable was surely in order. (It should also be noted that Dr. Weil further woke up experts by suggesting the importance of evaluating the collective GI formed by all foods consumed at one time, rather than scoring them on the basis of a single food.) According to Weil, it's a far more accurate measurement of the affect on blood sugar; unless of course, only one food is being eaten at a time.[17]

A few Finnish studies came along several years ago investigating the role of beta-carotene's potential in reducing the incidence of lung cancer in heavy smokers. The Physician's Health Study, the PHS Beta-Carotene and Retinol Efficacy Trial (CARET), and the Alpha-Tocopherol, Beta-Carotene Cancer Prevention Study (ATBC) appeared to simultaneously show that beta-carotene was a weak-kneed vitamin that failed to lower the rates of cancer in smokers with at least a pack-a-day habit. Beta-carotene, which is converted by the body to important vitamin A, suddenly became a "bruised" vegetable. Whether or not it could protect heavy smokers had little relevance in the minds of most non-smokers. Many abandon this important nutrient believing that beta-carotene simply failed to deliver.

A 1995 study of Eiserich et al., "Dietary Antioxidants and Cigarette Smoke-Induced Biomolecular Damage, a Complex Interaction" (*American Journal of Clinical Nutrition*), shows us how certain oxidants in cigarette smoke can interfere with lipid membranes, creating both lipid peroxidation and protein oxidation. By doing so, it may also inactivate crucial protective enzymes. But what the news media failed to report was that subjects with the highest levels of beta-carotene in their blood—measured before the ATBC study and the CARET study—went on to have fewer incidences of lung cancer. And researchers only gave the participants in the study *synthetic*, isolated trans fat beta-carotene supplements (void of fiber pectin and other nutrients), which are difficult to absorb, rather than whole foods rich in this antioxidant that are bio-available and replete with other nutrients that work synergistically to empower each other.[18]

But here's the great news that grew out of these studies. It became clear that the proven protection of using whole foods such as carrots and other beta-carotene rich foods was due, at least in part, to the action of *other* important nutrients. And this is precisely the point. Our limited knowledge is rapidly expanding. Nature's foods are complex. Some are particularly blessed. And carrots are one of them.

Several studies have shown that it may be the action of ***alpha-carotene*** and other carotenes, working in conjunction with beta-carotene, that effectively protect us against oxidative damage. Both of these and other carotenes are present in carrots, while neither the alpha version nor other carotene is present in *synthetic* beta-carotene.

Dr. Michiaki Murakoshi, research manager of the Oleochemistry Research Center of the Lion Corporation in Tokyo and a researcher in the department of biochemistry at the Kyoto Prefectural University of Medicine in Japan, showed that alpha-carotene had *ten-times* the ability to suppress messenger-carrying RNA to neuroblastoma cell lines than beta-carotene did (neuroblastoma is the most common cancer found in children). Incredibly, this suppression

SEVERAL STUDIES HAVE SHOWN THAT IT MAY BE THE ACTION OF ALPHA-CAROTENE AND OTHER CAROTENES, WORKING IN CONJUNCTION WITH BETA-CAROTENE, THAT EFFECTIVELY PROTECT US AGAINST OXIDATIVE DAMAGE.

occurred within only *eighteen hours* of treatment with alpha-carotene! Their research (*Journal of the National Cancer Institute*, 1989) also showed that after messenger RNA began recovering from alpha-carotene's knockout punch, these cancer cells resumed their normal cycle.

In an interview with Dr. Richard A. Passwater, PhD ("Alpha-Carotenes and Other Carotenoids"), Murakoshi refers to the work done by Dr. P. D. Mascio and colleagues who showed that the single oxygen-quenching anti-cancer ability of *alpha-carotene is higher than that of beta-carotene.* Two distinctly different findings of how alpha-carotene helps protect us against cancer. Almost *one third* of the carotene content in a carrot comes from this important nutrient. Yet, most supplements focus on the more popular beta version, excluding the important alpha version. (Similarly, as you'll soon see, the Packer Lab identified *three different* forms of vitamin E, each with distinctly unique capabilities.) But most supplement makers, as with carotene, focus only on the one form most abundant in our bodies, failing to recognize that various forms of these important antioxidants perform incredibly different functions.

The powerful protective mechanisms found in carrots don't stop here. *Falcarinol*, a compound found in carrots, which helps protect them against fungal disease, may prove to be an important cancer fighter as well. More human studies are required. Most of the available data at the time of this writing was gathered from research on lab animals or small human studies. For example, rats suffering from precancerous tumors (*Journal of Agricultural and Food*

Chemistry, 2005) showed greater than a 30 percent decreased risk in tumor progression when they were fed a diet rich in falcarinol versus those that were not—in just eighteen weeks! Dr. Kirsten Brandt, who led the team of researchers at the University of Tyne in England and Denmark, admits to eating plenty herself. She suggests we all eat at least one small carrot a day in conjunction with other fruits and vegetables. We look forward to more persuasive data from human studies to substantiate falcarinol's ability to fight cancer. In the meantime, there's sufficient credible evidence regarding other important compounds in carrots that support its role as a super-food.

Heating carrots appears to be the best way to break down its structurally tough cell wall and release the maximum amount of its carotene and other antioxidants. Even high heating was shown to increase concentrations of antioxidants when measured—by an astonishing 34 percent (*Journal of Agricultural and Food Chemistry,* 48: 1315–1321, 2000); but I suggest lightly steaming them. More intense cooking depletes other vital nutrients.

LOADED WITH MORE BETA-CAROTENE THAN ALL OTHER VEGETABLES, THE AVERAGE PERSON EATS ABOUT 10,000 CARROTS IN A LIFETIME.

Loaded with more beta-carotene than all other vegetables, the average person eats about 10,000 carrots in a lifetime. Carrots can trace their roots to Afghanistan where colorful varieties can still be found. As a taproot that grows into the ground and then swells, the Greeks used it as an aphrodisiac (a perverse logic here). According to history, Roman Emperor Caligua also embraced the hidden power of the taproot, frequently inviting the members of his senate to dine on carrots. Some say it was to make his merry men more potent. But why? By all accounts Caligua was a half a sandwich away from a picnic. This is the same guy who appointed his horse as consul of the senate, which may explain to us today this animal's love affair with this super-food.

There are many other orange and yellow foods, but in general, I would opt for their darker skinned counterparts.

Rutabagas, once the ancient symbol of a damned soul, were used as the first jack o-lanterns in the United Kingdom prior to the arrival of the pumpkin. Considered something only the most desperate ate as a last resort during World War I, they were generally regarded as a poor man's food. In the years 1916 and 1917, when crops such as potatoes and others failed, large numbers of the German population survived by eating little more than rutabagas. They also served as a coffee substitute, and even animal fodder. Still grown in Siberia and elsewhere, rutabagas are available in many colors, such as a yellow variety with a purple cast.

This member of the turnip family was crossed with a cabbage, and this root vegetable as well as others, such as maize, sweet potatoes, lima beans, and others, are goiterans. Excessive consumption can lead to hypothyroidism. They actually contain small amounts of *cyanide*, which eventually becomes detoxified. But the product of this detoxification, thiocyanate, can put the thyroid in danger as it impedes the transportation of iodine to that gland. Don't be tricked by this poor man's treat. They fell out of favor for good reason. Collard greens, mustard greens and turnips are lower in calories and are healthier alternatives.

PUMPKIN

Old ORAC: Not tested/listed.

New ORAC TAC (Total Antioxidant Capacity) score: 560

Serving size: 1 cup

TRAC (Total Realistic Antioxidant Capacity): 280- raw. Note: The researchers measured raw pumpkin only, which alone is impractical; so is 1 full cup.

Serving size: 1/2 cup

GI: 75

GL: 6—canned.

EWG: Not listed/tested.

Growing pumpkins can be good business, not only in our country but elsewhere in the world. They're grown in six of our seven continents (Antarctica, according to our last report, remains pumpkinless). In places such as Uganda, pumpkins can grow in only four months and both the business and the vegetable (it's actually a squash) are helping to fight poverty and feed both people and animals. The seeds are loaded with zinc and may protect the prostate against cancer. Once used as a cure for freckles, their L-Tryptophan is a natural antidepressive. One cooked cup contains a whopping 2,650 IUs of vitamin A (more than 50 percent of its daily value), and serves as an excellent source of important *lutein* and *alpha-carotene*, linked to lower rates of certain cancers. A recent study at the Harvard School of Public Health showed that still another carotene found in this fruit, beta-cryptoxanthin, may offer protection against lung cancer.

Pumpkin is a great source of magnesium (1/4 cup contains more than 45 percent of your daily value) and important bio-available carotenoids. It also contains high concentrations of important minerals such as manganese and phosphorous, as well as trace elements of copper and iron.

While generally regarded as a vegetable, pumpkins are actually a fruit (a member of the Cucurbita family, which includes the squash and cucumber). Consider lightly heated fresh pumpkin soup; it's an excellent way to release many of its highly prized nutrients. This super-food is loaded with one of the greatest combinations of phyto-nutrients, vitamins, trace elements, and minerals known to man.

Other orange and yellow fruits include apricots, butternut squash, golden kiwifruit, mandarin oranges, nectarines, oranges, orange peppers, peaches, persimmons, sweet corn, sweet potatoes, tangerines, yellow apples, yellow beets, yellow figs, yellow pears, yellow peppers, yellow summer squash, yellow tomatoes, yellow watermelon, and yellow winter squash.

WHITE, TAN, AND BROWN FOODS

Both allicin and saponins have been found to offer important protection against a long list of diseases. This is another area of research where findings have only just begun to unfold. A peek into their natural microbial activity is like unlocking the door to the magical land of Oz. The *interaction* of these molecules with a host of important enzymes seems to occur in a *determined fashion* designed by nature to protect the organism from many forms of potential invasion. In research led by student Allison Ellington, Mark Berhow, and Dr. Keith Singletary of the University of Illinois, soy saponins have been found to stimulate programmed cell death (autophagy) in colon cell cultures. Their research was based on a purified soybean extract (*Carcinogenesis*, 2004). While more research is warranted and planned, Dr. Singletary believes they are on the right path: "Whenever you're talking about a plant chemical or a nutritional compound, you have to ask whether this compound can reach the target tissue. In this case, it appears that soy saponins may actually reach the colon in concentrations that are cancer-preventive ... The saponins appear to block certain cancer signaling pathways in the colon cancer cells that control cell survival." Of course if you must eat soy, I would opt for the fermented variety; in products such as tempeh, miso, bean paste, and tofu. Not highly processed, unfermented soy, with additives. But the value of this color family doesn't stop here.

GARLIC

Garlic affords protection against several types of cancer while supercharging your immunity. Cooking it into foods improves not only the flavor, but the nutrient content as well. Rich in diallyl disulfide, researchers Manivasagam et al. at the Department of Biochemistry at Annamalai University (*Journal of Applied Biomedicine*, 2005) found that the compound contained in garlic oil normalized the liver in rats with hepatocellular carcinoma, a common and deadly form of cancer caused by tobacco smoke, preservatives in certain soft drinks, and in cured and fried meats.

In humans, garlic has been shown to inhibit vascular calcification. Its allium sativum appears to reduce unusually high levels of lipids in the blood. And garlic's ability to enhance immunity, reduce internal inflammation and arterial plaque, and help protect against damage from processed food additives is well documented. Its role in supercharging your body's ability to protect itself may explain why its devotees successfully fight off infection and viruses compared to those in control groups who don't. Fortunately, we eat more than 250 million pounds of garlic annually!

Ninety percent of the white skinned variety grown in the U.S. comes from the state of California (though the U.S only accounts for 2 percent of global production, in contrast with China's 75 percent). Otherwise known throughout the world as the *stinking rose*, allicin—its pungent sulphur-based organosulphur compound—is only released when enzymatic action occurs after the clove cells are broken (from cutting, peeling, or chopping). One of nature's true superheroes, allicin is endowed with the amazing ability to protect us against both bacterial *and* fungal infections. Garlic's powers range from its ability to lower LDL and blood pressure to reducing internal inflammation. But that's just the beginning of its ability to heal.

Recently, scientists across the world have discovered the unique power of *aged* garlic to heal us as well, in incredibly unique ways that distinguish its power from that found in raw or cooked fresh garlic. While aged garlic extract contains *no* allicin, according to an impressive study by Carmia Borek (*Journal of Nutrition*, 2001;131:1010S–1015S; "Antioxidant Health Effects of Aged Garlic Extract"), it contains far *more* antioxidant activity than both fresh garlic and non-aged supplements. The researchers' findings conclude that, "A substantial body of evidence shows that AGE (aged garlic extract) and its components inhibit the oxidative damage implicated in a variety of diseases and aging. These effects strongly suggest that AGE may play an important role in lowering the risk of cardiovascular disease, cancer, Alzheimer's disease and other age-related degenerative conditions, protecting human health and mitigating the effects of aging."

The same researchers also found that the compounds in aged garlic extract inhibit oxidation of LDL while reducing oxidative damage to endothelial cells. They conclude by stating that, "compelling evidence supports the beneficial health effects attributed to AGE, i.e., reducing the risk of cardiovascular disease, stroke, cancer and aging, including the oxidant-mediated brain cell damage that is implicated in Alzheimer's disease."

What's more, AGE is one of the only foods known to man that increases the production of an important antioxidant enzyme, *glutathione,* in our cells and tissue. The other is lactose-free organic whey. As we'll discuss shortly, even supplements of *glutathione* itself *fail to increase* its own presence in our cells, since it can't be absorbed when ingested orally. Though we *can* produce gluta-thione ourselves, our ability to do so substantially diminishes with age, which in turn causes us to physically age. That's why the amazing power of aged garlic extract is *that* important.

Combined with the whey isolate and an amazing supplement you'll learn about shortly, you will be able to accomplish what few in the world have ever managed to do before—*restore* one of the most incredibly protective mechanisms naturally produced by our bodies to defend our cells, *regardless* of our bodies' diminished ability to do so as we age.

But don't throw the baby out with the bathwater. Fresh garlic, loaded with allicin, has its own unique ability to heal. Both aged garlic extract and raw or cooked fresh garlic provide a one-two punch against the ravages of time, toxins, invasive bacteria, and microbes.

Other key foods in the white, tan, and brown family include coconut, cauli-flower, kohlrabi (same family as broccoli, cabbage, and brussels sprouts), lentils (which help control blood sugar), leeks (same family as garlic and onions but sweeter), pinto beans (they help detoxify sulfites), horseradish (be alert to its potential interaction with certain medications; pregnant women should avoid it), and *shallots* (they contain *five times* the amount of phenols found in onions and help detoxify the liver—a truly remarkable food).

As healthy as onions are, shallots are even healthier, and they're sweeter when used in cooking. Home gardeners, listen up. Unlike onions, shallots branch into a cluster of several compact bulbs making shallots the gift that keeps giving!

As far as other foods in this color group, dates and figs don't make the cut. While they're nutritionally dense, they also contain a good deal of sugar (particularly fructose), and are high in calories. The dried version of figs may also contain a good deal of sulfites.

Other members in the white, tan, and brown group include jicama (a legume with a nice texture and small amounts of fat and protein), garbanzo beans (high in glycation precursor galactose sugar, but loaded with fiber), great northern beans, mushrooms (they're a fungus), peanuts (which are okay unprocessed but allergy rates are accelerating and there are better choices), white corn, turnips, white potatoes (ugh), white nectarines, white peaches, and *parsnips* (another super-food that's even more dense with nutrients than carrots, and a wonderful source of soluble fiber). The latter are just a little ugly, and as Rodney Dangerfield might have said "they don't get no respect." But they deserve to.

There's one more important favorite white/yellow/brown food that's worth noting—*ginger root*. Ginger root has an amazing anti-inflammatory power. I grate it on my salads and soups, and more than occasionally nibble at the whole root. Long revered for its ability to relieve symptoms of painful gastrointestinal distress, its potent anti-inflammatory compound gingerol has been shown in clinical studies to relieve pain or swelling in arthritis, as well as those that suffer from muscle pain. A number of other studies consistently support its effectiveness in relieving nausea (*Obstet Gynecol*, 2001; 97:577–82, "Is ginger root effective for decreasing the severity of nausea and vomiting in early pregnancy?"). For example, one to two grams a day of ginger root powder caused a *significant* decrease in nausea and vomiting, according to the study. Particularly from sea sickness (*British Journal Anaesthesia*, 2000, Mar; 84(3):367–71; "Efficacy of ginger for nausea and vomiting: a systematic review of randomized clinical trials") and even morning sickness (*Journal of the American Dietetic Association*, Volume 95, Issue 4, Page 416; "Vitamin B-6 and Ginger in Morning Sickness") that often accompanies early pregnancy. As you can see, ginger root offers practical benefits that many can appreciate.

SPICES—TURBO-CHARGE EACH MEAL

It's not easy to surprise scientists. But researchers Wu et al. of ORAC testing fame (*Journal of Agriculture and Food Chemistry*, 2004) whose information helps fashion the USDA's nutrient lab database acknowledged that they were indeed surprised. The results from their analysis of the liphophilic and hydrophilic antioxidant activity in sixteen commonly used dried spices provided unexpected insight into the power of these foods. On the basis of weight (results were based on only 1 gram), *no foods* in any category scored as high in TAC as these! Topping the scoreboard were the following dried spices and their respective scored antioxidant capacity:

Cloves	3144
Cinnamon	2675
Oregano (leaf)	2001
Turmeric	1593
Parsley	743
Basil (leaf)	675
Curry Powder	485
Pepper (black, whole peppercorn)	301
Mustard Seed (yellow)	293
Ginger, Ground	288
Pepper (black, ground)	251
Chili Powder	236
Garlic Powder	67
Onion Powder	57
Poppy Seed	5

Note: All scores were rounded up or down to the nearest whole number.

The scientists were rightfully concerned about the difficulty in trying to determine the typical amount of these spices the average person will consume, which is generally small. But based on their findings, I recommend a mix of spice or herbs on all foods, boosting their value and density!

Parsley, for example, is easy to tolerate and might be considered as not only a delicious addition to salads and a munch between meals, but as an important pallet cleanser that can complement any meal, particularly one featuring garlic, onions, or any other foods with potent flavor. Avoid it if you're prone to kidney stones due to its oxalate content, and don't eat it with aspirin (if taken together, severe allergic reaction to parsley can occur). In addition to sweetening the breath, it's an anti-flatulent, anti-microbial, anti-rheumatic, and anti-spasmodic. A great source of potassium, it strengthens the ability of the urinary tract to resist infection as well.

CINNAMON

One of my personal favorites, with proven anti-microbial activity from the oil's principle constituent, cinnamic aldehyde, the ground version ranked second among all spices tested in Total Antioxidant Capacity (second only to ground cloves). Importantly, it dusted all other spices in its content of important hydrophilic (water-based) antioxidants, topping the charts with an H-ORAC score of 2,640 (umol TE/g), followed by dried oregano leaf at 2,001, and 1,533 for cloves. According to researchers, its rich proanthocyanidins and phenolic content might explain its amazingly high hydrophilic antioxidant activity.

This same cinnamic aldehyde (alternatively known as cinnamaldehyde) helps prevent the irregular clumping of blood platelets. Clotting is important when we cut ourselves or when we experience internal bleeding when our vessels are broken. They become sticky, change shape, and patch and repair the endangered area. In a truly amazing process, they signal and activate proteins such as fibrogen (known as "clotting factor"), normally deactivated but circulating in the blood to form a type of web when activated. This "fishing net" corrals more red blood cells as well as platelets to fortify the clot. At the same time, the platelets signal the surrounding blood vessel to constrict itself. It's another way they seal and fortify the barrier we call a blood clot. Cinnamic aldehyde actually hinders cell membranes from releasing inflammatory arachidonic acid. While its role in moderating blood sugar, reducing triglycerides, and lowering destructive LDL appears to be quite promising, further research with larger populations is required to say this with certainty. Research headed by Khan et al. (American Diabetes Association's *Diabetes Care Journal*, 2003) demonstrates that intake of 1, 3, or 6 grams of cinnamon per day reduces serum glucose, triglyceride, and LDL cholesterol. LDL decreased between 10 percent to 24 percent after forty days of subjects taking as little as 3 grams per day. After the same period of time, blood serum triglyceride levels decreased an astounding 23 percent to 30 percent.

Measurements also showed that a distinguishing feature of this group is that four of its members (clove, ginger, pepper, and turmeric) have a far higher content of fat-based (lipophilic) antioxidants than they do water-based (hydrophilic) antioxidants. According to Hu and his team of researchers, this suggested that "the essential oils in them contained considerable quantities of antioxidants … However, the other compounds responsible for these high values of antioxidant activity are unknown." That means exciting research will likely unlock other important constituents of these foods—powerful constituents that are currently unknown.

The study of what makes foods do what they do biochemically is still in its infancy. It's hoped that our understanding of the complex interaction within a given food will eventually extend to an understanding of the powerful interaction *between* all those foods in a given meal. One of the inherent shortcomings of some of these studies (as significant as they are) is their evaluation of foods *in vitro*. To truly understand the impact of foods upon us, their capacity will eventually need to be measured *inside* of us (in vivo).

THE WEIRDBERRIES

Our final discussion on food groups will include those we've all heard about but few have experienced eating firsthand. They were not included as part of the selected foods by color group since they don't meet the criteria for several reasons:

Organically Grown:

At the time of this writing and to the best of my knowledge, few are organically grown (the certification requirements for organic foods in foreign countries can be very different than ours).

Conveniently Available:

They're not. However, goji, which we'll soon discuss, is popping up in health food stores and on a host of internet sites, but the majority of the weirdberries are not, other than as sugar-laden juice.

Locally Grown:

At the time of this writing, only noni is grown in America (Hawaii), though some enterprising farmers are attempting to grow them in California.

Long-term clinical studies with reasonably-sized human populations are not available at this time. Not because they lack the value of other important foods, but only because, comparatively speaking, widespread acceptance has just begun. The type of data required to support any kind of recommendation isn't currently available (though goji and acai have been ORAC tested and received top honors). Only one of these three, noni, is grown in our country. Hopefully, more solid data will become available.

GOJI, ACAI, AND NONI FRUIT

As indicated, the ORAC values of some of the weird ones are off the charts. But unlike most consumers, you now understand why that's not reason enough to embrace them. Importantly, our over-reliance on a food's

ORAC score can be used as a tool by unscrupulous or uninformed marketers. They either know or should know that comparing an ORAC score of a dried fruit against that of a wet fruit is grossly misleading.

The wolfberry, also known as goji, refers to a closely related species of berries, lycium chinense and lycium barbarum. Used in traditional Chinese medicine for well over 2,000 years, they've been credited with miraculous healing powers. This includes their ability to enhance the immune system, protect the liver, boost sperm count, and increase vision.

At the time of this writing, the goji berry is one of the most aggressively marketed "superfruit" wannabes in the world. While it may indeed qualify as a wonder food in some people's minds, at the present time, it doesn't in mine. Yes, its ORAC value is far higher than even blueberries. But as you've learned, that's only one of the many criteria we use to properly evaluate the merit of a given food. And as you'll see, in this case, it can be a misleading one. Our foremost consideration is the ability of a food to prove its worth in well-constructed human trials.

Despite all the hype, a search on Pubmed Central revealed one human study involving wolfberrys (as part of a preparation used to study hemorrhaging in rats). But I owe it to the reader to get to the bottom of the purported goji super-fruit miracle.[19] So let's examine this lone study. We're told by this research that certain drugs do indeed perform better in combination *with* goji's polysaccharides than without them. That's when I learned that the subjects were divided into three groups (including a placebo group that received both drugs with no lycium barbarum polysaccharides), and enjoyed a positive variance when the two drugs with goji proved their effectiveness in 18 of 44 subjects treated. Of these 18 persons, *two* had complete remission. That's 2 out of the 44 subjects, or less than 5 percent. In essence, these numbers mean *nothing*. Sheer coincidence would have given us a better number than 5 percent. But if these studies are this weirdberries' best foot forward, why are we paying a small fortune for this stuff?

Contrary to marketer's claims, I believe it's unlikely they're receiving a crop of gojis harvested directly from Tibet or from the Mongolian Himalayas, as advertised. While it's a chant with a nice religious and even mystical ring to it, it seems ridiculous. At 10,000 feet above sea level, the Tibetan Plateau is a brutal, forsaken land with frost half the year. With cold nighttime temperatures and lousy soil, it's impossible to ship commercially from there. Tibet is an even more unlikely candidate as a food purveyor to the West. As the highest region on earth, it rests at an average elevation of 16,000 feet. Mongolia is landlocked. Bordering Russia on the north and China on the south, I'd love to know the name of trucking line we can count on to make its way through this perilous region to deliver these little berries to Wal-Mart.

It's more than likely that your gojis come from a plantation in the Ningxia Hui region in Northern China, which accounts for over 40 percent of the nation's almost 100 million pounds they produce. Used for medicinal purposes in China for almost 2,000 years, the claims touting their huge concentration of vitamin C value are quite exaggerated. In fact, goji's vitamin C content is considerably *lower* than other fruits recommended in this book. Some of these claims are made by comparing the vitamin C content in goji on a *weight-for-weight basis.* That means marketers are comparing the weight of dried goji fruit to the true weight of a watery whole food. As you've already learned, it's not a legitimate comparison. Comparing a dried fruit containing almost no water on a weight basis to a wet whole fruit is the marketing equivalent of a parlor trick. As Miek Kinnaird points out in the "Great Goji Juice Controversy" (April 2007), claims are made that goji trumps oranges in vitamin C. Determined to make a fair comparison, he compared goji to dried oranges and found that that the dried orange contained 402 milligrams of vitamin C, versus goji's 306 milligrams. And as you know, there are far better sources of vitamin C with higher levels than even oranges.

So, where does that leave the legendary goji berry? Rarely found fresh outside of the areas it's grown, this dried fruit has a whopping 4 grams of sugar per ounce (some 20 percent of its content or more).

IT'S ALSO SUGGESTED BY SOME THAT GOJI OFFERS PREVENTION FOR CERTAIN TYPES OF CANCER ...

It's also suggested by some that goji offers prevention for certain types of cancer, in part due to the goji's large concentration of important anthocyanins and germanium, a trace mineral that appears to have the potential to stimulate the body's immune response to unbridled tumor growth. But garlic also contains a good amount of germanium, and is available locally and even organically, and it contains no sugar. And it's cheap!

I've found no proof that this berry prevents cancer in any human trial. Before purchasing any new miracle food, ask for a copy of the human trial.

Other claims include the importance of gojis as a valuable source of carotenoids, particularly the antioxidant zeaxanthin, which research shows can help protect your retina from deterioration. But while reports of goji's content of zeaxanthin range from 25 to 160 milligrams per 100 grams, the amount in dried fruit drops considerably; and it's practically *absent* in the goji juice due to processing. On the other hand, kale contains almost 22 milligrams for the same weight, without all the sugar, and you can buy it far closer to home.

All of this, coupled with the fact that China's agricultural practices and standards vary a good deal from ours (and are even more dissimilar to our organic certification requirements), make this "over-priced garbage" in my book. According to Dr. Robert O. Young, Ph.D., D.Sc., drinking the juice of this and certain exotic fruits that are marketed today is one of the *worst* things you could do for your health. And he tells us (*Articles of Health*, October 2006) one of the reasons why: "The quantity of organic cations (protons or acids) from high sugar fruits and fruit drinks like Goji Juice significantly exceeds the number of free anions (bases or electrons). Therefore, a net acidification occurs in the blood and tissues."

A net acidification is precisely what we want to avoid.

Dr. Young is well versed on another important test that some say is far more important than the food's ORAC. Rather than targeting in on the *activity* outside of the body, it measures the actual *oxidizing potential* of food (ORP), or its chemical potential to give up electrons. Antioxidants are supposed to prevent oxidation by doing just that. A negative ORP value means it has plenty of electrons to spare. Active antioxidants stabilize free radical activity and are of great benefit to a human being. A positive ORP value means that it's already oxidized and has no chemical potential to give up electrons. According to Dr. Young: "Over the years I have warned people in my books and lectures to stay away from high sugar fruits or fruit drinks because they over-acidify the blood and tissues. This includes Himalayan Goji Juice."

After ORP testing of Himalayan Goji Juice he concludes: "The ORP of the Himalayan Goji Juice is +181.9 mV. The positive ORP of the Goji Juice indicates that this product has NO antioxidant potential or electrical potential and is saturated with protons. The increased protons from the Goji Juice will pull energy from the body rather than contribute energy to the body, in the form of electrons. Therefore, the Goji Juice is electrically dead and is not fit for human consumption." Young contends it will acidify the blood and tissue in much the same way acidic cola does, depleting the "alkaline reserves of the body which may result in bone loss, calcium stones in the brain, breast, liver, kidneys, and/or renal failure."

There are some positive nutritional characteristics of the whole fruit that warrant further investigation, such as goji's high content of important poly-saccharides. They've been shown in certain teas, for example, to reduce the stickiness of blood platelets, which can reduce the possibility that they will adhere to the walls of your arteries. The wolfberry itself *is* loaded with nutri-ents. When so many good things are present in one nutritionally dense food, it is likely that further research will provide a better understanding of how to properly utilize its potential. Until then, while the whole world appears to be hailing this as the next harbinger of long life, I won't. Not until it's proven over time in well-constructed human studies with good-sized populations, available locally and organically grown. Even then, I would have reservations about eating it, or any dried fruit that contained this much sugar (the same position I've taken on other dried fruit).

We embrace the romance of these exotic fruits with little information, other than that provided by multi-level marketing groups. Skilled marketers cleverly bundle bits of anecdotal information together and sell it to an eager public seeking the next quick fix. Often, no more than false hope in a bottle. In the end, the false statements of some, and commercially processed super-nonsense may be hiding a food whose basic nature has real benefit. But then again, it may not. Many of these companies will prey on those that will pay dearly for miracle foods. But the only real miracles, like those recommended in this book, are backed up by hard data. They may not be very exotic, but they've shown their colors in real studies over time. Maybe it's time multi-level marketeers turn their attention to something like broccoli. Boring to some, it's the real thing. But the weirdberries seem to appeal to our sense of adventure. Just don't fall off the perennial multi-tiered cliff.

ACAI PALM

Pronounced "a-sigh-ee," the black purple fruit bears a visual similarity to the grape and is grown in many countries throughout South and Central America, such as Brazil and Peru. They're full of healthy fat and important fiber. Indeed over 56 percent of its fat content is of the monounsaturated variety, the same healthy fat found in avocado, olive oil, coconut, nuts such as the almond and macadamia, and seeds such as sesame. With over one third of its weight consisting of important dietary fiber, eating acai makes it easier to achieve the recommended daily requirement of approximately 25 grams of fiber daily.

Acai also boasts an ORAC value almost ten times higher than lowbush blueberries (again, it's only one measurement, and based on drying, less than an accurate one). However, any way you slice it, its antioxidant activity is significant. Freeze-dried acai powder proved to be a formidable foe against superoxide, according to researchers Schauss et al. (*Journal of Agriculture and Food*, 2006). Superoxide is a highly toxic, extremely reactive free radical that has been linked to the onset of disease and premature aging; but it's neutralized by an amazingly powerful enzyme known as superoxide dismutase (SOD).

SOD busts up the heinous clod, swiftly knocking the wind out of this highly destructive paramagnetic ion. Superoxide produces highly reactive ancestor molecules. Not only does acai offer protection against this onerous precipitator of aging and disease, but among the findings of the study by Schauss and collegues, "The SOD of acai was 1614 units/g, an extremely high scavenging capacity for O_2—by far the highest of any fruit or vegetable tested to date."

The other good news: Since acai is too perishable (due to its high concentration of healthy fat) to export without running the risk of it turning rancid, its pulp is freeze-dried and certified as organic. According to producers at Sambazon, their method of flash freezing and dehydrated-drying within 24 hours of picking the berries creates a powder that retains all of the benefits of fresh acai.

According to legend, the company was founded by two surfers who experienced local acai with fellow sportsmen while travelling in Brazil in celebration of the new millennium. The company harvests through a fair-trade program, and their organic certification and packaging process gives me a high degree of confidence in using this product. The company offers their product on their online store at www.omnisupplements.com. Studies at the University of Florida's Institute of Food and Agricultural Sciences, headed by lead researcher Dr. Stephen Talcott and his colleagues (*Journal of Agricultural and Food Chemistry*, 2006), showed that acai extract created a self-destructive response in 86 percent of the leukemia cells they tested. While encouraging, the tests were conducted on human cancer cells in a cultured lab model. Talcott is the first to caution us not to conclude from this that acai "compounds are able to defeat or prevent leukemia within a human." In a soon to be published article (*Journal of Agricultural and Food Chemistry*, 2008, "Açai Human Consumption

Trial: Bioavailability of Anthocyanins Pharmacokinetics of Anthocyanins and Antioxidant Effects after the Consumption of Anthocyanin-Rich Acai Juice and Pulp in Human Healthy Volunteers") Talcott said: "We don't want to give anyone false hope. We are encouraged by the findings, however. Compounds that show good activity against cancer cells in a model system are most likely to have beneficial effects in our bodies."

Talcott believes he's on to something. According to a faculty bulletin from the Department of Nutrition and Food Science (June 15, 2007), a provisional patent application was filed with the United States Patent and Trademark Office on behalf of Texas A&M University and Dr. Steve Talcott of the Department of Nutrition and Food Science. The invention describes methods of extraction and the unique chemical composition of a 100 percent acai oil product, suitable for food, dietary supplements, and cosmetic applications.

We are anxiously awaiting the fruit of this outstanding researcher's labor. Should the data warrant it, updates will be published on our web site.

Of all the weirdberries studied, acai seems to have the most established value. But I suggest staying away from any sugary juice. The organic freeze dried powder is a far healthier choice. Its capacity to scavenge toxic superoxide is most encouraging.

NONI

Some Noni producers (not all) sell groundless hope to those eager for miracles. Preying on the desperation of ill people looking for a solution, snake oil salesmen have made billions of dollars lying to you and making unsubstantiated claims, ritualizing their mantra to a cult of multilevel salespeople. Make no mistake about it, for some, it's all about separating you from your money.

In 2004, the FDA issued a warning letter to Flora Inc. They found that Flora made numerous health claims regarding noni juice, all of which were unfounded, and promoted the consumption of noni by touting its medicinal properties. The FDA's Federal Food, Drug and Cosmetic Act (21 U.S.C and 321 (g) (1)) requires that any such claims be supported by clinical safety testing proving these claims. The year 2005 was a revealing one for noni growers and processors. Both the *Journal of Natural Products* and the *European Journal of Gastroenterology & Hepatology* reported that the consumption of noni juice caused acute hepatitis.

A 2008 meta-analysis of noni's value, based on medical research from three databases by Rolf Johansen entitled "The health food product Noni—does marketing harmonize with the current status of research?" (*Tidsskr Nor Laege-foren*, 2008, Mar 13;128(6):694–7) concludes as follows: "***There is no scientific basis*** for claiming that patients will benefit from using noni for any diseases. The way this product is sold has several worrying aspects."

While some makers have touted the fruit's miraculous power to heal, I found no evidence to support this. Hoping to legitimize their sensational claims, the makers of Tahitian Noni® Juice submitted their product to the scrutiny of the Scientific Committee on Food of the European Commission on Health and Consumer Protection for public safety testing. According to committee notes, the owners had recently filed a patent for a dietary supplement to reduce cellular damage within the human body. After an extensive evaluation and review of the data, the committee found *nothing* to suggest that noni was substantially different than any other fruit. In fact, the only nutrient other than sugar it scored high in was vitamin C … with considerably less than can be found in a single orange. It also contained far *more* calories than the latter, and considerably more sodium. And its high content of potassium poses a risk for those on potassium restricted diets. The committee concluded: "The data supplied and the information available to the Committee provided no evidence for special health benefits of Tahitian noni juice, which go beyond those of other fruit juices."

What troubles me the most are the number of people struggling with disease who have worked throughout their lives to earn every dime they have, only to pay upwards of $40 for a 32-ounce bottle of this baloney to a multilevel sales-person who conned them. In fact, I just did a store check in the new health food section at our local grocer and found one 32-ounce bottle of Tahitian Trader Bio Noni Juice retailing for more than $37—with a label making incredible claims that are not necessarily supported by human studies. Many of these same folks wouldn't feel good about robbing a bank, but separating you from your money based on these claims appears to be all in a day's work. Don't mistake their passion and enthusiasm for knowledge.

On August 26, 1998, the attorney generals of four states (Arizona, California, New Jersey, and Texas) announced a settlement with Morinda, Inc., a multilevel sales company that made unsubstantiated claims about Tahitian Noni Juice. They distributed marketing material claiming their product could treat, cure, or prevent everything from depression and arthritis, to diabetes and more. Other promoters of Tahitian Noni appeared on a Los Angeles TV show claiming that the juice miraculously cures everything from dementia to lupus.

Despite fines, the company continues making false claims elsewhere in the world. Warnings issued by respected authorities (like Dr. Philip S. Chua, MD, currently the Chairman of Cardiovascular Surgery of the Cebu Cardiovascular Center, Cebu Doctors' Hospital, Cebu City, Philippines), or the complete ban by Finland on the sale or importation of this product, does little to deter us from buying this weirdberry. One salesman told CBS undercover reporters that "every 1.7 seconds somebody buys a bottle of Tahitian Noni juice" (CBS Los Angeles, 2006, "Miracle Or False Hope In A Bottle?" David Goldstein).

To those purchasing noni for its miraculous healing power, I say no-no.

END NOTES

1. The trend shows no signs of slowing down according to the Department of Health and Human Services (Center for Disease Control and Prevention Report, November 17, 2007), who compared rates based on data from two different NHANES (National Health and Nutrition Examination Surveys) from two different periods of time. The study found that the prevalence of obesity increased from 15.0 percent (in the 1976–1980 survey) to 32.9 percent in the later 2003–2004 survey. Those classified as overweight more than doubled in children ages 2–5 (from 5 percent to 13.9 percent), almost tripled for children ages 6–11 years of age (from 6.5 percent to 18.8 percent), and more than tripled for children in the 12–19-year-old group (from 5 percent to 17.4 percent).

2. Capacity limits of information processing in the brain. Rene Marois, January 2005

3. Interfaces, 65, pp. 6-7, Winter 2005, the brain and the web - a quick backup in case of accidents, www.hcibook.com/alan/papers; A. Dix

4. Dr. Anne Kulze points out in her excellent book, *Dr. Ann's 10-Step Diet* (Top Ten Wellness and Fitness, Charleston, South Carolina, 2004), a precipitous drop in your blood sugar quickly ensues. And the cycle continues. "Our brains have learned that these same white carbohydrates will rapidly satisfy its immediate need for more glucose." So, a repetitive and terribly unhealthy cycle ensues as your brain again signals your appetite centers to find more of these quick hits.

5. www.nutritiondata.com

6. Two other forms of starch (rapidly digesting and slowly digesting) are broken down in earlier stages of digestion. They are not shown here. The percentages for total dietary fiber represent the amount of dry matter in each ingredient that is considered in the fiber.

7. Cancer Epidemiology Biomarkers & Prevention ; 2007; 16, 2304, November 1, 2007. A Prospective Study of Dietary Acrylamide Intake and the Risk of Endometrial, Ovarian, and Breast Cancer; Hogervorst et al.

8. American Journal of Clinical Nutrition,May 2008, Volume 87, Number 5, Pages 1428-1438;Dietary acrylamide intake and the risk of renal cell, bladder, and prostate cancer ;J.G. Hogervorst et al.

9. http://fnic.nal.usda.gov./fnic/foodcomp

10. According to Brittany Sauser, "The most notable example: in Mexico, which gets much of its corn from the United States, the price of corn tortillas has doubled in the past year, according to press reports, setting off large protest marches in Mexico City" (*Technology Review, 2007*).

11. James Bovard. Opening statement. Executive summary of policy analysis, written for the CATO Institute.

12. Extention Toxicology Network; A Pesticide Information Project of Cooperative Extension Offices of Cornell University, Michigan State University, Oregon State University, and University of California at Davis; http://pmep.cce.cornell.edu/profiles/extoxnet/carbaryl-dicrotophos/copper-sulfate-ext.html

13. Public Campaign, USAction, Campaign for America's Future, the Association of Community Organizations for Reform Now (ACORN), and locally by WV Citizen Action (a USAction affiliate) and the WV People¹s Election Reform Coalition (PERC-WV)

14. A study published in 2007 by Glinska and colleagues from the Department of Plant Cytology and Cytochemistry at the University of Lodz in Poland demonstrated the protective action of the ATH-rich extract from red cabbage leaves against heavy metal toxicity.

15. In earlier work, researchers Seddon et al. in the Eye Disease and Case Study Control Group (*JAMA*, November 1994;272(18):1413-20: "Dietary carotenoids, vitamins A, C, and E, and advanced age-related macular degeneration") studied the effect of these and other nutrients on advanced-stage AMD. The experimental model included 356 case subjects and 520 control subjects. The scientists concluded that: "A higher dietary intake of carotenoids was associated with a lower risk for AMD. Adjusting for other risk factors for AMD, we found that those in the highest quintile of carotenoid intake had a 43 percent lower risk for AMD compared with those in the lowest quintile ... Among the specific carotenoids, lutein and zeaxanthin, which are primarily obtained from dark green, leafy vegetables, were most strongly associated with a reduced risk for AMD."

16. "... offers protection to brains cells against oxidative stress," *Experimental Neurology*, 2005, and "... may retard cognitive behavioral defects," *Journal of Neuroscience*, 1998.

17. For example, a ripe banana has a high glycemic load of 120. But combining it with a low glycemic food such as peanut butter diminishes it's impact on blood sugar.

18. Patrick N.D.'s thoughtful review, "Beta -Carotein: The Controversy Continues," touched on this and other issues regarding the beta-carotene research with heavy smokers: "In both observational and case control studies, the intake of carotenoid-rich fruits and vegetables has been found to be inversely correlated with risk for cardiovascular disease. Numerous retrospective epidemiological studies have established an inverse relationship between dietary carotenoid levels and the incidence of specific cancers. Numerous animal and laboratory studies have substantiated— carotene's ability to inhibit tumor cell growth and the progression of carcinogenesis."

19. The most impressive research I could find was conducted by the Second Military Medical University, Department of Microbiology, Shanghai, China, comparing the effectiveness of drugs LAK/IL-2 both alone and in combination with lycium barbarum polysaccharide on 75 late stage cancer patients. The site correctly stated, "The response rate of patients treated with LAK/IL-2 and LBP was 40.9 percent while that of patients treated only with LAK/IL-2 was 16.1 percent."

20. The Health Effects of High Fructose Corn Syrup. American Medical Association. Report #3. Council on Science and Public Health.

CHAPTER 4

THE FRANKENFOODS

"Genetic engineers don't make new genes, they rearrange existing ones."
— Thomas Lovejoy

Scientist's newfound ability to unravel the genetic code has permitted them to construct diagrams known as "genomes." A genome is essentially a roadmap that enables researchers to determine the specific location of a gene. A gene is a hereditary unit consisting of a special sequence of coded instructions made of transmissible material known as "deoxyribonucleic acid" or DNA. This instruction is matched up to one or more amino acids. Amino acids are, as you've already learned, the building blocks of protein. Your genetic code contains hereditary instructions necessary for the creation of the protein in your body. The characteristics of each of these proteins, and in turn the way they express themselves, are largely determined by the sequence in which your particular genetic code is written. Like a musical composition, the precise sequence in which this coded material plays out determines its unique characteristics, and to a large extent, yours (though your external environment and choices you make are capable of profoundly modifying or completely changing this predetermined programming).

DNA is the hereditary substance that scientists have successfully manipulated; they accomplish this by removing a gene from one organism with a particular trait and insert it into another. By doing so, they're literally changing life as we know it. Genes are coded to produce one or more proteins and proteins are the building blocks of life. Change their code and you change the genetic expression of the gene and the protein it's programmed to effect.

Each of these genes with its specific sequence of DNA code sits on a thread-like strand of material found in the nucleolus of every cell (except red blood cells), called a chromosome. These chromosomes always come in pairs; the exceptions are the two original germ cells that were used to create you. The latter contain just one strand of DNA from the mother and another strand of coded information from the father. This produces an embryonic cell with one complete set that contains each of these two chromosomes. This special embryonic cell with its complete set of chromosomes then divides into two identical copies. Then it divides over and over again. By doing so, each of the 100 trillion cells in your body ultimately contain identical genetic material.

So, why do tissues in your body look and act so *differently*?

According to Michael Fumento, author of *The Bio Evolution: How Technology is Changing our World* (2003, Encounter Books), it's because some of our genes are switched on while others are switched off. That's why different tissues in our body with the same DNA behave so disparately.

NOW THAT SCIENTISTS CAN CREATE ROADMAPS OF GENE LOCATIONS IN PLANTS AND ANIMALS, THEY CAN MODIFY THEM.

Now that scientists can create road maps of gene locations in plants and animals, they can modify them. Today, researchers have the power to literally change our lives by altering our genetic code. Through the help of something called a "restriction enzyme," capable of initiating cleavage of DNA, scientists can genetically cut and paste a gene, as it were. By doing so they're rewriting our preprogrammed genetic software; software that evolved over billions of years that can now be modified in minutes. Genes can now be altered that enable us to combat almost every disease known to man, from cancer to arthritis. The benefits to mankind are astounding, and at the same time—potentially onerous.

But it doesn't stop there. Unlike cross-breeding or selective breeding—the centuries-old processes of mating two members of the same species with different characteristics—known as genetic manipulation, knows no such boundaries. Today, we have the technology to actually combine one or more genes from one organism into the chromosome of an entirely different species. Often referred to as "transgenic" engineering or gene splicing, the end product of recombining a gene in this way is known as "recombinant DNA." The latter term is often used to refer to genetic modification that takes place when creating medicines, pharmaceuticals, or biceuticals; it's typically used when referring to the genetic manipulation of a botanical.

On the other hand, when discussions center on an animal as the host organism, the term "transgenic" is often evoked. The consequences involved in applying this technology have created a host of ethical challenges and moral consternation. Few topics are as contentious and highly charged with such emotion as genetic manipulation (GM). Countless ethical, social, political, biologic, ecologic, moral, psychological, legal, industrial, economic, etiologic, and agricultural issues beg for resolution. Big biotech companies such as Monsanto wanted in, and wanted in now. So, it should come as no surprise to you that, although we're never polled or consulted, more than 75 percent of the processed foods available today have already been genetically modified.

So where's the FDA? The watchful eye of the country that produces two thirds of the world's genetically modified foods has decided not to require any labeling of these products. There are none of the same safety reviews required for food additives. So, you have no way of knowing if the food you've been chowing down has been altered or not. This potentially protective arm of the United States government knows no bounds. In fact, two more watchdog agencies are involved in this important issue as well. It's the USDA's job to require that all GM crops are regulated for their potential as pest plants. They allow companies to market whatever GM seed they want, as long as they can show they're not pest plants. That's like asking King Kong to prove he'd look silly in heels.

The third government agency that presides over the marketing of genetically altered seed is the EPA. This agency is responsible for evaluating plants to ensure that they're "environmentally" safe, and for safeguarding other human health issues. Every conventional pesticide sprayed on crops must also be licensed by the EPA to every pesticide producer and grower. This agency is tough. More than one farmer has been imprisoned, significantly fined, or had a license revoked when an EPA inspector popped in to ensure compliance.

While they've done a great job at establishing strict limits on residue levels and tolerances for conventional pesticides, they've established no such tolerance testing or criteria for plants that have been genetically modified with biocides. This means they've done nothing to monitor the internal effect on your health of genetically modified plants with the power to repel insects.

While productive in certain areas, the combined effect of all three of these agencies is little more than keystone copping an issue of such importance. Genetic engineering is here now. It's time to put together an all-star panel of experts to focus on it. Today, over 123 million acres of land in the United States is devoted to growing genetically modified food. If you're like the average American, you didn't have a clue. This isn't science fiction. It's already here. Of the more than

617 million acres of land in the world presently cultivated, approximately one third is devoted to the growth of genetically modified foods. Today, 93 percent of all canola (in the United States) has been modified to resist herbicides.

Estimates also suggest that almost 90 percent of all soybeans grown in the United States are genetically modified, and soybeans are found in the vast majority of all processed foods. However, you'd never know it, because the FDA requires no producers to label their GM products accordingly to tell you so. They clearly don't feel you need to be advised in order to make an informed choice. They appear to be more concerned that if you were made aware, you may not purchase these products, because you might perceive the label as a warning of sorts.

By 2004, based on the National Agricultural and Statistics Service (NASS) Acreage Report, nearly 80 percent of the total crop land in the state of South Dakota (almost 2.9 million acres of the 4.2 million total available farm land) was used to raise GM crops, making South Dakota the leading grower in the United States. Other states in the Midwest are right up there. The bowels of our corn belt, traditionally the most bountiful, lead the world in the production of genetically altered crops.

Canada's principal GM food today is none other than canola oil. And more than 90 percent of all Canadian canola oil is genetically modified. The leading company selling the seed used for this is Monsanto. It's now called "canola seed," despite the fact that you've never seen a canola plant, let alone a transgenic canola plant, rustling in the highlands.

Just ask Canadian farmer Percy Schmeiser, who spent years fighting Monsanto, claiming that he illegally planted GM corn without the company's permission. Schmeiser had planted rapeseed plants for use in canola oil on his 1,400 acres of land for over forty years. However, this time, he noticed some small patches of plants that refused to die after spraying them for weed protection with Monsanto's powerful herbicide, Roundup®. Monsanto, owners of what is purportedly the largest biotech center in the world in St. Louis, Missouri, had successfully introduced what they call "Roundup Ready Canola," a rapeseed that resists destruction *by its own herbicide*. Think about that—Roundup Ready® Transgenic Canadian Oil.

First introduced in 1995, Roundup Ready has become the Canadian farmers' preferred choice for weed control. Monsanto modified the rapeseed, called canola seed, to tolerate glyphosate, the active ingredient in their leading herbicide. This means that farmers can now yield more produce at less cost by spraying less pesticide. Drift from seed is quite common, and Schmeiser contends that the wind carried the patented seed genes into his fields. Monsanto sued claiming Schmeiser knowingly replanted the seed without paying them a royalty. The low court, Supreme Court, and Court of Appeals all ruled in Monsanto's favor. Schmeiser harvested and captured those seeds as he did all seeds each year for many years. Based on the high percentage of Schmeiser's crops that now contained the Roundup Ready altered gene, coupled with the fact that Schmeiser knowingly harvested and replanted them, the court ruled against him.

So, it's really just a matter of time until the seed that's not GM becomes GM. It's already spreading like wildfire. Not only through drifting, but quite by accident. Just ask more than a few European farmers and Advanta (a joint venture of AstraZeneca and Cosun U.A), headquartered in Kapelle in the Netherlands. Advanta sold some of its GM rapeseed mixed with non-GM rapeseed to farmers in France, Sweden, and Germany. Unlike the United States and Canada, the European community has cast a guarded eye on GM seed. Those products that are approved after long-term research must be labeled as such if over 0.9 percent of their ingredients are modified.

SO, IT'S REALLY JUST A MATTER OF TIME UNTIL THE SEED THAT'S NOT GM BECOMES GM. IT'S ALREADY SPREADING LIKE WILDFIRE.

Greenpeace believes that over 2.5 million acres of farmland in the European Union (EU) were contaminated by GM crops in the year 2000 alone. The German government acted quickly, demanding the immediate destruction of GM-contaminated rapeseed plants. France and Sweden also demanded the GM-contaminated crops, now being grown inadvertently throughout Europe, be destroyed.

It was too late. Just as many of us are now beginning to consider our position on GM, the seeds they are sowing have already infiltrated nearly every aspect of our food supply. Irresponsible governments that sanctioned companies to go for it are responsible for flooding our planet with whole new life forms, living things that did not evolve, nor prove themselves genetically over millions of years of natural selection. Natural selection has been dismantled by unregulated biotechnologists and given way to "super natural selection." Unregulated technologists working for giant biofood companies for profit yield a powerful wand that appears to have gone largely unchallenged. No long-term studies by the FDA were required. In fact, no testing of any sort was obligatory. Even organic-certified farmers who are prohibited from using genetically modified proteins in their seed have their reputations and certification at risk. The world's largest producer of GM crops in the world, the United States, apparently feels that it's in your best interest not to know it. The FDA used the law of similarity to condone the use of this new technology. Apparently, proteins in GM food appear similar enough to those in non-GM engineered food, according to our watchdogs.

Dr. John Hagelin, director of the Institute of Science, Technology & Public Policy, appears concerned about the lack of labeling: "Soy used in infant formula has genetic material and bacteria never before ingested by the human race." Hagelin told Newsweek.com *(Food Fight,* June 17, 1999) that "we are rewriting the genetic library of the earth in only three to five years. This is just the tip of the iceberg."

Proponents of GM site a brave new world—a world where technologists have the power of creation and natural selection at their fingertips. All they need do is cut and paste. Take a few genes out of one living organism and place it into another. Much like the promise of "Golden Rice," developed by the Rockefeller Foundation as an inexpensive solution to end vitamin A deficiency in third world countries. What began as an act of benevolence in the private sector became a money grab for big business.

AstraZeneca, the powerful biotech company in the U.K. who owns over seventy patents on Golden Rice, signed an agreement to sell this genetically modified food (the word "golden" refers to the beta-carotene contained in the outer sheath of the rice) to India. Because the third world eats polished rice because they have to, introducing this genetically modified miracle food is supposed to eradicate blindness and related vitamin A deficiencies in developing nations. However, the facts suggest otherwise.

As it turns out, the amount of beta-carotene that this rice presently contains (which gets converted by the body to vitamin A) won't make a dent in the minimum daily requirement. To do so would require the person to eat more than practically possible. But, is this a legitimate indictment of a promising technology, as its critics suggest?

While *drift* can carry seed from genetically modified crops to fields where they weren't present, is that a bad thing if the seeds are engineered to present no danger? But how is that possible?

The answer is a simple one. If genetic seed makers were regulated, long-term testing could be required before a product is introduced. For those that would remain skeptics, seed companies could simply be required to engineer crops with sterile pollen. We need to carefully review logical objections to a technology with such promise, when it appears almost too good to be true.

Theoretically, a gene from a piranha could be spliced into a human being. Pretty scary, huh? One can only imagine the potential danger if other equally shocking variations were ever engineered and introduced to our world. Yet just as theoretically, an airplane could be made to have a weakness in a wing, if it were engineered by evil and misguided wrongdoers. Does that make avionics a bad thing? Of course not. The potential for any technology to be used for evil exists, but we have found countless ways to ensure that the potential to do so is remote.

THE POTENTIAL FOR ANY TECHNOLOGY TO BE USED FOR EVIL EXISTS, BUT WE HAVE FOUND COUNTLESS WAYS TO ENSURE THAT THE POTENTIAL TO DO SO IS REMOTE.

On the flip side, a gene from a fish that has the ability to resist freezing can now be placed into a chromosome of a vegetable. The transplanted gene will do exactly as it was originally programmed to do, transmitting its special properties into its new host. This vegetable, once prone to early death from frost, is no longer susceptible. Now there can be enough of this food to feed the many who are starving for it nutrients.

How can that be a bad thing? It's important that we examine all sides of this multifaceted issue, to help us sanely and responsibly resolve a seemingly irresolvable issue. Gene transferring permits scientists to solve many age-old problems that have plagued mankind for billions of years and now beg for resolution. Today, using this technology, food can be produced where it couldn't before, at a lower cost, and in less space. Scientists can even grow bone where it's needed, and where it never existed (for example, in a child who was born without a breastplate). Should we condemn a technology that holds such incredible promise?

Genetic modification is just one of many exciting branches of the biosciences that are utilizing life science technologies to improve the structure and behavior of living organisms. The term "bioscience" refers to any of the natural sciences dealing with living organisms. This includes all technologies that use living things to vastly improve our way of life.

Fumento describes some of the exciting advances being made, which includes phytoremediation, a technology that takes advantage of the need of certain plants "to remove, destroy or sequester hazardous substances from the environment." This includes the ability to efficiently and effectively clean contaminated water by using plant roots to uptake contaminates. It also includes the use of plants to reduce the mobility of contaminants in the soil. To illustrate the power of this technology, Fumento cites an article by Dan Johnson ("Flowers that Fight Pollution," *Futurist*, April 1999) that chronicles the work of a company known today as EdenSpace systems of Reston, Virginia. They actually used sunflowers to absorb 95 percent of the deadly radioactive elements found in groundwater close to a small pond near the Chernobyl nuclear plant. An amazing accomplishment, particularly given the fact that it was completed in just ten days!

Fumento notes equally amazing accomplishments through advancements made in a number of other biosciences, including the use and science of biopesticides. These are naturally occurring substances such as bacteria with pesticide activity that kills insects (for a fraction of the cost farmers pay for pesticide protection) but are not toxic to birds, mammals, or fish, nor does it persist in the soil. With over 120 insecticidal proteins, it's an example of one such bacteria that's been recombined successfully into modified plant genes for some time.

Today, seeded cotton, potatoes, and corn all have built-in protection against predators. This method is also making the environment safer, crop yields higher (less land is required to achieve the same results), and labor costs lower. In a nutshell, it's a more effective, more productive, and far safer approach than using many hazardous, conventional pesticides.

So, is GM the demon its detractors would have you believe? A report published in 2006 by the National Center for Food and Agricultural Policy confirmed the significant benefits of GM crops that have been continually embraced by American growers in the preceding decade. In 2005, eight genetically modified crops (canola, sweet corn, feed corn, squash, soybeans, cotton, papaya, and alfalfa) were planted in our country on 123 million acres of land that fortified these crops with resistance against insects, herbicides, and/or viruses. The impact of doing so was extraordinary. In 2005, it resulted in

8.3 billion additional pounds of crop production, and a reduction of some 69.7 million pounds of pesticides.

Such amazing increases in productivity, coupled with a subsequent reduction in the costs required to protect their crops from infestation, improved these growers' net returns by some two billion dollars. Other biotech solutions appear equally promising, including amazing advances such as the use of monoclonal antibodies and antisense technology to fight disease. These solutions will rapidly solve many of the gravest problems facing our world, and will do so efficiently.

Today, genetic modification allows us to improve the flavor, healthfulness, and availability of the food we eat and the environment we share. Less land will be required to feed far more people less expensively than we currently believe possible. Plants and animals will be saved, most diseases we know today will be eliminated, and the poor will be fed.

This is no fairy tale. Many such miracles are being performed while hundreds more are in final trial stages in laboratories across the world. Our world is filled with a good deal of despair for many. The Worldwide Success Organization estimates that today 1.2 billion people survive on less than $1 a day, and that the top 1 percent of the world's richest people earn as much as the poorest 57 percent. We will soon be capable of gene splicing a host of perfect foods. Good foods (white rice with the amount of beta-carotene being added isn't one of them) that will feed the hungry. Detractors should balance the reality of the poor with the hope that our food system will be capable of feeding them.

THE WORLDWIDE SUCCESS ORGANIZATION ESTIMATES THAT TODAY 1.2 BILLION PEOPLE SURVIVE ON LESS THAN $1 A DAY, AND THAT THE TOP 1 PERCENT OF THE WORLD'S RICHEST PEOPLE EARN AS MUCH AS THE POOREST 57 PERCENT.

Today it won't. Only a miracle will—and that miracle will be found through the genetic modification of our food. If the technology was available to you for your starving child nearing the end of his or her young life, would you dwell on the shortcomings of GM, or advocate ways to improve it? There are shortcomings with this new technology, as there are with all new technologies, to be sure.

The first is the lack of required labeling. Why is a *toy* company required to warn the consumer about potential hazards of their products, but *food* companies selling us stuff we count on for survival are not? If a food has been modified, manufacturers should be required to state so, and to explain exactly how they did so. The FDA allows certain health claims be made, because they know suppliers use it for the sole purpose of marketing their product. However, they don't require the complete truth in labeling, nor any labeling of GM foods at the time of this writing. If there are potential allergens, say so. If the bacteria used might pose a potential risk for those of us with certain diseases or health conditions, say so. If there *is* potential for any modified food to interact with any medication, then tell it like it is. The same should hold true for foods containing preservatives and additives. While they're required to be listed, food makers are not required to spell out their potential impact on our health.

Why? After all, even drug companies are required to list the potential side effects of their products. Is the FDA afraid that doing so would be too costly? Or that special interest groups from some of these companies might be upset, because such warnings might scare away their consumers? I, for one, believe such a warning could accomplish exactly that. Holding the maker's feet to the grindstone with this kind of accountability would force many of these suppliers to stop adding certain preservatives and additives to our foods.

The Keebler company did just that, after one brave American took out ads about the trans fat content in some of their products. Keebler found a way, because they had to. The other guys will as well, but only if they have to.

While the lack of labeling is one problem, the lack of testing is another. No retailer will accept a product from a toy manufacturer that's not tested for potential hazards to a child, and they're required to perform these tests at an independent lab. However, the government has no such requirement for *food* makers. GM foods are actually tested for any allergy potential in the manufacturer's *own* labs.

... PHARMACEUTICAL MAKERS ARE REQUIRED TO TEST FOR ANY POTENTIAL HAZARDS. BUT THEY'RE NOT REQUIRED TO USE INDEPENDENT LABS.

Similarly, pharmaceutical makers are required to test for any potential hazards. But they're not required to use independent labs. They're permitted to use their own labs, or labs *they* select. That's okay with the FDA. If the drug proves faulty and people become ill or die, the FDA simply slaps their hands with a fine and recalls it. Before a drug is approved, clinical trials are required to be performed by makers which must be reviewed by the FDA. But drug manufacturers are permitted to fund and select the researchers they choose to perform crucial stage 3 clinical trials. Though not necessarily flawed, the potential for conflicts of interest are great.[1] They're free to design tests that favor their own product.

In an article entitled "Third Party Quality Assurance: Why External Control Is Better?" author Yun Zheng, writing for the International Biopharmaceutical Association puts this practice into perspective," GlaxoSmithKline, maker of the antidepressant drug Paxil, is being sued by the State of New York for fraud. The drug company is accused of withholding negative results and distorting study data in order to get Paxil approved for the treatment of children.

While toy makers must use truly independent labs to design and perform their own trials; pharmaceutical makers sponsor researchers to design their own.

In addition to labeling and testing, certification is non-existent for many products and claims (such as using the word *natural*, except as previously mentioned); regulation is often absent as well. The FDA is powerless for example, to make a drug maker test a product at all after it's been given approval.

Today, anyone with the right knowledge can create a modified plant. Anyone. Plant seeds can drift or be forced to drift, with potentially adverse consequences. The lack of regulation in this area is frightening and Congress needs to address it without further delay. I share the same concern on this subject as Karl Klaus (one of the biggest critics of the aerial age of flight) did on a similar one. The deceased Vienna journalist was one of the harshest critics of the airplane. He believed that while people were clever enough to create sophisticated machines, they often lacked the intelligence to use them properly. Which begs an answer to an important question … who should we choose to certify and regulate genetically modified material?

In the case of our food products, local farmers are the most qualified for the job. The federal government has proven it has no desire, talent, ability, or fortitude to protect you and your children. The reasons to buy locally grown foods go far beyond your wish to help the local farmer. They're about helping *you*. Genetically grown food, with the support of the people, will turn the need to eat ORGLOC (Organic, Locally Grown) into the need to eat *GORLOC* (Genetically Modified, Organic, Locally Grown). Genetically modified foods should be all about the local farmer. Which makes the argument for eating locally grown foods even more compelling—when many of these foods can be provided and sold by them.

As our genetic food revolution rapidly evolves, the average farmer in any part of the country will be able to plant a far greater variety of crops, without the need to be concerned about soil erosion from the lack of crop rotation; growing foods more economically, with bountiful yields and require considerably less land. Biopesticides will accomplish much more for much less, reducing the cost of labor for the local farmer. (Strange as it may seem, in one area of Africa, the government is opposed to the introduction of GM foods on the grounds that while it may put an end to starvation, it could hurt the locals who are paid to pull the weeds!)

GENE SPLICING WILL ALLOW CROPS THAT WERE EITHER COLD OR HEAT RESISTANT TO SURVIVE IN AREAS THEY COULDN'T HAVE BEFORE ...

Gene splicing will allow crops that were either cold or heat resistant to survive in areas they couldn't have before, while crops the locals currently grow with great difficulty will flourish with relative ease. Now, changing the food supply chain will make more sense than ever. There will be no need for countless middle men such as grocery chains and long-distance food purveyors, nor manufacturers who supply machines that rapidly and artificially complete the maturing/ripening process of our foods after they're prematurely harvested.

The destiny of our poor, and of the rest of the population, lies in the hands of the local farmer. Yes, it's hard to believe, but we *can* completely change the way we currently approach the way we receive and distribute our food.

We did so once before. That's precisely how we got ourselves into this mess, putting our food supply in the hands of giant food processors. As the GM revolution evolves, and buying GORLOC becomes the only way to solve our problems of health and hunger, the few courageous farmers that are left are going to need your support. So will food co-ops, and food programs in our schools.

It starts with you.

It ends with certification from the *state* for GORLOC foods that pass independent lab testing based on a host of important criteria. The requirements themselves would be determined by a national independent GORLOC Council, focusing on improved affordable, and more available foods, locally grown by council certified farmers. The council would consist of fourteen members with two representatives from each of the following areas:

- Agricultural researchers from major universities
- Genetic researchers from leading hospitals or universities
- Seed corporations involved in biotech food modification
- Researchers or authors focused on preventative health with a focus on food

In addition to these eight council members, the remaining six representatives would consist of:

- Two school superintendents
- Four local farmers who practice organic farming

The council chairman would nominate no less than three candidates for each slot (not less than thirty-six persons). The voting would be done by the head of the Department of Agricultural, representing each county in the United States. The chairman of the *council of fourteen* would not be a government official, and would be required to have no commercial affiliation with any business enterprise involved in any aspect of the food supply chain. This citizen would be elected from a list of known humanitarians and benefactors who have demonstrated that helping others, without a profit motive, is an important part of their life's work.

A list of ten such candidates for the chairman's position that fit these criteria would be developed and submitted by the council. The final selection for the position of chairman would be made by the head of the Department of Agriculture from every county in America, who would subsequently vote on the chairman's nominees. Licensing would be the responsibility of each state, based on the rules drafted by the council. Supervision and annual compliance would be enforced by every agricultural department in each of the over 3,100 counties in the United States.

But who would fund this new group of county-level regulators? The junk *food processors,* who seek to sell their food in that county, that's who. Yes, this is a terrific sin tax. I feel no remorse for the impact it would have on its makers. Yes, they will be forced to raise their product costs accordingly or live on less gross margin, or a combination of each. Yes, "users" will have to pay more for *junk food,* just like those who have had to pay through the nose to smoke cigarettes. In the end, this will only help the local farmer and support their efforts to do everything they can to sell us healthier products. Along the way, maybe more than a few of us will change the way we choose to eat. And what about those that don't? In the end, we'll have to thank them. Their bad habits, could help us support our good ones.

No specific recommendations for solving problems can be made without evoking criticism, and mine will be no exception. But it's a real plan, with the genuine potential to improve the lives of us and our children. We must make our health an issue for our elected officials. After all, what should take precedent over *our* health, and the safety of our children? This is no fantasy. It's a reality that I hope all of us and the officials we elect truly work toward. There's a lot at stake here. Unless you'd prefer to remain *Misinformed About Food*.

END NOTES

1. *WEBMD Health News*; April 15, 2008 ; Can Drug Clinical Trials Be Trusted? Quote from interview by Daniel J DeNoon with Catherine D. DeAngelis, Editor-in Chief of the Journal of the American Medical Association.

CHAPTER 5

THE SOS SUPPLEMENTS

"The best vitamin for making friends ... B1."
—Doyle Brunson

There's a great deal of confusion regarding the *use* of supplements, which generally contributes to their *misuse*. There are those that feel that supplements are a waste of your time and money. And, that if we just eat properly, there's no need for them. But I believe such people are misinformed. And so are several of the leading makers that produce them. While the focus of this book is whole foods, supplements are required to optimize the fuel in our tanks. While they are that important, make no mistake about it—supplements are no *substitute* for foods rich in important nutrients.

In fact, in contrast, they're more often than not an inferior source of nutrients. That's why isolated sources of vitamins or minerals are known as supplements. Many studies referred to in this book show the value of other constituents found in whole foods that work collectively to provide far more than any single nutrient can on its own. But often, it's simply not possible to eat enough of them to fight or reverse certain conditions and disease (particularly given the depleted nature of our food supply). The following discussion illustrates the importance of supplementation.

Few of us eat *properly;* even those that make a genuine effort may fail. As you know, we are what we eat—ate. And what our *foods* are eating today is degraded soil in contrast to the nutrient laden earth their ancestors ate.

In 2003, the *Journal of Nutritional Health* published a study by Dr. David Thomas that analyzed follow-up data from a study that first began in 1927. That study, first undertaken at Kings College at the University of London, was designed to provide dietary recommendations to diabetics. Over successive generations the scope of the study grew to include identification and measurement of the mineral and biological content of foods.

The fifth edition, published in 1991, captured fifty-one years of comparative data collected since the original study began. By using this information, Thomas was able to compare the mineral content in a number of foods over a good deal of time. The results show an alarming loss of minerals and trace elements during these periods. Spinach, for example, lost 60 percent of its iron and 70 percent of its phosphorous, while carrots lost 75 percent of its magnesium and broccoli lost 75 percent of its calcium. Dr. Thomas was kind enough to send me data from his latest study published in 2007, which confirmed the fruit and vegetable analysis of his previous work while expanding the investigation of those foods he previously reviewed.

Unfortunately, the affect of super-farming and the corresponding reduction of its important nutrients remains alarming. The trend remains intact. Produce more and receive less. As Dr. Thomas remarks: "What a dilemma we have found ourselves in. Research from all over the world has demonstrated the reality of the loss of micronutrients from our foods and provides evidence that micronutrient deficiencies significantly undermine our health, contributing towards chronic physiological and psychological illness in people of all ages."

Is there anything of value left in commercially produced food? Yes there is. But it's important to understand that eating, alone, may not be enough to help us overcome all the obstacles we face in life. Preventing a frontal attack is not the same thing as averting a full-scale invasion.

... OUR PUSH TO PRODUCE LARGER CROPS IN A SHORTER PERIOD OF TIME HAS RESULTED IN OUR PLANTS' DIMINISHED ABILITY TO GRADUALLY ABSORB HIGH QUALITY ORGANIC NUTRIENTS FROM TOPSOIL.

Author Brian Halweils' critical issue report, written for the Organic Center (September 2007, "Still No Free Lunch: Nutrient Levels in U.S. Food Supply Eroded by Pursuit of High Yields"), further illustrates the impact of mushrooming crop yields on the corresponding erosion of nutrients in our food. Clearly, our ability to increase production of food in a given amount of space has come at a price. As Halweils points out, our push to produce larger crops in a shorter period of time has resulted in our plants' diminished ability to gradually absorb high quality organic nutrients from topsoil. Instead, they've come to depend on chemical fertilizers that are quickly broken down from highly watered ground, where plants compete for organic matter in crowded quarters. They were densely planted to increase yield on the same amount of acreage.

In the end, advances in agricultural practices have succeeded in yielding far more produce in the same amount of space with considerably less value. Now, ship it 1500 miles, gas it, store it, expose it to light and heat, and then refrigerate it. As a people, we are eating a greater amount of food but receiving nutritionally less.

To that end, I'm pleased to quote a passage from Dr. Thomas' conclusion in his most recent 2007 study (*Nutrition and Health*, 2007, Volume 19, pp. 21–55): "There is clearly still a long way to go and the next step will be to insist on the proper nourishment of the soils on which our food is grown and reared, preferably through organic, bio-dynamic and other sustainable farming methods, so that it will necessarily provide the minerals and trace elements that are essential for our future health and well being."

Dr. Thomas clearly understands that we are what we eat—ate. *Soil is the food for our food.* And sadly, we continue to take advantage of mother earth. Crowded planting and over-watering, combined with mega doses of pesticides, fungicides, chemical fertilizers, and root stimulators produce cattle-like food that's all talk with little walk. Like gerbils on a treadmill, our bodies work harder to go nowhere.

According to the United Nations Food and Agriculture Organization, the average American eats 3,790 calories a day (for the period between 2000–2002), compared to 3,480 (for the period between 1979–1981). The trend is clear. We continue to eat more, and benefit less. It's also important to note that some of the startling benefits reported in studies regarding the intake of certain nutrients were a result of concentrated doses or extracts of that vitamin or mineral, rather than from the normal consumption of the whole foods they're found in. This doesn't take away from the value of eating the right foods. But it underscores the importance of supplementing to achieve the higher-octane performance we're after. Topping off the tank is affordable insurance.

According to researcher Diamsao Hornero-Mendez (Chemistry and Biochemistry of Pigments Group, Department of Food Biotechnology, Instituto de la Grasa), less than 5 percent of carotenoids are released from our food. To put the value of a supplement in perspective, Lester Packer points out in his book *The Anti-Oxidant Miracle* (1999, Lester Packer PhD and Carol Colman, John Wiley and Sons, Inc.) that in order to receive his recommended amount of vitamin E (500 I/ Us daily), one would need to eat 125 tablespoons of peanut butter, or 100 pounds of broiled liver.

Dr. Timothy J. Smith, MD (1998, *Renewal: The Anti-Aging Revolution*, Rodale Press) compares supplements in human diets to fertilizing plants. While both can generally get by with the basics in their initial period of growth, those with nutrient-dense diets flourish in later stages of life. He contrasts the RDA of vitamin E, which was designed to prevent us from deficiency, to with what he calls the ODA, or optimum amount of nutrients required in the opinion of leading nutritionists. As you may have guessed, there's much disparity between these numbers.

The RDA has traditionally focused on the least amount of a nutrient required to prevent a deficiency, while the ODA (optimal daily allowance) is the amount a professional in the field feels is necessary to maximize the potential of a given nutrient. Dr. Smith's ODA for vitamin E, for example, starts in the range of 400 IUs daily. To achieve this with vitamin E-dense foods alone would require you to eat the equivalent of 2 pounds of wheat germ, or 33 pounds of spinach. Finally, he reminds us that allergies, smoking, infection, and stress further deplete our nutrients.

Vitamin C is also diminished in persons taking aspirin, birth control pills, and other drugs. Injury and trauma result in larger losses of this important nutrient, a fact you need to be aware of if you or a loved one experience either. Hopefully I've succeeded in convincing you that spending money on the *right* supplements is money well spent. The problem is trying to determine what's right.

If you're like most people, you've done what someone else suggested you do. We generally don't have the time to research these recommendations, and often find ourselves accepting what we've been told. But, more often than not, the people that gave this advice, received it the same way they're providing it to you. As a result, most of us are supplementing with things we don't need to, in ways we don't have to, or know how to. The purpose of the book is to assist you, by researching the researchers. It's also why we developed our Informed Living "Super-Multiple", providing real protection morning and night, based the ODA's found here.

We only have to turn again to Dr. Lester Packer, senior scientist at the distinguished Lawrence Berkeley National Laboratory. As a member of UCLA's Department of Molecular and Cell Biology, and head of its famed Packer Lab, one of the leading antioxidant research centers in the world, Dr. Packer has devoted five decades of his life in research designed to further our understanding of these important vitamins and minerals.

THE IMPORTANCE OF VITAMIN C: THE WATER-SOLUBLE WONDER

You can believe what you've heard from someone else, or you can rely on hard data from solid research garnered by one of the true icons in the field. There are a few people, and a few nutrients, whose reliable information is noteworthy. Dr Packer is one. His discovery of the role of lipoic acid as the quarterback to help rebuild a team of important nutrients is critically important. We'll return to this significant discovery shortly.

There are other researchers who are also authorities in the area of supplementation. Collectively, their recommendations based on real science, in whole or in part, have been incorporated into the SOS Super-Nutrient program. But his belief and the belief of many others, which has gained a good deal of steam, is that the body has a low threshold before your tissues are saturated with vitamin C. This issue is the subject of much debate. He cites research that shows that when subjects took a 180-milligram supplement, half of this amount was expelled in the urine. And *90 percent* is excreted if you take a 2000-milligram supplement. Packer believes that if you take more than your body needs, the body simply won't accept it.

Today, while opinions still vary, there is a groundswell of support for the less is best notion regarding vitamin C; which stands in direct opposition to Linus Paulings' research on mega-doses of this important nutrient.

While Packers' finding regarding lipoic acid and other nutrients are groundbreaking, I respectfully disagree with his position on our bodies' low threshold of saturation for this nutrient. You see, much of the "less is best" notion stems from two different studies performed by the National Institutes for Health. A 2001 study coauthored by NIH researchers (Biofactors, 15: 71–74, 2001) concluded: "Furthermore, the concentration of ascorbic acid (the technical name for vitamin C) in blood plasma never exceeds much more than 70–85 micromole per deciliter of blood regardless of the dosage of vitamin C consumed."

Their April 15, 1996, press release based on an earlier study (National Institute of Diabetes and Digestive and Kidney Diseases) states that "at 200 milligrams oral intake, blood plasma had more than 80 percent maximal concentration of vitamin C and tissues were completely saturated. Doses of 500 milligrams and higher are completely excreted in urine."

Unfortunately, these studies have also been used to establish a basis for the RDA of vitamin C in the U.S. But, according to authors Dr. Steve Hickey and Dr. Hilary Roberts (*Ascorbate: The Science of Vitamin C*, May 2004), the research was flawed. Their argument—they failed to account for the half-life of this nutrient. You see, vitamin C disappears from blood plasma after approximately 30 minutes (fortunately, Dr. Packer's discovery of the role of lipoic acid, however, is that it helps us rebuild this and other important nutrients). Hickey contends that NIJ researchers waited until it was gone, retested, and concluded that since it was eliminated, the body had reached its saturation point.

The NIH must feel that way too. Because in 2004 NIH researchers coauthored another Study (Archives of Biochemistry and Biophysics, 423, 109–115, 2004) on vitamin C's bioavailability, which completely contradicted their own work. This time, they showed that *plasma* concentrations *did increase* with progressively higher levels of oral intake. In fact, doses of 2000 milligrams showed corresponding plasma concentrations of 143 micromoles. Now remember their conclusion from previous studies in 2001: "Blood plasma *never exceeds much more than 70-85* micromole per deciliter of blood regardless of the dosage of vitamin C consumed." And in 1996 … "At 200 milligrams oral intake, blood plasma had more than 80 percent maximal concentration of vitamin C and tissues were completely saturated. Doses of 500 milligrams and higher are completely excreted in urine."

This time the researchers concluded that "optimizing vitamin C intake appears warranted." We can all give thanks to vitamin C pioneer and Nobel Laureate Linus Pauling who was operating on the right track. And, to doctors Hickey and Roberts for keeping him there.

Vitamin C is an electron donor. It gladly gives up an electron to an unstable molecule to stop it from further oxidizing. Like so many other molecules we've already discussed, free radicals are both good and bad. In fact, without free radicals, we'd have no life. They do everything from fight infection to signal our genes to turn on and off. A natural by-product of oxidation, too many free radicals, the result of excessive oxidation, ages us and results in chronic inflammation, thus promoting disease. Too few prevent our blood from flowing properly, and diminish our ability to protect ourselves against dangerous bacteria and viruses. Some are messengers, such as nitric oxide, that signal our vessels to expand and are helpful. Others, like hydroxyl radical, are dangerous and hurtful. The key, as always, is balance. The right balance to protect ourselves from *excessive* oxidation.

Oxidation is a normal process of life. But life has surrounded us with an excessive amount of free radicals that promote excessive internal oxidation that must be countered. Antioxidants, in the form of certain vitamins and nutrients found in food and supplements, thwart oxidation, stabilizing highly reactive molecules by giving up an electron. While mega-dosing can cause the wrong balance to occur, proper dosing can create equilibrium.

How do we know if our balancing act is right or wrong? There are various tests that are important to take, to develop a baseline that can be periodically monitored. The upcoming SOS chart will get you there.

Vitamin C is a powerful antioxidant, and a major player in the Synergy of Super-Nutrients program. While most animals can synthesize it by converting glucose, we've lost our ability to do so somewhere along the line in the evolutionary process (so did guinea pigs and birds). Vitamin C is an electron donor to eight different enzymes. And when you're frightened, it's your adrenal gland that protects you by producing hormones such as adrenaline, histamine, corticosterone, and cortisol. Collectively, they create that

VITAMIN C IS AN ELECTRON DONOR TO EIGHT DIFFERENT ENZYMES.

flight response in all of us—to react to and avoid imminent danger. Without a sufficient supply of vitamin C, the adrenal gland is incapable of doing so.

And to that end, an intricate system evolved to stimulate them to do so. Our brain first signals our pituitary gland to secrete a substance known as adrenocorticotrophic hormone (ACTH). This prompts the adrenal glands to get going. All of this occurs as a normal response to stress; a condition we're all too familiar with in life. And each time this occurs, the vitamin C present in our adrenal glands is further diminished by not only the amount required to produce these hormones, but by the effect of ACTH itself.

Since we can't produce vitamin C, it needs to be on hand. But we're just as incapable of storing it as we are producing it. Goats can. In fact, they're capable of producing a whopping 15,820 milligrams of it. But so what? Have you ever seen a stressed out goat? And while we're all affected by stressors in our external environments that are chemical, behavioral, and social, we're also receiving a good deal of internal stress from drugs, poor food choices, and toxins in our environment. Some of us are more prone than others to perceive and intensify stress. For such individuals, insuring an adequate intake of vitamin C may be even more critical.

While its role in protecting us from external events is huge, its primary function is to keep us from becoming unglued. Not just cognitively, but physically;

and not just figuratively, but quite literally. That's right—vitamin C is required to form collagen, the glue that actually holds us together. The major protein in our body, it's required for cartilage, tendons, connective tissue, teeth, and facia (type of connective tissue all over our bodies). This protein provides our skin its elasticity; and as it diminishes, the signs of wrinkles and aging become increasingly evident. It's also used medically to create artificial skin for burn victims.

So if we can't produce enough of this very important nutrient, we have to continually replenish by eating it. While some studies suggest vitamin C has a serum life of only 30 minutes, others show it can last in us for longer periods of time. In vitro, scientists Smith et al. (*The FASEB Journal*, 2002;16:1102–1104; "Vitamin C matters: increased oxidative stress in cultured human aortic endothelial cells without supplemental ascorbic acid") showed that epithelial cells replete with vitamin C enjoy significantly less oxidation and experience a substantial increase in nitric oxide production. And that C lasted in this tissue for far longer than previously thought. According to the study: "We show that providing vitamin C results in uptake into cells and intracellular vitamin C levels are maintained for at least 6 hours before declining. Thus, vitamin C supplementation results in a transient yet marked improvement in intracellular ascorbic acid levels despite the potential for oxidation or hydrolysis occurring in the media."

The number of studies proving the incredible value of this life altering nutrient are too numerous to mention. It's been credited with its ability to help us prevent just about everything detrimental to our health. According to a meta-analysis of 13 clinical studies that included 14 groups of subjects with elevated blood fat, daily doses of approximately 500 milligrams a day on average, for periods ranging from three to twenty-four weeks, were responsible for a reduction in pro-inflammatory triglycerides of an incredible 8.8 percent (*Journal of Chiropractic Medicine June*, 2008, Volume 7, Issue 2, Pages 48–58, "Vitamin C supplementation lowers serum low-density lipoprotein cholesterol and triglycerides: a meta-analysis of 13 randomized controlled trials"). Contrast that with the 40,000 milligrams a day (40 grams), which was the amount taken daily by Lineus Pauling, often referred to as the father of vitamin C. He also recommended 10,000 milligrams (10 grams daily) to others, based, at least in part, on the amount synthesized by most other animals capable of producing this oxidant daily. Pauling believed we lost our ability to do so as we evolved, after our early ancestors began eating plants that were rich with this nutrient.

But where does that leave us, given our modern diet? The RDA remains a paltry 60 milligrams a day for adults. Remember, all RDAs are based on the minimum amount of a nutrient required to avoid disease, such as scurvy, which occurs in those who have an insufficient intake of this vitamin. In the past, this disease plagued many a pirate and sea captain at sea for long periods without sufficient intake of fruits and vegetables. It wasn't until James Linds' book *A Treatise of the Scurvy* was published in 1753 that we learned of experiments with citrus fruit that remedied this situation. Fresh lemons were such a godsend that they soon earned the nickname "scurvy grass." On the other hand, the Royal British Navy opted for limes on board when at sea, and soon the term "limey" was born.

ON THE OTHER HAND, THE ROYAL BRITISH NAVY OPTED FOR LIMES ON BOARD WHEN AT SEA, AND SOON THE TERM "LIMEY" WAS BORN.

But low levels of vitamin C are characterized by less spectacular trauma that should also signal danger, such as joint pain, nosebleeds, frequent infection, easy bruising, gingivitis, bleeding gums, swelling, dry skin and hair, and anemia. And the majority of Americans fall woefully short of receiving an optimum intake of vitamin C. While contrary to claims, C has not been conclusively shown to prevent cancer as Pauling and others contend (Pauling lived to be 93 years old before dying of pancreatic cancer, which he claimed was postponed twenty years by this mega dose regimen). But some studies indicate a substantial reduction in the *incidence* of certain cancers for those with a high intake of vitamin C—those eating dense fruits and vegetables as opposed to those eating minimal amounts of them. But other research, including the respected *China Study*, shows that regular consumption of high fiber foods (such as leafy vegetables), as well as beans and whole grains, were associated with correspondingly lower rates of colon and rectal cancer (*The China Study*, T. Colin Campbell, PhD, Thomas M Campbell 11, page 92). Were the results showing a reduction in the incidence of certain cancers from the C itself, or from the fiber in the foods that contained it?

Vitamin C has been associated with lowered risk of other chronic conditions, such as stroke. But a good deal of these studies, while well constructed and longitudinal, were based on the dietary records provided by participants who were subject to their recall or a more favorable recollection of good versus bad decision-making. One such study (*BMJ*, 1995;310:1563–1566; "Vitamin C and risk of death from stroke and coronary heart disease in cohort of elderly people")

ACCORDING
TO THE STUDY:
"MORTALITY
FROM STROKE
WAS HIGHEST
IN THOSE WITH
THE LOWEST
VITAMIN C
STATUS."

conducted by researcher Catherine R. Gale and colleagues followed the dietary habits of 730 men and women with a history of stroke, atherosclerosis, or CHD over a twenty-year period. According to the study: "Mortality from stroke was highest in those with the lowest vitamin C status." Note that 643 subjects died during this twenty-year period—124 deaths were from stroke.

They found no such correlation with heart disease. They also attributed the potentially life saving benefits of vitamin C as much to the consumption of fruits and vegetables as they did to supplements, which only a few of the participants had taken on a regular basis. But, another respected study that *did* focus on supplementation found that supplementation of vitamin C *did* indeed reduce the risk of heart disease in women (*Journal of the American College of Cardiology*, 2003; 42:246–252, doi:10.1016/S0735-1097(03)00575-8; "Vitamin C and risk of coronary heart disease in women"). The team of researchers, led by Stavroula K. Osganian, MD, concluded: "Users of vitamin C supplements appear to be at lower risk for CHD." A number of other studies support this. Clearly, vitamin C intake in foods and supplements is that important, and sufficient consumption can protect you from oxidation, certain stress related trauma, heart disease, and stroke.

However, researchers have found that *post-menopausal* women who were *diabetic* actually *increased* their risk of cardiovascular disease from high doses of vitamin C (*American Journal of Clinical Nutrition*, Vol. 80, No. 5, 1194–1200, November 2004; "Does supplemental vitamin C increase cardiovascular disease risk in women with diabetes?"). But keep in mind that their blood plasma and hormonal deficiency varies a great deal from those in normal healthy subjects.

Vitamin C has also been shown to help eliminate toxins, such as lead in our bloodstream. In a study headed by Earl Dawson, he and his colleagues showed a dramatic reduction in lead in the blood plasma of smokers after only one month of taking 1000 milligrams of ascorbic acid (*Journal of the American College of Nutrition*, Vol. 18, No 2, 166-170, 1999; "The Effect of Ascorbic Acid Supplementation on the Blood Lead Levels of Smokers"). Researchers believe that vitamin C may accomplish this by reducing our kidneys' ability to absorb toxins such as lead. This also has implications for the reduction of lead and other pollutants in those of us exposed to second-hand smoke and other airborne industrial pollutants.

Vitamin C absorbs iron. Too much iron is a risk factor for heart attacks. As a water-soluble vitamin, it also serves to protect fat-soluble vitamins E and A. This important antioxidant is available in many different forms such as mineral ascorbics.

Other forms of ascorbic acid that involve attaching vitamin C to certain minerals (like calcium, chromium, magnesium, potassium, and zinc) are generally buffered and easier on your stomach (and often more expensive). But you'll need to take into consideration the decrease of C per milligram reduced by the amount of the mineral it's attached to. According to one of the world's leading experts on vitamin C, Dr. Robert Cathcart, MD, *mineral* ascorbates are not able to achieve basic ascorbate acid's ability to quench free radicals. As he explains in an interview with *Medline News Today* (January 24, 2005; "Vitamin C Foundation to Offer Best Vitamin C"), a molecule of ascorbic acid reacts with two free radicals, while mineral ascorbates only react with one free radical per molecule (they're already bound to the mineral ion that delivers them). That means you'd need to use twice as much to accomplish the same results. My suggestion: stick with ascorbic acid. While some brands tout special formulas of mineral ascorbate such as the Ester C® brand, large-scale studies proving it's more absorbable are, at the time of this writing, not available.

Made primarily of calcium ascorbate with small amounts of other vitamin C metabolites, the company indicates that a human study shows it's more bioavailable, while another small study found that this was not the case (Oregon State University, Linus Pauling Center, Micronutrient Research Center; The Bioavailability of Different Forms of Vitamin C). Vitamin C from natural food sources, such as rose hips or sago palm, is typically more expensive. Many brands featuring the former need to be examined carefully. Rose hips, the pomaceous fruit of the rose plant, are generally present in supplements. I've never seen any brand that contains 100 percent rose hips—probably due to the very high cost of processing them. So makers can put in any amount they wish and label their product as vitamin C, with Rose Hips. Even a hint will do.

So again, the greatest vitamin C for the buck remains the popular ascorbic acid form of vitamin C. Its contribution to our health and immunity can't be underscored. The key is how to conveniently take the right amount of it affordably. And as importantly, how to take the right amount, and get it to last as long as possible; since we can neither manufacture nor store it. The answer is to supplement twice a day with 500 milligrams of ascorbic acid—in conjunction with the other supplements that "empower" it, which we'll discuss shortly. And, eat the recommended SOS foods. Doing both will insure a steady supply of this important nutrient throughout the day. And for those of you who feel you need more, due to stress or the other extraneous situations discussed above, increase your intake gradually. The best evidence to determine when your body has had too much C is to listen to your body. Stomach cramps and diarrhea are signs that you're probably taking too much too fast. It's referred to as bowel tolerance. If you choose to increase your intake and experience any discomfort, cut back until you find the right amount your body can comfortably assimilate. There is no *one* amount that is right for everyone.

Take vitamin C or other vitamins with food to increase their absorption. Drink plenty of non-fluoridated spring water. Surprisingly, researchers haven't determined the optimal amount we require. While the notion that we all need eight glasses is unproven, I believe we need more. At a minimum, we need to replace the amount we lose daily. That's 64 ounces for the average adult. Tea, coffee and food *do* count toward satisfying our requirement. Drink an hour or so before and after meals. You'll avoid diluting nutrients and hindering their absorption.

Recall that vitamin C is poorly stored in our body. If there is no yellow color in your urine, your tissues aren't fully saturated. I'd rather see that color than not. It means I've done my job, and protected my body as fully as I can with this important nutrient. Of course, all of life is a matter of degree. The amount listed in the SOS program is just enough to get me there. And there's another benefit. The excess amount of vitamin C producing that healthy yellow color actually acidifies the blood, reducing your risk of urinary tract infection.

VITAMIN E: THE FIRST FAMILY OF NUTRIENTS AND PROTECTOR OF THE HEART AND IMMUNITY

A powerful antioxidant, what we often refer to as vitamin E, is actually an entire family of eight different fat-soluble vitamins; not just a single compound as is commonly thought. One group of these is known as tocopherols. The other group is known as tocotrienols. Each of these two groups consists of four different isomers: alpha, beta, gamma, and delta, respectively.

As you'll recall, isomers are molecules that share a similar chemical composition, but these same chemicals are structured differently. As a result, each isomer has a different role to play, effecting in a uniquely different manner. Exciting research involving both the tocopherol and tocotrienol families, as well as their isomers, has shown us exactly that. By focusing on the first group—the tocopherols (the type most commonly sold in this country)—at the exclusion of the others means we've missed out on the powerful healing ability of the second group—the lesser known tocotrienols.

Furthermore, most of the vitamin E tocopherol supplements that are sold today generally consist of the alpha variety only. So we've not only missed out on the wonderful benefits of the entire tocotrienol family, but of the other three isomers in this family as well. Makers principally focus on alpha tocopherol, which is understandable. First, according to Dr. Lester Packer, our liver seems to prefer to utilize this particular form. A special protein in our liver chooses alpha tocopherol more than it chooses any other isomer to travel in lipoproteins, which allows it to nourish each cell in our body. So our tissues contain more alpha tocopherol than any other form of vitamin E.

Since it's the most abundant source found in the human body, products were developed to provide more of what we appear to need most. Secondly, it's only in recent times that researchers have discovered the powerful role of the other isomers. And manufacturers have recently begun to make those available as well. Today, it's possible to purchase vitamin E in many forms. The principle ones are as follows:

Alpha tocopherol—the most popular sold today

Mixed tocopherols—which includes all of this family's isomers

Tocotrienols—the second lesser known class, with all *its* isomers.

All forms are available as a natural or synthetic supplement. Natural vitamin E is produced from plants and has the preface *"d."* Synthetic vitamin E is produced from oil and has the preface *"dl."* So, for example, a *natural* supplement of an E isomer, say gamma-tocopherol, would be properly labeled: *d* gamma-tocopherol. The synthetic version would be correctly labeled *dl* gamma-tocopherol. In general, natural sources, derived from natural molecules, are your best choice. And making the right choice is important.

An estimated 80,700,000 Americans (one in three) have one or more types of cardiovascular disease (CVD), according to the American Heart Association/American Stroke Association (Heart Disease and Stroke Statistics, 2008 update). Each year, approximately twelve million people die from cardiovascular disease in our world according to World Health. To put it in perspective, by the time you're done reading this short paragraph, another person will die of CVD (approximately one person every 37 seconds).

Now, the facts. A brief synopsis of only a few of the many impressive *human* studies:

ALPHA TOCOPHEROL

1. Boosts immune response in the elderly

Subjects: 88 people age 65 and older, divided into three groups

Dose: Group 1—60 IU, Group 2—200 IU, Group 3—800 IU,
   Group 4—Placebo

Study Origin: Tufts University-Jean Meyer USDA Nutrition Center on
   Aging at Tufts University (*Journal of the American Medical Association*,
   1997, May 7; 277:1380–6. Issue number 17).

Duration: Four months.

Results: **Stronger immune response** than control group to hepatitis B, marked increase in T and B cells that fight infection. Subjects also self-reported 30 percent less infection than those in study that did not supplement. Those taking 200 IU had a six-fold increase in the amount of antibodies in the blood to defend themselves against hepatitis B (shown on lab test known as titer). Interestingly, those taking 800 IUs only had a 2.5-fold increase. And the 200 IU group had a 65 percent increase in something known as DTH in contrast to the 800 IU group who only had an increase of DTH of 49 percent. It appears that, once we cross a certain threshold for alpha-tocopherol, in this case 800 IUs, our benefits are diminished.

DTH (delayed-type hypersensitivity skin response) is a measure of the body's ability to react quickly to opportunistic infections, such as HIV, hepatitis B, pneumonia, etc. and to develop antibodies to protect us against them.

2. Significantly reduces risk of heart disease in women

Subjects: 87,245 female nurses, ages 34–59.

Dose: Various—Those taking 30 IU or more enjoyed reduced risk, but the
   highest reduction was found in subjects taking more than 100 IUs daily.

Duration: Up to eight years for most subjects.

Study Origin: Harvard University ("Vitamin E Consumption and the Risk
   of Coronary Disease in Women," Volume 328:1444–1449, May 20,
   1993, Number 20), Meir J. Stampfer et al.

Results: **41 percent lower risk for heart disease for those supplementing for at least two years,** versus those in the study who did not supplement. Note, this study was a follow-up based on questionnaires, so while indicative, it can't be construed as definitively causal.

3. Significantly reduces risk of heart disease in elderly
Subjects: 11,178 people between the age of 67–105
Dose: Varied. Estimated at 100 IUs or more for best results.
Duration: Nine-year follow-up study based on data gathered in The
   Established Populations for Epidemiological Studies of the Elderly.
Study Origin: Epidemiology, Demography and Biometry Program,
   National Institute on Aging, Bethesda, MD (*American Journal of
   Clinical Nutrition,* 64(2):190–196; Aug 1996; "Vitamin E and
   vitamin C supplement use and risk of all-cause and coronary heart
   disease mortality in older persons: the Established Populations for
   Epidemiologic Studies of the Elderly"), Katlin Losonczy et al.
Results: **40 percent lower risk for heart disease** versus those taking the
least amount of E.

4. Reduces risk of heart disease in subjects previously diagnosed with CHD
Subjects: 2002 persons
Dose: 400 IU or 800 IU daily; 1035 subjects, 967 placebo group
Study Origin: Department of Medicine, Cambridge University (*Lancet,*
   1996 Mar 23; 347(9004):781–6; "Randomized controlled trial of
   vitamin E in patients with coronary disease: Cambridge Heart
   Antioxidant Study," CHAOS); Stephens et al.
Duration: 510 days
Results: Either dose **reduced progression of coronary artery atheroscle-
rosis in men** with previous coronary artery bypass graft surgery.

5. Reduces risk of coronary heart disease in men
Subjects: 39,910 male health professionals 40 to 75 years of age, free of
   diagnosed diabetes, heart disease, and hypercholesterolemia.
Study Origin: (*New England Journal of Medicine*; Vol; 328:1450–1456;
   May 20, 1993, Number 20) Eric B. Rimm et al.

Duration: Four-year follow-up study

Dose: Group 1—60 IUs daily, Group 2—100 IUs, Group 3—7.5 IUs
each day for at least two years

Results: Both 60 and 100 a day IU groups had almost the same substantial results when compared to those taking only 7.5 IUs a day. **A reduction of 36 percent and 37 percent, respectively, in relative risk for CHD** compared to the control group.

At this point it's worth pointing out my frustration when some authorities suggest to their readers that there is no real need for supplements if they just eat properly. In their book *The China Study*, coauthors Dr. T. Colin Campbell, PhD, and Thomas A. Campbell II (Benbella Books, 2005) tell us: "Vitamins and nutrient supplements do not give you long-term protection against disease." While everyone is entitled to his or her opinion, my job is to make sure that yours is informed. Our growing body of knowledge regarding the role that vitamins and other supplements play in allowing us to prevent disease is compelling.

GAMMA-TOCOPHEROL: PROTECTS US AGAINST NITROGEN FREE RADICALS THAT THE ALPHA FORM CAN'T

As researchers have begun to discover the important role of lesser known (but important) alpha tocopherol isomers, one in particular has really jumped out of the starting gate of Super-Nutrients. In a prospective study, men with the highest plasma levels of gamma-tocopherol (the top quintile) had only one fifth the risk of prostate cancer compared to the men with the lowest plasma levels (*Journal of the National Cancer Institute*, December 20, 2000; 92(24):2018–202, "Association Between Alpha-Tocopherol, Gamma-Tocopherol, Selenium, and Subsequent Prostate Cancer"). According to Dr. Packer, gamma-tocopherol, not alpha-tocopherol, levels are significantly diminished in patients with cardiovascular disease. But sufficient supplementation can help us prevent not only heart attacks and stroke, but high blood pressure as well. In a provoking review of the findings on this important antioxidant ("Newly Discovered Benefits of Gamma Tocopherol"; *Le Magazine Life Extension Foundation*, 2002), the authors note gamma-tocopherol's ability to protect us from dangerous nitrogen-based free radicals. Alpha-tocopherol is unable to do so. Highly inflammatory free radicals lay the groundwork for Alzheimer's, cancer, heart disease, and other disorders.

Importantly, they caution we bear in mind that large doses of alpha tocopherol actually *diminishes* the amount of gamma-tocopherol in our blood serum. Other data further suggests that alpha tocopherol, as important as it is, may inhibit the action of other important isomers that are found in lesser amounts in our body. For this and other reasons, it's important that we supplement with not only d alpha tocopherol, but *mixed* tocopherols containing all the "other" important members of this family as well—at different times of the day. Because alpha is by nature also found in the mixed family of isomers, we need to find sources that maximize the ratio of d gamma in the mixed family taken at a different time of day than pure alpha. But you'll be hard pressed to find it in a daily program. A maker would need to inventory two different formulas. So I devoted years to create it. (You can find this product at www.RKInformedLiving.com.)

Of all the mixed vitamin E family isomers beyond alpha, it's the *gamma form* that's been shown to be far and away the most effective for the prevention of heart disease. To focus on alpha alone, in light of today's research, is short-sided. Proper protection requires us to supplement with each. But gamma-tocopherol is even more costly and far more difficult to isolate.

The ultimate program would consist of a morning dose of alpha (the powerful reactive *oxygen* scavenger), and an evening dose of harder to find gamma (the powerful reactive *nitrogen* scavenger) kicked up in a mixed tocopherol formula. While alpha provides the most abundant form of *anti-oxidant* protection, researchers at the University of California/Berkeley have shown the amazing power of gamma-tocopherol to heal by neutralizing inflammatory toxic peroxynitrite and other hazardous *nitrogen* based oxides.[7, 8] According to the University, "Peroxynitrite is a powerful mutagen, reacting readily with DNA, proteins and fatty compounds called lipids, and causes extensive cell damage". Not surprisingly, studies have consistently shown that low concentrations of gamma not alpha in heart tissue closely correspond with a higher incidence of heart disease.

Vitamin E was first discovered by Berkeley scientists more than 80 years ago. These researchers' findings support the importance of increasing the amount of d gamma-tocopherol in our diet.

On a different note, research by Robert V. Cooney (Cancer Research Center of Hawaii), shows that gamma-tocopherol detoxifies nitrogen dioxide, the yellow gas found in smog, more effectively than alpha-tocopherol. Californians, take note!

Now that scientists have begun expanding their research to the other forms of this important antioxidant, we'll be able to more properly harness the true power of vitamin E, as different forms are positioned for different events.

THE OTHER FAMILY OF E: THE TOCOTRIENOL FAMILY

The amount our bodies contain of these guys is chump change next to all that alpha-tocopherol. And based on some recent findings, there "appears" to be *some* justification that supplementing with tocotrienols makes sense, under certain conditions.

Unlike tocopherols, present in vegetable oils such as canola and soy, tocotrienols are naturally present in cereal grains such as rice, barley, and oats. But the largest commercial sources are crude palm and rice bran oils. It's also found in coconut oil, which is a less dense source.

Though synthetic forms (with a prefix of *dl*) of vitamins may soon be available, at the time of this writing tocotrienols are only available in their all-natural or *d* forms. We'll skip the three blind mice and other animal studies to start, though we will mention one in particular, in the best interest of the animals studied (not as a testimonial to its effect on humans).

Supplementing with tocotrienols has been shown to help prevent coronary vascular disease in *some* studies. But few are large or valid. Packer reports (page 65, *The Anti-Oxidant Miracle*) tantalizing results in studies performed by Dr. Marvin Beirenbaum (1995; *Lipids* 301179–83; "Antioxidant effects of tocotrienols in patients with hyperlipidemia and carotid stenosis") that supplementing with tocotrienol can *reverse carotid stenosis by clearing out* blockage in arteries.

While its sister tocopherol has the power to reduce the risk of heart disease, it's never been shown to help reverse it. But *apparently* tocotrienols can. Yet a thorough review of this study left me somewhat nonplused. Not that there wasn't value in this research; there was. It apparently was effective in reversing stenosis in 7 of the 25 people in the group supplementing with tocotrienol.

Please note the following information below:

1. **Reverses blockage in carotid stenosis**
   Subjects: 50 high-risk adults already diagnosed with carotid stenos
   Study Origin: Kenneth L. Jordon Research Group (Lipids; 1995, 30(12): 1179–1183) Tomeo et al.

Duration: 18 months

Dose: 240 milligrams daily

Results: Bilateral duplex ultrasonography revealed apparent carotid atherosclerotic regression in 28 percent of the group taking tocotrienol supplements. But that was only 25 people. The other half of the group did not. Now 28 percent is pretty impressive. Remember, we're talking about *reversing blockage*. I would have preferred data from a larger group. And two members of this group actually saw further *progression*.

While there appears to be important benefit here, broader human studies are required before this can be touted as anything more than potentially helpful. While I don't like to rely on the results of one study such as this, if I had carotid stenosis, I would probably supplement with tocotrienols anyway. But there are few additional *human* studies and no broad ones I am aware of that have followed up on the above.

A second but important claim is this family's ability to actually lower harmful LDL. Up until now we've found little, outside of diet, drugs, and exercise, that shows it has any proven ability to lower pro-inflammatory LDL. One important study showed that subjects taking tocotrienol showed reductions in total serum cholesterol of 15 to 20 percent (which as you know I regard as unimportant), but the majority of that drop was in destructive LDL. Reducing serum levels of a pro-inflammatory such as this is a powerful testimonial. And it occurred in humans as well as in lab animals.

2. Reduces serum cholesterol and LDL

A. Reduces serum cholesterol in hypercholesterolemic humans

Subjects: Ninety hypercholesterolemic human subjects

Study Origin: Advanced Medical Research; Madison Wisconsin (Atherosclerosis, 2002 Mar; 161(1):199–207). Quereshi et al.

Duration: 35 days

Dose: 100 IU from rice bran

Results: **20 percent drop in total cholesterol, 25 percent drop in LDL, 12 percent drop in triglycerides.**

B. Hypercholesterolemic pigs fed palm cholesterol experienced a 44 percent drop in total cholesterol and a 60 percent reduction in LDL (*American Journal of Clinical Nutrition*, Vol 53, 1042S–1046S; "Dietary tocotrienols reduce concentrations of plasma cholesterol, polipoprotein B, thromboxane B2, and platelet factor 4 in pigs with inherited hyperlipidemias"). I site this study because I believe you are what you eat— ate. Less pro-inflammatories in animal sources of food means healthier choices for humans.

I believe both of the above studies are quite impressive. I'm anxious to tout the next coming of a Super-Nutrient that can extend our chances of surviving life better and longer. But dig deeper. A more recent study led by Vicki Mustad et al., completely contradicts the results of studies such as the Advanced Medical Research study above (*American Journal of Clinical Nutrition*, August, 2008; "Supplementation with 3 compositionally different tocotrienol supplements does not improve cardiovascular disease risk factors in men and women with hypercholesterolemia"). Using 200 IUs, the group suggests that a mixed tocotrienol supplement failed to reduce risk for vascular disease, and might even be harmful by *increasing* pro-inflammatory LDL.

According to the randomized, double-blind, parallel design study of 67 healthy hypercholesterolemic men and women: "The results of this study show that daily supplementation with commercially available tocotrienol supplements at a level of 200 milligrams total tocotrienols/d has no measurable beneficial effect on key CVD risk factors in highly compliant adults with elevated blood cholesterol concentrations. These results suggest that the mixed tocotrienol supplement from palm oil may even have a *negative* effect by increasing LDL-cholesterol concentrations. Unexpected given that our study design, subject population, and dosage and composition of tocotrienols were nearly identical to those in 3 double-blind, placebo controlled studies by Qureshi et al. (10–12) that showed substantial cholesterol reduction. In contrast, the results from the current study did not show any blood cholesterol or glucose-lowering response, even in those subjects who had the highest serum concentrations of tocotrienols and, thus, greater absorption." It's also worth noting that the Quereshi used a commercial brand of palm oil known as Palmvitee®. While this product intrigues me, the subject group was quite small. It appears that its ability to perform this magic is due in large part to its high content of d gamma-tocopherol (82 milligrams), and a high content of palm fatty acid distillate. According to the company, it's "a sap-like by-product of palm oil, rich in tocotrienol." Their unique formula warrants further testing in larger populations. Until that time, I fall short of being able to wholeheartedly endorse it.

It's clear that there is more to vitamin E than alpha-tocopherol. And, that other tocopherol isomers, such as gamma, are of equal importance. We've also learned that the alpha form can actually inhibit the effectiveness of gamma. The best course of action is to supplement with d alpha in the morning, and mixed tocopherols (kicked up with gamma) at night. I can't suggest supplementing with tocotrienols at this time, unless you're at high risk for stroke or have been diagnosed with carotid stenosis. If so, or if you're on blood thinning medication, please consult with your physician before taking any form of vitamin E.

VITAMIN K: DO YOU NEED TO BONE UP?

Vitamin K is a compound of vitamins that builds special proteins required for blood to coagulate (K1-phylloquinone), and for the creation of special Gla proteins essential to properly metabolize calcium in bone matrix (K2-menaquinone). The average person appears to have enough K1. But research shows that supplementing with K2 can improve bone mineralization and density in post menopausal women. While no upper level has been set, any amount interferes with blood thinning agents like warfarin. Research shows that supplementing with 15 milligrams daily can increase bone mineralization, and that 45 grams daily increased bone density in post menopausal woman.

GLUTATHIONE: TEAM CAPTAIN. MOST ABUNDANT WATER-SOLUBLE ANTIOXIDANT PRESENT IN OUR CELLS

Few substances provide as valuable a marker of oxidative stress as this important antioxidant. It's present in our body in two forms: *Reduced*—serving as a donor of electrons to unstable molecules, and *oxidized*—which is potentially harmful. But in a healthy body this form is converted to glutathione disulfide, which is not harmful. If you're well, 90 percent of it is found in its harmless reduced form. And it remains this way until your body becomes challenged.

When you're ill, for example, the ratio of the reduced versus the oxidized form becomes imbalanced—a powerful bio-marker for increased oxidative stress. As Lester Packer tells us, AIDS patients with the lowest levels of glutathione have the highest risk for death. And low levels are found in lung tissue of those suffering from respiratory disease such as asthma, as well as in chronic pathological lung disease such as cystic fibrosis (*Journal of Applied Physiology*, 1993, Dec; 75(6):2419–24; "Systemic deficiency of glutathione in cystic fibrosis"). Roum and colleagues from the National Institutes of Health (Pulmonary Branch, National Heart, Lung, and Blood Institute, National Institutes of

Health) also found a marked reduction of glutathione in the blood plasma of those with cystic fibrosis. Low levels of glutathione indicate a serious decline in every aspect of immunity. High levels are associated with optimum health. Not surprisingly, feeding your blood with a steady supply of this antioxidant is an important component of the SOS program.

While far more plentiful in our cells than other antioxidants such as vitamin E, it's also in tremendous demand. Dr. Packer, whose distinguished work in this area (along with that of his former colleague, the late Anton Meister), advises us that additional production is triggered by the body *whenever* it undergoes oxidative stress. Unfortunately, our levels of gluta-thione, the foremost antioxidant found in our cells, are diminished as we age. According to Calvin Lang (*Journal of Anti-Aging Medicine*, Volume 4, Number 2, 2001; "The Impact of Glutathione on Health and Longevity"), deficiency is most pronounced in adults between the ages of 60 and 79. In a study of clinically healthy subjects between the age of 40 and 94 (levels of 20 to 39 served as a baseline), almost half those deficient were found in this age group, though deficiency increased with age from 40 to 79. Lang suspects that the reason those 80 and older had a lower incidence of defi-ciency than those 60–79 is due to the death of those more frail by the time they reach this age.

It's every cell's job to produce a sufficient supply of glutathione to fend off oxidation. And it's our job to help them do so. If we fail to provide our cells with the nutrients they require to produce the larger amounts they need as we grow older, the more rapidly we age. Every stressful intrusion in our lives, including but not limited to illness, stress, and lack of sleep, all contribute to further diminished levels of this small but important protein.

Unfortunately, simply supplementing with glutathione doesn't appear to work. According to several leading authorities, the molecule is quite large and doesn't get efficiently absorbed. Though small amounts may survive the diges-tive process and find their way into our bloodstream, experts believe it's not a sufficient amount.

And though it's produced in cells by three amino acids—glycine, glutamic acid, and cysteine—and eating foods high in these amino acids is important, supplementing with other nutrients (not glutathione itself) helps get us over this important hump. The SOS foods highest in these amino acids include pasteurized chicken and free-range bison, sesame seeds and eggs (glycine), cottage cheese, free-range buffalo, pasteurized turkey (glutamic acid), onions, red peppers, broccoli, and brussels sprouts (cysteine).

But research at the Packer Lab has shown that the best way to increase your level of glutathione is to supplement with 100 milligrams of lipoic acid daily. It bears a good deal of similarity to glutathione and, according to Dr. Packer, its most important role may be its powerful ability to boost glutathione's production in our body. That's why you find exactly that in our Super-Multiple (RKInformedLiving.com)

Supplementing with 500 milligrams daily of amino acid N-Acetylcysteine (NAC) has also been shown to boost the production of glutathione. According to Dr. Lyn Patrick, ND (Alternative Medicine Review 2000 (Aug); 5 (4): 290-305; Nutrients and HIV: Part Three—N-Acetylcysteine, Alpha-Lipoic Acid, L-Glutamine, and L-Carnitine): "N-acetylcysteine has been demonstrated to have heavy metal chelating capacities for toxic metals, as well as for copper, zinc, and boron. Several studies support evidence that NAC increases gluta-thione levels in vivo and in vitro; there is also evidence NAC may boost cellular immunity directly."

Research has also shown a couple of additional ways to supplement your diet and increase your glutathione level. A particular brand of whey protein known as Immunocal® is clinically proven to increase glutathione levels by as much as 35.5 percent (most published research on whey has used this specially formulated whey).

Aged garlic extract (AGE), that we discussed in Chapter 3, is also proven to increase the level of this important antioxidant. Research shows that daily supplementing with AGE increases the production of glutathione in endothelial cells (in vivo), and in humans (*The Journal of Nutrition*, 36:821S–826S, March 2006; "Aged Garlic Extract Has Potential Suppressive Effect on Colorectal Adenomas in Humans").

A diet rich in important SOS foods, along with 100 milligrams of lipoic acid and AGE, is a great place to start. I also drink two tablespoons of whey mixed in water daily. And though I've tried to tolerate AGE and couldn't, don't let that stop you. Clearly, increasing your body's level of this important master antioxidant is one of the most important things you can do to slow aging and bolster immunity.

LIPOIC ACID (MORE COMMONLY ALPHA LIPOIC ACID): THE ENABLER, AND THE ULTIMATE PROTECTOR OF OUR CELLS

(Note: Don't confuse lipoic acid or alpha lipoic acid with the parent fat ALA, alpha linolenic acid, that we discussed in Chapter 2. In its alpha form they both share *the same ALA* acronym.)

We've previously discussed this organic compound's amazing ability to increase the uptake of cysteine, which in turn helps boost our ability to produce important glutathione —whose absence or deficiency is a huge biomarker for disease. But research has shown its ability to improve our health in a number of other important ways.

According to Dr. Lester Packer of Packer Lab Fame and the coauthor (with Carol Colman) of *The Anti-Oxidant Miracle* (1999, John Wile and Sons, Inc.), lipoic acid is not only one of five network antioxidants (Dr. Packer's term for those that work together to rebuild and empower each other), but it's the master antioxidant that boosts the production of glutathione. Recall that low levels of glutathione peroxidase (the form found in every cell in our body) are a key marker of disease and imminent death. Low levels precipitate aging, and correspond with high levels of oxidative stress. According to Packer, the level of this antioxidant is "dramatically depleted in people with chronic illnesses such as AIDS, cancer and autoimmune diseases (such as rheumatoid arthritis and lupus) leaving them seriously antioxidant-deficient." Conversely, optimum levels correlate with a peak state of well being. Our principle weapon of defense against the ravages of oxidation from the dangerous hydrogen peroxide free radical, this powerful scavenger also thwarts other pernicious, highly reactive molecules, such as ascorbyl, and chromanoxyl. Its action has been shown to help protect us against such illnesses as stroke and heart disease. But like other important nutrients, our levels decline as we age. And since directly ingesting glutathione supplements is ineffective (it's broken down and degraded before it's absorbed), the discovery of lipoic acid's role in boosting its production can't be underscored.

NOT SURPRISINGLY, MS VICTIMS HAVE BROKEN BLOOD-BRAIN BARRIERS, ALLOWING WHITE BLOOD CELLS UNCHALLENGED ENTRY.

Unlike all other antioxidants we've discussed, which are either fat- or water-soluble, lipoic acid is *both*; with the unique ability to act in fat as well as tissue fluid. Dr. Packer references the work of long-time colleague Dr. Bruce Ames (*Proceedings of the National Academy of Sciences*, Feb. 19, 2002, 99,

4:2356–61, 2002, 99, 4:1876–81, 2002, 99, 4:1870–5, 2002) who has shown that in combination with the amino acid L-carnitine, lipoic acid is capable of revitalizing mitochondria.

Scientists at the Linus Pauling Institute and College of Veterinary Medicine at Oregon State University, and the Department of Medicine at the University of Washington, found that supplementing with lipoic acid reduced the formation of atherosclerotic lesions in two types of mice widely used to study cardiovascular disease by 55 percent and 40 percent, respectively (Oregon State University, 2008, January 17; "Lipoic Acid Could Reduce Atherosclerosis, Weight Gain," *ScienceDaily*).

Not surprisingly, the Packer Lab found that lipoic acid protected rats from stroke-related brain injury and free radical oxidation. According to Dr. Packer, it proved to be one of the few substances capable of crossing the brain's blood barrier (BBB); a truly incredible mechanism. Semi-permeable, it protects brain cells from toxins and other hazardous substances that would otherwise enter and infect them. Dense endothelium cells keep large molecules such as bacteria and potentially hazardous chemicals out. While permitting important molecules the brain requires, such as oxygen and glucose (which hitchhike on special transporter molecules to gain access) to enter easily.

Unfortunately, the BBB also protects cells by blocking the entry *of other* foreign objects in the blood that we may wish could enter, such as antibiotics, making any infection in the brain difficult if not impossible to treat.

When chronic inflammation of the membrane that protects our brain and spinal cord (known as meningitis) does occur, this miraculous, seemingly impenetrable barrier is broken. It's clear that oxidative stress precipitates this inflammation. Viruses (that include HIV) also pass through the BBB effortlessly. Attacks such as body injury open the door as well. And while glycated beta amyloid peptides can't penetrate this bio-force field, Dr. George Glenner of University of California in San Diego believes that a precursor of amyloid tangles, "a short chain of amino acids" known as A-4 peptide, can.

Not surprisingly, MS victims have broken blood-brain barriers, allowing white blood cells unchallenged entry. Once inside, they work to destroy protective fatty sheaths known as myelin that insulate the flow of electrochemical nerve impulses (voltage) from brain cells to other parts of our body; disrupting their ability to communicate with the rest of our body laying the groundwork for neurological disease.

While water-soluble substances can't pass the brain's fatty reef, molecules that dissolve in fat appear to fare far better. Dr. Nicholos Bodor and colleagues at the University of Florida in Gainesville, have shown just that (*Science*; December 18, 1981:Vol. 214. no. 4527, pp. 1370–1372; Site-specific, sustained release of drugs to the brain).

While further research is hoped for, it's clear that free radical oxidation, caused by obvious and lesser known stressors, creates internal inflammation. A bridge of fire that burns through the protective membrane leaving brain cells vulnerable to attack. I believe that in time we'll discover that many of today's increasingly common auto-immune and neurological disorders will be linked to a door that first opened here.

In animal studies, lipoic acid has been shown to protect brain cell membranes from free radical damage while boosting the ability of their mitochondria to produce the energy required to protect itself from plaque. And in a study by Schreibelt et al. (*The Journal of Immunology*, 2006, 177: 2630-2637; Lipoic Acid Affects Cellular Migration into the Central Nervous System and Stabilizes Blood-Brain Barrier Integrity), the researchers concluded that "the antioxidant LA is an effective reducer of monocyte migration across the BBB and stabilizes the BBB in vitro, making it a potent inhibitor of cerebral inflammation and a promising therapy for the treatment of MS."

Though we can't conclude lipoic acid has this same effect in human beings, further research is likely to discover a broader role that's played by this important Super-Nutrient. While a number of studies have shown its ability to positively affect human cells in vivo, I look forward to solid broad-based research in humans to further illustrate its ability to protect our health in other important ways. But its power to rebuild key antioxidants makes it unique and worthy of the MVP award.

In addition to its amazing power to regenerate glutathione, Dr. Packer further demonstrated its capacity to rebuild important vitamins C, E, and CoQ-10 (*Free Radical Biology and Medicine*, 19: 227–250, 1995; "Alpha-Lipoic acid as a biological antioxidant") as well.

After freely giving up electrons to stabilize free radicals, these antioxidants become unstable free radical versions of themselves (though considerably less unstable than those they originally surrendered them to). For example, vitamin C becomes the free radical known as ascorbyl.

Packer's discovery, that these nutrients can also be restored, has powerful implications for optimizing our health. Not only for prolonging their value, but by countering their ability to propagate another cycle of additional free radical destruction.

It's possible to do more harm than good to yourself if you take mega-doses of antioxidants. After the electron exchange, they become unstable—but only as unstable as the free radical they helped to balance. Fortunately, certain antioxidants, what Packer and co-author Carol Colman call "network antioxidants," actually *rebuild* each other. And lipoic acid is the grand master in this regard.

Following the SOS food plan provides a sufficient amount of the vitamins and nutrients *not* highlighted in this section.

We've previously discussed the important role of proper methylation, CoQ-10 and vitamin D. But some additional information is worthy of note, followed by a brief discussion regarding the importance of folic acid, selenium and other powerful supplements. Collectively, these nutrients, along with those available from foods, will propel you to a far healthier, longer life.

TMG—THE BIG DONOR PROMOTES HEALTHFUL METHYLATION

The importance of your body's ability to properly "methylate" can't be under-scored. This exchange of a methyl group (three atoms of hydrogen attached to one atom of carbon), occurs billions of times a second throughout your body. The process is one of nature's most powerful and pervasive methods of repairing and protecting our cells. When it's disrupted or broken, the potentially deadly by-product known as homocysteine aggregates. While low levels of this naturally occurring amino acid are indicative of healthy methylation, high levels pose a real threat.

Its role as a solid predictor of heart disease is indisputable. But now high levels, and what were formerly considered normal levels, have been implicated in not only stroke, but every form of chronic disease precipitated by inflammation of blood vessels, including Alzheimer's and Parkinson's disease, as well as dementia, depression, osteoporosis and more. Levels that were formerly considered acceptable are now proving they're not. As Dr. Miller explains, "a person with a "normal" homocysteine level of 10 umol/L of blood has twice the risk of heart disease as someone with an optimal level of 6.3 umol/L or lower."

The U.S. Physicians Health Study of 14,916 physicians showed that those with "high" levels (H Level/Zone) had three times the risk of heart attack over a five year period of time than those with low levels (Life Extension Magazine,

November 2003; starling new findings About Homocysteine). They also report the findings of another important study that found that each 3-umol/L increase in homocysteine caused a *35 percent increase* in heart attack risk (*American Journal of Epidemiology*:1996 May 1;143; 9:845-59. Homocysteine metabolism and risk of myocardial infarction: relation with vitamins B6, B12, and folate).

TMG (trimethylglycine), an organic compound naturally produced in our body, is the chemical name for betaine (found in sugar beets). It's widely considered the greatest methyl donor of them all. Study after study shows the value of supplementing with 1500 milligrams of TMG daily to lower homocysteine levels and keep them there. By donating methyl groups, TMG facilitates the conversion of homocysteine back to methione, diminishing the magnitude of disruption. 750 milligrams daily should help you maintain healthful levels, coupled with 1200 micrograms of folic acid, most of us can bring our body into a healthy "H Zone" (below 7, and ideally just over 6) in only 30–90 days. While this one two punch is more than enough to work its magic for most of us, a couple of vitamins help complete the process by restoring and enhancing our ability to rid ourselves of excessive amounts of this potentially hazardous residue.

TO B OR NOT TO B

Life Extension Institute has also found, after an extensive review of the published studies, that homocysteine aggregates at higher levels as we age, because the system our body uses to rid itself of this amino acid "becomes defective." While folic acid helps restore patterns of methylation we enjoyed in younger years (and provides numerous other important benefits), and TMG gives us the ability to generate the optimal number and improved efficiency of methyl exchanges, vitamins B12, and B6 are equally important. The Institute recommends 600 micrograms a day and 5-10 milligrams respectively to its members. They add: "For those whose homocysteine levels remain above 7-8 umol/L despite taking the recommended oral doses of folic acid, TMG, and vitamins B12 and B6, a weekly 1-milligram vitamin B12 shot is strongly recommended."

COQ-10: THE ENERGIZER AND STABILIZER

CoQ-10 (ubiquinone, which means "found everywhere") is another powerful member of Dr. Packer's *network* antioxidants. Research has shown it's proven its ability to impact numerous aspects of our health, which includes production of the energy in our mitochondria and the strengthening of our muscle tissue.

Importantly, it has also been shown to protect our proteins against the ravages of oxidation. Again note that statins inhibit the production of this essential compound. While our bodies produce both of these antioxidants, the production of both goes down with age. So we must get more from our food and our supplements.

Like almost everything else that's important to sustain us, our bodies' production of CoQ-10 diminishes with age; typically after the age of *twenty*. It's a primary component of our electron transport chain, and without it, our bodies are unable to meet its energy requirements. Not surprisingly, it's most heavily concentrated in the mitochondria in those organs with the greatest requirement for *energy*—the liver, pancreas, and heart (not surprisingly the heart is a CoQ-10 hog, needing sufficient energy to beat 100,000 times each day). This critical nutrient actually *becomes* essential when elderly or impaired persons are incapable of producing enough of it to sustain themselves.

First isolated in 1957, statistically significant low levels of CoQ-10 are found in victims of breast cancer (*International Journal of Clinical Pharmacology*, 36 (9): 506–9, 1998: "Plasma coenzyme Q10 concentrations in breast cancer: prognosis and therapeutic consequence"). But that's a far cry from being able to suggest that taking a sufficient amount of this nutrient cures breast cancer. As of this writing, there's no solid evidence in human trials that suggests it can do so.

Low levels of CoQ-10 are also common in those suffering from other forms of cancer (*Biochemistry and Biophysical Research Communications*; "Activities of Vitamin Q10 in Animal Models and a Serious Deficiency in Patients with Cancer"; 234 (2): 296–9, May 19 1997), including lung, prostate, kidney, pancreas, colon, and even lymphoma. But as was the case with breast cancer, this doesn't mean taking CoQ-10 will prevent these cancers. Further broad studies in humans are required before we can conclude a cause and preventative relationship between this supplementation and any form of cancer. The next time you hear a leading authority suggest it does, challenge them (a simple Google search reveals more than three million articles on CoQ-10 and cancer.)

We've also been told that supplementing with CoQ-10 prevents heart disease. While there are a few broad studies on humans, they're not as controlled as I would like to see. I've highlighted two of the larger studies most frequently used to support its value in fighting coronary heart disease:

1. Oral supplementation significantly improves the ability of the heart to fight back

Subjects: 424 adults with any of six various forms of heart disease

Dose: Depending on the classification of their disorder (either ischemic cardiomyopathy, dilated cardiomyopathy, primary diastolic dysfunction, hypertension, mitral valve prolapse, valvular heart disease) doses range from 75 IUs to 600 IUs a day.

Study Origin: University of Texas Medical Branch, Galveston, Texas (Molecular Aspects of Medicine; 1994; 15 Supplement: 165–75. Usefulness of coenzyme Q10 in clinical cardiology: a long-term study) Langsjoen et al.

Duration: Over eight years; but the patients entered at different intervals. On average, they were monitored for just under one and a half years (17.8 months)

Results: Of 424 patients, 58 percent improved in a one class of New York Heart Association (NYHA) Functional Classification, 28 percent by two classes, and 1.2 percent by three classes. These classifications are as follows: Mild symptoms and slight limitation during ordinary activity. Comfortable at rest: Marked limitation in activity due to symptoms, even during less-than-ordinary activity. Comfortable *only* at rest: Severe limitation: Experiences symptoms even while at rest.

Does reading the above cause you to question the value of this study? Of particular significance is the 28 percent reduction in two classifications in 17.8 months. But *what dose produced which results in what period of time?* Using an *average* length of time subjects were monitored, or the *average* amount of CoQ-10 administered, is less than predictive. I also have a problem with the design of the study itself. Using criteria like "comfort" is too subjective. And similar studies have used similar methods. If this is the best foot forward for advocating its use to prevent heart disease, I'm less than convinced.

Another large-scale study, with a couple of the same objections sited above, is a bit more impressive:

Researchers showed (*The Journal of Clinical Investigation*, 1993; 71; 8 Supplements: S145–9) that 80 percent of 2500 Italian heart patients from 174 different medical centers with previously diagnosed chronic heart failure (diagnosed at least six months prior to the study) received daily supplements of between 50 to 250 milligrams of CoQ-10 a day. The number that saw marked, clinically-diagnosed improvement after such trauma was impressive. At least on the surface.

According to the study, after only three months of supplementation, the percentage of those showing clinical improvement ranged from 81 percent of those with cyanosis (abnormal hemoglobin lacking oxygen and causing bluish coloration in mucous membranes) to 76.9 percent of those with edema (damage to heart causes too much or too little transfer of fluid to tissue). And 49.3 percent saw improvement for those with enlargement of the liver, while 81.5 percent improved with jugular reflux, 54.2 percent with dyspnea (abnormalities of breathing), 75.7 percent with palpitations, 82.4 percent with perfuse sweating, 62 percent of those with arrhythmia, 60.2 percent of insomnia sufferers, 73 percent of those diagnosed with vertigo, and 50.7 percent of nocturia victims (frequent need to wake up in the night and urinate). While the amount of supplements varied by condition (from 50 to 50 milligrams daily for some), 78 percent of those in the study received only 100 milligrams a day for three months.

Okay, but define *clinical improvement*?

This doesn't mean CoQ-10 is not of value; it is. But there is not a single human study, despite all the hype, that proves that supplementing with CoQ-10 prevents cancer or heart disease. But it *does* appear to have some benefit in mediating an imbalance of blood pressure:

2. CoQ-10 supplementation reduces systematic hypertension (high blood pressure)

Subjects: 83 adults (46 men and 37 women) with isolated systolic hypertension; the most common form of hypertension in the elderly (aged 65 and up), according to Dr. Norma M. Kaplan, MD (*Circulation*, 2000; 102:1079, "New Issues in the Treatment of Isolated Systolic Hypertension")

Dose: 120 milligrams of CoQ-10 orally (60 milligrams twice daily)

Study Origin: Research Service, Department of Veterans Affairs Medical Center (*South Med J*, 94(11):1112–1117, 2001, 2001 Southern Medical Association) Burke et al.

Duration: Twelve weeks (randomized, double blind, placebo-controlled study)

Results: **55 percent** of those receiving supplements saw an average corresponding drop in systolic blood pressure of 17.8 mmHg. On average this represented a decrease of between approximately 8–11 percent). It's also been shown to benefit those who intensively train.

3. CoQ-10 has also been shown to lower oxidized stress and improve recovery time following endurance training in adults.

Subjects: 41 adults. Approximately half were aerobically trained while the other half were not.

Dose: 200 IUs daily (100 IU—morning and 100 IU—evening)

Study Origin: Exercise & Sport Nutrition Lab; Center for Exercise, Nutrition and Preventive Health; Department of Health, Human Performance & Recreation; Baylor University (*Journal of the International Society of Sports Nutrition*, 2008, 5:8doi:10.1186/1550-2783-5-8; "Effects of acute and 14-day coenzyme Q10 supplementation on exercise performance in both trained and untrained individuals"), Cooke et al.

Duration: 14 days

Tests: Isokinetic knee extension endurance test, a 30-second wingate anaerobic capacity test, and a maximal cardiopulmonary graded exercise test interspersed with 30-minutes of recovery with baselines established prior to each event.

Results: **Marked decrease in exhaustion time** (likely due, according to the study, to the heightened level of CoQ-10 in blood plasma) and substantially improved muscle performance.

So, why write about CoQ-10?

First, because many of us have been misinformed. Human studies may eventually support its value to help us guard against cancer and heart disease. But they haven't at this time. Not in my book. And while the correlation between low levels of this nutrient and disease is worthy of note, *several* important nutrients are found to be at minimal levels in our body when challenged. Many cancers, for example, are characterized by correspondingly low levels of zinc in those afflicted.

CoQ-10 is also quite expensive. That's largely because a good deal of it's in a form that's patented by the Japanese. First discovered in 1957 by researchers at the University of Wisconsin-Madison, it was the late Karl Folkers who would later determine its chemical structure. Folkers worked for Merck at the time, but the pharmaceutical giant had little use for a product that could not be marketed as a drug. There was no money in it. But the Japanese, a resourceful people, thought otherwise.

But while its value in preventing cancer and heart disease is unproven, its role in the production of energy can't be underscored (nor can its ability to scavenge free radicals, mediate blood pressure, and protect our DNA).

And in a landmark human study, CoQ-10 was shown to reduce the functional decline of subjects with Parkinson's disease (*Archives of Neurology*, October 2002, Vol. 59, No. 10, pp. 1541–1550; "Effects of coenzyme Q 10 in early Parkinson disease: evidence of slowing of the functional decline"). This important finding, along with the discovery that CoQ-10 improves our endurance and response to physical stress, further emphasizes its important role in improving the function of important mitochondria—the power plants of our cells that convert oxygen and certain nutrients into adenosine triphosphate (ATP).

ATP is the fuel that powers the metabolic activity of every cell in our body. Without mitochondria, we can't survive. And CoQ-10 has the power to protect mitochondria from degrading and improves its ability to function (*Journal of Biological. Chemistry.*, Vol. 278, Issue 30, 28220–28228, July 25, 2003; "Coenzyme Q10 Prevents Apoptosis by Inhibiting Mitochondrial Depolarization Independently of Its Free Radical Scavenging Property"). Because statin drugs inhibit the production of this important nutrient, users are at risk for weakening muscle tissue in important organs that need energy the most. That's also why muscle pain and weakness is a frequently reported side effect of statin drug use.

While there's currently no compelling evidence, despite all the hype, validating CoQ-10's ability to safeguard us from heart disease or cancer, it's clear that the tissue surrounding these important organs depends on this co-enzyme to protect its integrity. Without an optimum amount of energy, the cells and the tissue surrounding them deteriorate. Since the highest amount of CoQ-10 is found in red meat (best to buy grass-fed) and organ meat which is rarely eaten, and our ability to produce it declines significantly as we age, supplementing with CoQ-10 is the answer (you'll receive 100 mg a day in our Super-Multiple).

FOLIC ACID: GUARDIAN OF THE CENTRAL NERVOUS SYSTEM, AND THE KING OF HEALTHY CELL MEMBRANES

Folic acid is the number one nutrient required to normalize our homocysteine level. As we've learned, this measure is forty times more powerful as a predictor of heart disease than your total cholesterol level. It's also the principal nutrient that led researcher Lucy Wills to identify it as the corrective substance in brewer's yeast that reversed anemia, in 1931. And its important role in the development of new cells and their ability to replicate their DNA is second to none. That's why a deficiency of this particularly important water-soluble B vitamin has been associated with everything from miscarriages in pregnancy to congenital birth defects, such as spina bifida. Pregnant woman are advised to take additional folic acid and eat vegetables and fruits rich in this nutrient; foods identified in the Synergy of Super-Nutrients program, such as turnip greens, spinach, beans, and more.

The list of credible research in humans demonstrating its important role in maintaining a healthy nervous system is pervasive. A drug-induced deficiency of folic acid has been implicated in a wide range of cognitive disorders, including "depression, apathy, psychomotor retardation and dementia," according to neurologist E. H. Reynolds (*BMJ*, June 22, 2002; 324: 1512–1515; "Folic acid, aging, depression and dementia").

The current recommended allowance of 400 to 600 micrograms daily (the latter, for pregnant women) is woefully deficient. Dutch researchers have recently confirmed the incredible power of an 800-milligram supplement daily (*Lancet*, 2007 Jan 20; 369(9557):208–16; "Effect of 3-year folic acid supplementation on cognitive function in older adults in the FACIT trial: a randomized, double blind, controlled trial").

In a well designed study, 818 adults ages 50 to 70 who supplemented with this amount daily for three years showed marked improvement in a number of cognitive dimensions that typically decline as we age, including the ability to remember and the ability to more rapidly process information. And their homocysteine level fell a whopping 26 percent!

The list of benefits that accrue from eating a proper amount of folic acid in the form of SOS foods and folic acid supplementation is endless. A case-controlled perspective study of 1224 woman (half the group breast cancer victims, the other half the control group) conducted by lead researcher Zhang et al. (*Journal of the National Cancer Institute*; 2003 95(5):373-380; doi:10.1093/jnci/95.5.373; Plasma Folate, Vitamin B6, Vitamin B12, Homocysteine, and Risk of Breast Cancer) concluded that: "Higher plasma levels of folate and possibly vitamin B6 may reduce the risk of developing breast cancer. Achieving adequate circulating levels of folate may be particularly important for women at higher risk of developing breast cancer because of higher alcohol consumption."

In addition to SOS foods, I personally supplement with 1200 micrograms each day (the amount you'll find in our Super-Multiple). Of course, requirements vary with age and conditions that put increased levels of stress on our nervous system—such as pregnancy, illness, and emotional duress.

VITAMIN D: THE ANTI-CANCER KING OF SUPER-NUTRIENTS

The Dr Pepper® of supplements, it's without a doubt the most misunderstood of all the Super-Nutrients, yet one of the most important. Due at least in part to our lack of information, over one billion people throughout the world are deficient in this fat-soluble pro-hormone.

In an excellent review, Jane Higdon, PhD, of the Oregon State University's Linus Pauling Institute (Micronutrient Information Center, Vitamin D, March, 2004), cautions us that these deficiencies are associated with everything from aching bones and sore muscles, to more chronic disease such is as hypertension (high blood pressure), type 2 diabetes, osteoporosis, osteomalia (soft bones, typically in adults), rickets (the failure of bone to mineralize in children and infants), hyperparathyroidism (mineral imbalance characterized by calcium-decreased blood levels of phosphorous, and kidney stones), autoimmune disease (such as multiple sclerosis (MS), rheumatoid arthritis (RA), and diabetes mellitus), and appears to be involved in a number of different cancers—not surprisingly, since according to Dr. Higdon, citing the work of M. F. Holick: "The active form of vitamin D, $1,25(OH)_2D$, inhibits proliferation and stimulates the differentiation of cells." (*American Journal of Clinical Nutrition*, 2004; 79(3):362–371, "Vitamin D: importance in the prevention of cancers, type 1 diabetes, heart disease, and osteoporosis").

Vitamin D deficiency has also been shown to strongly correlate with intellectual disabilities, and many hypothesize a link, yet unproven, between low levels of this nutrient and autism.

According to Dr. John Jacob Cannell, of Atascadero State Hospital's department of psychiatry and executive director of the Vitamin D Council (*Medical Hypothesis*, 2008; 70(4):750-9, "Autism and vitamin D"): "Children with vitamin D deficient rickets have several autistic markers that apparently disappear with high-dose vitamin D treatment ... Calcitriol down-regulates production of inflammatory cytokines in the brain, cytokines that have been associated with autism. Consumption of (vitamin D containing) fish during pregnancy reduces autistic symptoms in offspring." (Note: A 3.5 ounce serving of wild red salmon contains a whopping 988 IUs, far more than any other food.[2] Contrast this to the 245 IUs found in farm-raised salmon).

In a study published in the prestigious *Journal of Epidemiology and Infection* (Cambridge Journal; "Epidemic influenza and vitamin D"; August 5, 2006), Cannell and his associates, in a review of the literature, discussed the profound role played by vitamin D in our immune system. According to their study, once activated, vitamin D modulates the ability of inflammatory cytokines (created in response to pathogens, and required to activate our immune response) to increase the ability of protective white blood cells, known as macrophages, to "burst" *after* they've *already* eaten invading organisms. This action (known as an oxidative burst), is a good thing. It's the biological equivalent of "shock and awe" (like throwing a hand grenade to insure that foreign invaders can't get up again after they've already been surrounded). Macrophages provide an important line of defense in the immune system. They gobble up germs that permit disease or illness to fester. They also stimulate important white blood cells, known as lymphocytes, that usher an immune response to protect us from virus and tumors. Bursting them after they've gobbled up the enemy is like carpet bombing them—delivering a one two punch from our immune system to would be assailants. The ability of vitamin D to empower our troops to do so can't be underscored.

ACTUALLY, IT'S NOT A VITAMIN AT ALL BUT A PRECURSOR TO A SECO-STEROID HORMONE ...

The researchers also cite vitamin D's role in triggering the expression of powerful anti-microbial peptides, which protect our lungs from infection. They conclude: "Vitamin D deficiency predisposes children to respiratory infections. Ultraviolet radiation (either from artificial sources or from sunlight) reduces the incidence of viral respiratory infections, as does cod liver oil (which contains vitamin D). An interventional study showed that vitamin D reduces the incidence of respiratory infections in children."

I'm not a big fan of cod liver oil, though I take it occasionally in place of fish oil during prolonged winters that are overcast; winters that keep me from getting sunshine. While overdoses from oral ingestion of vitamin D are rare, and appear to occur in adults taking more than 40,000 IUs daily, it occurs more frequently from over-consumption of cod liver oil. More often than not, that's due to its enormous concentration of vitamin A (not D), which has been found to be more toxic.

From boosting immunity, to preventing chronic disease, and insuring bone mass and health, vitamin D is indeed one of the real kings of Super-Nutrients. Unlike CoQ-10, there is no shortage of solid human study supporting a number of important roles played by supplementing with this Super-Nutrient.

Actually, it's not a vitamin at all but a precursor to a seco-steroid hormone, which "inhibits proliferation and induces differentiation of malignant cells including those of the hematopoietic system"[3] and targets over 200 genes in the human body. In 1921, an enthused scientist by the name of Elmer McCollum mistakenly called it a vitamin (the fourth to be discovered, he named it D).[4] It converts to an active hormone (known as calcitriol—actually a steroid hormone) after it's transported in an amazing and complicated process.

The inactive form we receive from sunshine has two important stops to make. First, it's brought to the liver where a chemical action takes place that converts it to an active form. From there, it circulates to the kidney where an enzyme turns it into the most powerful form of this nutrient. Disorders of the liver or kidney can hinder our body's ability to convert it to its active form and absorb it.

In addition to adults and children, infants that are breast-fed may have a real need for additional vitamin D. First, because it's not present in breast milk, and next, because many doctors advise parents to protect their newborns from exposure to sunlight. Skin pigment, formed by compounds known as melanin, protect our body from harmful exposure to the sun. The darker the skin, the longer it takes for vitamin D to be synthesized. That puts darker skinned persons at greater risk for vitamin D deficiency. The clinically obese are also at greater risk. They typically have less circulating in their blood plasma. In fact, a study by Wortsman et al. found that after exposing human subjects to whole body radiation for 24 hours: "the incremental increase in vitamin D3 was 57 percent lower in obese than in non-obese subjects."[5]

D3 (also known as cholecalciferol) is one of the two primary forms of vitamin D. It's the only form produced by our skin after exposure to the UVB ultra-violet light in sunshine. The second major source, known as vitamin D2 (three other forms—D3, 4, and 5—have also been discovered), also known as calciferol, is found in growing plants as well as in fungus. While supplements are available in both forms, and thought by many experts as being biologically equivalent, a study by Houghton et al. has shown us otherwise (*American Journal of Clinical Nutrition*, Vol. 84, No. 4, 694–697, October 2006; "The case against ergocalciferol (vitamin D2) as a vitamin supplement"). Researchers showed that *only the D3 form* should be considered useful for supplementation, which was proven to be far more potent than D2. This is something few professionals are aware of. But now you are.

WE MUST HAVE A SUFFICIENT AMOUNT OF VITAMIN D TO EFFICIENTLY ABSORB CALCIUM. IF WE DON'T, CALCIUM AND OTHER MINERALS ARE LEACHED FROM OUR BONES TO BUFFER ACIDITY.

As discussed, those living farthest from the equator, and in areas with prolonged cloud-covered winters, are typically more deficient in vitamin D than those living in areas permitting more frequent exposure to sunshine. In addition to the numerous studies outlined in the previous chapter, a broad meta-analysis of over four million persons with either skin cancer or non-skin cancer, involving 13 different reporting facilities, found a striking correlation between *increased* rates of a number of cancers in *cloudier* countries such as Canada, Denmark, Finland, Iceland, Norway, Scotland, Slovenia, and Sweden, versus far *smaller* rates in *sunnier* countries such as Australia, Singapore, and Spain.[6] The researchers conclude: "Vitamin D production in the skin seems to *decrease the risk of several solid cancers*, especially stomach, colorectal, liver and gallbladder, pancreas, lung, female breast, prostate, bladder and kidney cancers." Still want to block sunshine and inhibit your skin's ability to produce vitamin D?

The list of cancer studies that further support vitamin D's ability to prevent many forms of this disease are too long to list here. Just recently, Northwestern University researchers completed a large meta-analysis involving 120,000 people from two long-term health surveys and found that subjects taking even the small US recommended daily allowance reduced their risk of pancreatic cancer by an incredible 43 percent!

Those at risk include slatherers, who cover their face routinely with lotions containing SPF (sun protection factor) of 8 or more. It causes 95 percent of the light we need to be blocked from synthesizing into vitamin D. Not a problem, if a significant portion of the rest of their body remains exposed and unprotected.

Unsurprisingly, our ability to convert the pro-hormone calcidol (vitamin D in its inactive state) to the active hormone diminishes with age. Our reduced ability to mobilize its precursor results in greater deficiency and a corresponding increase in the amount we require from other sources.

We're told to supplement with calcium to prevent bone loss, but a lack of vitamin D3, K2, estrogen, and resistance exercise, coupled with poor food choices, are the real culprits. Research suggests that mega-dosing with calcium is misinformed. Over-consumption results in the irregular distribution of calcium in our body, without these other nutrients. The discovery that bone building osteoblasts line the walls of artery (not just bone), and express calcified atherosclerotic plaque[7], is eye opening. Too much, from sources other than food, destroys matrix building osteoblasts in bone, which continue to flourish, and deposit calcium elsewhere. The leaching of calcium is nature's way of balancing highly acidic blood. Your parathyroid gland regulates and moderates that flow. Reduced bone density and the increased potential for obstruction of vessel from calcified plaque may follow. This helps explain why osteoporosis is often accompanied by athererosclerosis. Such strangely linked bedfellows of disease, created by the haphazard distribution of calcium, are known as the "calcium paradox". In a meta-analysis involving over 20,000 people, scientists concluded: "Calcium supplements (without co-administered vitamin D) are associated with an increased risk of myocardial infarction"[8].

Our greatest potential source of vitamin D is UVB ultraviolet radiation emitted by the sun. It's the type of radiation that sunscreen makers focused on blocking out. Think sunburn. This is the shorter wave UV light that damages the outermost layer of our skin, known as the epidermis. But the majority of UV radiation (98.7 percent) that reaches us is in the form of more deeply penetrating UVA light. Think tanning, it's the primary cause of melanoma.

Until recently, sunscreens failed to protect us against UVA. We believed that applying them liberally insulated us from the damaging effects of over-exposure. Today, more skin cancers are being diagnosed than ever before, due at least in part, to prolonged, unprotected exposure to longer wave UVB light. Sunscreen makers are under fire for giving fair-skinned persons a false sense of security.

A study of 1,621 adults over a four and half year period showed that while a broad spectrum sunscreen *did* lower the risk of developing squamous cell carcinoma by 40%, they failed to significantly lower the incidence of basil cell carcinoma and melanoma (*Cancer Epidemiology Biomarkers & Prevention* 16, 1921–1922, October 1, 2007).

According to a recent report by Julie Henry (NBC 17), "Kids get eighty percent of their lifetime sun exposure before the age of 18." So the earlier we begin to receive protection, the better; after all, some protection is better than none. Just make sure they receive at least 15-20 minutes of unprotected exposure first, or simultaneously on some body part that's varied each time they're outdoors. In those that are at such a risk that even this amount of sunlight on any body part leaves them prone to disease, supplementing with vitamin D, and eating foods high in vitamin D may be the only answer. Studies are now underway to develop compounds that protect us from sun burn damage from the inside out. But to date, there's no evidence in broad human studies that show they're effective.

UVB only penetrates the thin outer epidermal layer of our skin (it has a shorter wavelength than UVA). While UVA penetrates glass, UVB cannot. Therefore, to receive an optimum dose of UVB each day, we must be outdoors. In perfect conditions with little cloud cover close to the equator (the US is not), exposure for only 15–20 minutes a day can produce the equivalent of 10,000 IUs in supplement form. There's no evidence of overdosing on vitamin D from too much sunshine. This pro-hormone simply degrades as the body synthesizes the precise amount (only) of the radiated light it requires. Dosages as high as 100,000 IU, given once every four months for five years (15 times per subject), failed to result in acute toxicity in the 2,686 subjects that participated in the study (*The British Medical Journal*; 2003; 326: 469–75; "Effect of four monthly oral vitamin D3 (cholecalciferol) supplementation on fractures and mortality in men and women living in the community: randomized double blind controlled trial"). There are also decreases in their risk for hip, forearm, wrist, and vertebrae fractures by 33 percent over the control group.

Keep in mind that the subjects only took 15 doses in five years. That doesn't mean this level would be safe daily. But the optimum daily dosage is the subject of much debate, and it does put the amount required for a toxic overdose in some perspective.

So how much vitamin D do we require? Since most of us are woefully deficient, it would appear that as a people, we need a good deal more than we thought. But just how much more? After all, it's fat-soluble and an overdose can be dangerous. It also depends on a number of other factors, including where you live, how much sunshine you get and when, your ability to metabolize it, your age, and more.

In a 2007 meta-analysis (*Archives of Internal Medicine*, 2007;167:1709–1710, 1730–1737; "Vitamin D Supplementation and Total Mortality; A Meta-analysis of Randomized Controlled Trials") led by Autier et al., that studied the results of 18 randomized trials involving more than 57,000 people, researchers found that a mean daily dose of only 528 IUs substantially reduced mortality rates by 7 percent.

Fortunately, there *is* a way to make sure you don't overdose. It's a simple blood test available in most labs known as 25-hydroxy D. It will provide you with a baseline that you can monitor. I took one myself and learned that my initial reading, typical of other men my age, showed only a 40 percent level of the amount the lab regards as safe and effective. Despite the fact that I supplemented with a fair amount of D, and received at least 20 minutes of sunshine daily, I was just about as deficient as others my age.

In an excellent review article, authors John J. Cannel, MD, and Bruce W Hollis, PhD (*Alternative Medicine Review*, Volume 13, Number 1, 2008) recount numerous well-constructed studies that sought to determine optimal levels required to accomplish correspondingly healthful results. They recount results from Lappe et al. that showed a *60 percent reduction* in certain cancers when subjects supplemented with daily doses of 1,100 IUs. According to Cannel and Hollis, the recommended daily allowance of 400 IUs for adults will do nothing to prevent a deficiency—nor will the paltry 100 IUs per 8-ounce glass of milk. The authors recommend that breast-fed infants receive at least 800 IUs daily (400 IUs for formula fed newborns), and 1000–2000 IUs daily, depending on other factors such as body weight, for young children and toddlers who don't receive regular exposure from the sun. Some pregnant women, according to their research, require as much as 5000 IUs a day and as much as 7000 IUs for lactating moms.

They recommend that the average adult, barring other health problems, maintain their 25 (OH) D levels they tested for in the range of 40–70 ng/mL, which can be maintained in otherwise healthy patients with supplements of between 2000–7000 IUs per day.

However, I suggest you walk before you run. Get your levels tested, and if you choose to supplement, stay in the range they prescribe. I began supplementing with 1600 IUs a day but my levels increased only moderately. I've now increased my dosage to 3200 IUs daily (more than the 1800 IUs daily I'm comfortable suggesting to others). While that may seem like a lot, the researchers point out that 1000 IUs of vitamin D is equal to just 25 micrograms (or .025 milligrams). Again, the key is to maintain test levels of between 40–70 ng/mL in your blood. Twenty minutes in the sun, without sunscreen, is a good place to start. I make it a point to exercise outdoors, whenever possible, several times a week.

In closing, it's likely you're deficient. But there's always a danger in overdoing any supplement, particularly one such as vitamin D (that's fat-soluble). Before paying for a test, make up your mind to get more sunshine each day. Try getting out there for 15 to 20 minutes a day, or more. Start eating natural foods high in vitamin D (there are only a few) such as wild salmon, eggs, and shrimp (high in vitamin D -not Omega-3). Vital Choice now offers Oregon Pink Shrimp that the company claims are caught in clean, fresh water off the Oregon coast—then flash frozen without the additives used in most shrimp to avoid discoloration. Forget about fortified foods that will do little (other than prevent rickets perhaps, based on regular consumption). *Then* determine how much additional supplementation you require. Take the test to get a baseline, and periodically monitor it.

If you think that's too much work, consider the value! It may very well save your life.

EVENING PRIMROSE OIL

We previously discussed this important nutrient in detail in Chapter 2. 500 milligrams daily.

CARNOSINE: THE GREAT PROTECTOR-THE MINIMIZATION OF GLYCATION

Gunk, the type that floats around in our brain and elsewhere, occurs when a small portion of certain sugars we eat (the remainder are metabolized) combine with fat or protein molecules in our bloodstream, as previously discussed. Advanced glycated end products (AGE—not to be confused with the same acronym for garlic extract) are one of several destructive morphed molecules that accumulate as we get older. A primary member of the collective body of toxic garbage that destroys the function of healthy cells, glycation is an inevitable consequence of life. AGEs precipitate inflammation, create cellular confusion, damage or destroy collagen (resulting in premature aging of the skin and a loss of elasticity as well) eye crystalline (leading to cataracts), brain cells, vessel and nerves (which may lead to depression, dementia or Alzheimer's). The cross linking of protein or fats to sugar is, in the end, catastrophic. As previously noted, it lays the groundwork for most chronic disease, gluing together nerve endings, and disrupting and even suffocating cells. It causes a loss of collagen, and subsequent loss of elasticity in our skin, and even contributes to a loss of vision. But carnosine has been shown to help us minimize cross-linking. Miller indicates it protects us against cataracts, and even protects our brains against glycated damage to small blood vessels that often precipitates Alzheimer's disease. No supplement has shown carnosine's ability to protect collagen and prevent wrinkles, while helping our skin maintain its vitality. It's also proven to protect us against vessel damage, particularly in the heart and brain.

In addition to supplementing with this amazing antioxidant, it's clear that other molecular gunk, equally crippling, builds up over time. For the most part, these substances accrue with age, damaging our ability to live what we think—and to think as we live. Clumps of debris appear to form cumulatively. It's important to reduce the glue; to avoid simple sugars found in food, to the extent that's possible. In my opinion, calorie restriction makes the accumulated damage from a lifetime of consuming simple carbohydrates, protein and fat, even more minimal. In a nutshell, the more food we eat, the more damage we accumulate over time. Eating SOS foods will further reduce glycation. But by all means, contrary to what a leading health authority recently claimed, all simple sugars are unhealthy. They increase glycation and contribute to the formation of other molecules that interfere with our ability to live. Why in the world would we caramelize our insides by eating sugary foods? While we can be thankful for carnosine, the rest is up to you.

THE FLAVONOIDS

The Packer lab has shown us the tremendous importance of this antioxidant family. In particular, Gingko Biloba and Pycnogenol. According to Dr. Lester Packer and Carol Coleman, in their book *The Antioxidant Miracle*, Gingko was shown to do everything from speeding up the recovery rate of a heart attack, to preventing the oxidation of LDL. It's even been shown to prevent the primary cause of most male impotence-atherosclerosis by mediating nitric oxide.

The author's further reference studies in Europe showing Gingko's ability to improve memory. But that research has since been contradicted; more recently by the results of a study sponsored by the National Institute on Aging (*Journal of the American Medical Association: Volume 288; 835-840; No. 7: August 21, 2002;* Gingko for memory enhancement: a randomized controlled trial). Their conclusion: "When taken following the manufacturer's instructions, ginkgo provides no measurable benefit in memory or related cognitive function to adults with healthy cognitive function."

Unfortunately, this knocked the importance of Gingko down a good deal in the minds of its followers. But it shouldn't have. While additional studies are warranted, Gingko's value has been continually proven in a number of other important ways.

Its ability to improve the balance of nitric oxide, enhance blood flow and according to Dr. Miller "inhibit the formation of platelet aggregation factors" (which precipitates a hemostatic plug or thrombus/clot in vessel) are reasons enough to make Gingko an important part of our self-defense arsenal. The fact that it may not have yet be shown to improve memory does not overshadow its importance in increasing blood flow to the brain (and other important organs).

And flavonoid Pycnogenol was found by Packer to boost and recycle vitamin C. In fact this mixture of over 40 antioxidants found in Pine Bark, has more activity than all others he's researched (in more than three decades) at the helm of the famed Packer lab. He also found that not only does it also protect against platelet aggregation, the precursor to blood clots, but also greatly strengthens our immunity.

Notably, scientists have recently proven its ability to protect those suffering from ADHD. Research lead by Dr J. Trebaticka from the Department of Psychiatry at the University of Slovakias Comenius University, showed that supplementation of 1 milligram of pycnogenol daily had the amazing ability to naturally relieve the symptoms of ADHD in children. The researchers concluded, "Results show that 1-month Pycnogenol administration caused a significant reduction of hyper-activity, improves attention and visual-motoric coordination and concentration of children with ADHD." (European Child and Adolescent Psychiatry (2006 Sep;15(6):329-35. Epub 2006 May 13; Treatment of ADHD with French maritime pine bark extract, Pycnogenol). Other studies have shown its ability to protect us from the ravages of osteoarthritis; and even symptoms of menopause such as fatique and vaginal dryness (*Journal of Obstetrics and Gynecology*, 2007). I believe research showing even more benefit of this powerful flavonoid is just around the corner. I take 20 milligrams of Pycnogenol daily and 60 milligrams of Gingko Biloba (the same as in our Super-Multiple).

OTHER SUPPLEMENTS

The above are some of the giants. Trace amounts of others, such as selenium, identified with lower rates of cancer, may also be helpful depending on where you live and the selenium content in the soil. But, for the most part, eating locally grown SOS foods will supply you with all the other nutrients the average healthy person needs (some soils, depending on where you live, are deficient in selenium).

AGE—Aged garlic extract. Use as directed.

Isolated Whey—(both are capable of boosting your important level of glutathione) 2–3 tablespoons in water daily.

Psyllium—A natural supplement of fiber; take as needed.

Baby Aspirin—One coated 81-milligram tablet daily. But for protection against stroke, recent indications call for 2–3 times as much. Take one 81 milligram tablet morning *and* night.

Pharmaceutical Grade Fish Oil—I use the Zone Omega/Rx® brand Dr. Sears recommends (*The Omega Rx Zone: The Miracle of the New High Dose Fish Oil*, Harper Collins, 2003) two to three teaspoons a day (or 8–16 capsules) for enhanced brain function, reduced chronic inflammation, and improved cardiac health. Or for general maintenance, 1 teaspoon or 4 capsules daily. I prefer to hold my breath and simply drink the oil or put it in the Vitamix. The capsules are tasteless when taken with food.

After reviewing the research, it's difficult to understand why any authority in the field would discount the need for supplementation when levels of important nutrients, given the proper consumption of whole foods, may fall short of the amount required to optimize health. The food and supplements detailed in this books are all Super-Nutrients; substances painstakingly identified that will empower you. Now that you understand precisely why each was selected, it's time to review the powerful plan that's based on all we've learned.

END NOTES

1. Harold M. Schmeck, *New York Times*, Friday, October 17, 2008, Blood-Brain Barrier Begins to Yield.

2. (*Archives of Biochemistry and Biophysics*, Volume 460, Issue 2, 15 April 2007, Pages 213–217, "Factors that influence the cutaneous synthesis and dietary sources of vitamin D")

3. Cancer Research 61, 3361-3368, April 15, 2001;24-Oxo Metabolites of Vitamin D_3 Analogues; Disassociation of Their Prominent Antileukemic Effects from Their Lack

of Calcium Modulation

4. McCollum was the first person to say it prevented rickets disease.
5. *American Journal of Clinical Nutrition*, Vol. 72, No. 3, 690–693, September 2000; "Decreased bioavailability of vitamin D in obesity"
6. *European Journal of Cancer*, Volume 43, Issue 11, July 2007; "Does solar exposure, as indicated by the non-melanoma skin cancers, protect from solid cancers: Vitamin D as a possible explanation"
7. J Clin Invest. 1993 April; 91(4): 1800–1809, Bostrom et al.
8. BMJ 2010; 341:c3691, Bolland, et. al.
9. *Proceeding of the National Academy of Sciences*;1997 Apr 1;94(7):3217-22; gamma-tocopherol traps mutagenic electrophiles such as NO(X) and complements alpha-tocopherol: physiological implications. Christen et al.
10. *American Journal of Clinical Nutrition,* Vol. 74, No. 6, 714-722, December 2001; γ-Tocopherol, the major form of vitamin E in the US diet, deserves more attention Jiang et al.

CHAPTER 6

THE SYNERGY OF SUPER-NUTRIENT PROGRAM

"Let your food be your medicine, and your medicine be your food."
—Hippocrates

I f you've come this far, you've acquired a great deal of knowledge and a profound understanding of both food and supplements. You have the information that few do in this, our new field of self-defense. Now it's time to put all this to work and harness the power of the Synergy of Super-Nutrients. Following the SOS plan is easier than you think. Mobilize this knowledge and you'll live longer, grow stronger, and feel vital. Though aging is inevitable, many of us show signs of aging prematurely. And you'll significantly slow down its progression. Follow this plan and you'll substantially reduce the likelihood that this will happen to you. Other signs will begin to fade away. I'm pleased to present the most comprehensive program ever introduced, which will enable you to maximize your potential for healthier living. A remarkably easy-to-follow method of living and eating that really works!

(Disclaimer: The following is based on my needs. You may have to tailor them to best meet your own. I walk the talk and follow the program the best I can each day. Please consult your health practitioner before adding any of the following foods or supplements to your regimen. Your age, prior medical history, present state of health or illness, weight, life circumstances, allergies, and potential for drug interaction can all effect the way what I do for me may need to be tailor-made for you.)

Remain open-minded. There are several easy ways to get those 5–7 servings of healthy fruits and vegetables recommended daily. Just eat three meals at your normal mealtime. At breakfast and dinner eat at least one cup of salad mixed from the five color group salad you made enough of the night before. A vegetable at lunch. And now, the hardest part for those of you on the run. Train yourself to pack your bag. Put that attaché case or backpack to good use. Throw in a small bag of snack carrots, a 6-ounce bottle of vegetable juice (best if you make your own which takes *seconds* or stop at a juice bar) and perhaps a small fruit like a plum. That's it … a little time taken for much time given.

1. THE GOALS

The cornerstones of the SOS plan, and the keys to achieving optimum health through Super-Nutrient intake, are to:

Increase:	Balance:	Reduce:
Glutathione	Insulin	Homocysteine
Antioxidants	Fats	Glycation
Anti-inflammatories	Food Intake	Omega-6s
Vasodilation/NO	Metabolism	Internal Inflammation
Omega-3s	Cortisol	Internal Oxidation
Energy production		Vasoconstriction

2. THE TESTS

Before starting on this program, consult your health care professional and ask him to prescribe the following lab tests. It's generally less expensive to pay your health care professional directly for the tests than paying the lab. Ask. The following tests are the minimum required to be successful. Some tests, particularly those measuring fat-soluble vitamins, should be followed up on after weeks or months of changing your level. It's imperative to monitor to maximize health and minimize risk. Your blood should be measured for the following:

- Homocysteine Test: Simple blood test. Shop around for best price. (Ideal level- 6.3- 7.2)
- Vitamin D: Test: 25 -Hydroxy Vitamin D Test (Ideal level- 40 ng/ml)
- Inflammation: Test: C-Reactive Protein. According to Dr. Miller* (Ideal :Men: Less than .5 milligrams/l. Women: less than 1.3 milligrams/L. Though lab test may indicate standard range of 4.9 milligrams/L
- Inflammation: General: Lab test-:AA/EPA (Ideal level: Ideal Ratio- approx. 1.5)**
- Cholesterol: The ratio is the most important factor. The total level is a poor indicator.

LDL/HDL ratio: (Ideal: Men Less than 2: Women: 2-3)*

TG/HDL ratio: (Ideal: Less than 2 for Men of Woman)*

- DHEA/ Cortisol- (Ideal: Woman:15-25 for Men or Woman)*

* Information from *The Life Extension Revolution*, Dr Phillip Miller, MD and the Life Extension Foundation (Bantam Books, May, 2006)

** Information from Dr. Barry Sears (DrSears.com-the Official Site of the Zone Diet, September 28, 2008; www.DrSears.com)

3. THE PROGRAM—PART 1: THE SOS SUPPLEMENTS

Note: The concept of IU measurement was developed to reflect the amount of activity in a nutrient. But that standard is inconsistent due to differences in processing and procuring. For that reason, labeling the content of a vitamin is more properly accomplished by measuring it in milligrams. Unfortunately, the majority of makers continue to use IUs as a measurement for vitamin E and other compounds. So, I will list the dosages I take in IUs where applicable, the measurement we continue to be most familiar with. However for your reference: "The conversion is 1 IU natural vitamin E equals 0.67 milligrams d-alpha-tocopherol and 1 IU of synthetic vitamin E *equals 0.45 milligrams d-alpha-tocopherol." (Source: Memorial Sloan Kettering Cancer Center.)*

The following are daily dosages for the basic elements of my program, a good place to start. Most multiple vitamins provide a smattering of nutrients that, while useful, fail to provide the optimum levels required to achieve the results we've examined. It's simply not possible to get the dosages we require to optimize our health in one pill. They would be too large. Fifteen hundred milligrams, plus fillers and binders, is the most we can practically receive in a single pill that's easy to swallow. Since most of us are hard pressed to take even one a day, they're compromised solutions to help us avoid deficiency. But most fail to do so in all the areas we require them to. Few include important vitamin D for example. And more often than not, most contain one type of vitamin E, allowing makers to save cost and inventory by putting *both* forms of this important nutrient in one tablet. The nutrients listed below and the additional supplements on the optional list below it, in combination with the SOS food program that follows, are more than enough to provide the power required to super-charge immunity.

But I take a good deal more. Some to further assist me in restoring cell structure and performance, others to truly enhance intra-cellular function, improve cognitive ability, further reduce the effects of aging, and further assist in clobbering internal inflammation. Since few would take the number of pills required to do what I do, I've spent a great deal of time working with industry leaders to develop a powerful, yet easy to use program that offers an optimum intake of Super-Nutrients. A multiple program that considers the alpha as well as the beta form of carotene, mixed and gamma tocopherols taken separately from alpha tocopherol, and the amount of other important nutrients that allows us to truly capture their power. I refused to compromise. After years of work, the ultimate daily multiple program is now available. All information is available on our website at www.RKInformedLiving.com. It's the most powerful program of its kind. But the following *basic* program is life changing. Be sure to consult your doctor prior to starting any new health regimen.

Morning Supplements
Alpha Lipoic Acid–50 milligrams
Vitamin C–500-1000 milligrams[1]
Vitamin E *d* alpha tocopherol–400 IU[2]

Vitamin D–900 IU[4]
L Carnosine–500 milligrams
Folic Acid–500 mcg
CoQ-10–50 milligrams
Pharmaceutical Grade Fish Oil–2-3 Tsp[5]
*Pycnogenol®–20 milligrams
Baby Aspirin–81 mcg[6]

Evening Supplements
Alpha Lipoic Acid–50 milligrams
Vitamin C–500- 1000 milligrams[1]
**Vitamin E mixed *d* tocopherols–150 IU[2,3]
    (with at least 60% as *d* Gamma)
Vitamin D–900 IU[4]
L Carnosine–500 milligrams
Folic Acid–500 mcg
CoQ-10–50 milligrams
EPO–500 milligrams
Ginkgo Biloba–60 milligrams
Baby Aspirin–81 mcg[6]

*This is a product name that is registered. However, high quality pine bark may be substituted and will likely cost less. ** The National Research Council requires all forms of E other than alpha be restricted as milligrams.

1. Ascorbic acid form
2. Consult your health care professional before using. Particularly if you are pregnant or nursing, or take blood thinning/anticoagulant medication, according to PDR health (Physicians Desktop Reference)
3. Mix should contain at least 60–70 percent or more of *d* gamma-tocopherol
4. Fat-soluble vitamin, consult your health care professional and test blood before using. Then, periodically monitor.

5. Those taking anticoagulants/blood thinners should avoid. Consult your physician before use. Diabetics, those prone to easy bleeding, and asthmatics should avoid.

6. Some research has begun to suggest considerably more. Two 81 mcg. tablets appear to afford more protection against stroke. Consult your physician. Those with Reyes Syndrome or any viral infection, or on medication of any kind, should consult their physician before usage.

Again, I take many more supplements than the above and below, and can now do so simply.

Optional:

To further boost Glutathione levels:

N-Acetylcysteine (NAC)–50 milligrams daily

Isolated Whey–Two tablespoons mixed in water

AGE–300-600 milligrams AM and PM

Pink grapefruit–limonoids boost its *production*...so do other SOS foods such as asparagus, garlic, broccoli, avocado and spinach.

Curcumin–1 gram AM and PM-Increases glutathione biosynthesis[1]

For regularity/additional fiber if required:

Psyllium 2 teaspoons or more periodically

If H Level (homocysteine) remains normal to high:

TMG–375 milligrams AM and PM

B12–500 mcg. AM and PM

B6–5 milligrams AM

If soil where you live has low levels of selenium:

Selenium–100 mcg. AM and PM

To further lower LDL:

Brisk walk or other cardio–30 minutes or more 5 days a week.

Niacin–250 milligrams AM and PM

Teaflavin®–One 375 milligram tablet daily

Cognis Vegapure®–1.3 grams daily

One red grapefruit daily, unless contradicted by drug use.

(Decrease LDL oxidation: The right EVOO is proven to do so.

Gingko Biloba–slightly increase Gingko intake)

Ground Cinnamon–3 grams a day

To further raise HDL:

Niacin therapy–250 milligrams, AM and PM. "Niacin can raise HDL—the "good" cholesterol—by 15 percent to 35 percent. This makes niacin the most effective drug available for raising HDL cholesterol," according to Dr. Gerald Gau, M.D., a Mayo Clinic preventive cardiologist and a specialist in internal medicine and cardiovascular diseases.[2] Again, you may need to simultaneously increase your intake of folic acid.

Aerobic exercise–15 - 20 minutes to strengthen the heart 4 - 5 times a week. But to raise HDL, 40 minutes 3 - 4 times weekly, results in 2.5 milligrams /L increase in HDL, according to a meta-analysis by Kodam et al. (*Archives of Internal Medicine*; 2007, 167:999-1008; Effect of aerobic exercise training on serum levels of high-density lipoprotein cholesterol). While the increase may appear modest, scientists have determined that our risk for heart disease drops approximately 3 percent for every 1 milligram/L increase in your HDL level. This amount of exercise can equate to as much as a 7.5 decline in risk!

EVOO: Ours contains far more Polyphenols than the most polyphenol-dense EVOO. Shown to boost HDL in the important 2006 *Annals of Internal Medicine* study (Annals of Internal Medicine; The Effect of Polyphenols in Olive Oil on Heart Disease Risk Factors; 2006 ; Volume 145,(5); 333-341).

1 to 2 glasses of red wine daily (organic)–The drier the better. Those using the skin and pulp of the muscadine grape (don't try to eat these, they are tough as leather and require fermentation), native to the southeastern portion of the United States, are the healthiest and offer protection against heart disease, reducing the stickiness of red blood cells and in doing so, increasing blood flow, according to Dr. Al Sears. In fact, muscadine grapes have been found to contain as much as 40 times more resveratrol than other grapes! Resveratrol is one of the most powerful anti-inflammatories known to man. In other animals, a number of studies have shown its ability to prevent skin cancer as well as age-related decline in mice. Resveratrol (highest in Pinot Noir from upstate N.Y.)[3] is a natural antibiotic and antimutagen[4] produced by plants and toxic to invading organisms such as fungi and bacteria. Certain California wines are higher in sodium fluoride from use of the

pesticide Cryolite.[5] Buy organic wines from N.Y, Texas or Europe.

To further help reverse age related fatigue and brain function:

L-Carnitine–1000- 2000 milligrams per day.[6]

Phosphatidylserine (PS)–800 milligrams AM and PM

Freeze dried organic blueberry powder–as directed. Shukitt et al. showed that diets containing high concentrations of blueberry actually reversed age related decline in the hippocampal area of the brain.[7]

Choline–Promotes methyl transfer and an important precursor to the neurotransmitter acetylcholine. Best sources are lecithin and egg yokes.

Gingko biloba–As previously discussed. Increases the brain's circulation, reduces its fatigue and enhances memory.

To further assist your brain's ability to absorb nutrients:

Phosphatidylserine (PS)-100 milligrams AM & PM. PS is the most highly concentrated fat in the brain, comprising almost 70 percent of nerve tissue mass, according to Life Extention Magazine (September, 2002). Citing a study by Paris M. Kid (Kidd PM. A review of nutrients and botanicals in the integrative management of cognitive dysfunction. Altern Med Rev 1999 Jun;4(3):144-61) their report concludes: "Research has shown that dietary supplementation with phosphatidylserine can slow and even reverse the decline of learning, mood, memory, concentration, word recall related to dementia or age-related cognitive impairment in middle-aged and elderly subjects."

Phosphatidylcholine: 1500 milligrams daily. Facilitates intra-cellular communication.

To lower high levels of Cortisol (fight or flight hormone):

Relax. Yoga and meditation, and more sleep.

DHEA: Men - 25 milligrams AM and PM, Women - 10 milligrams AM and PM

Phosphatidylserine (PS)–Studies, and one large study in particular, have shown its ability to lower cortisol levels in athlete's recovery after endurance training after only 10 days of supplementation *(European Journal of Clinical Pharmacology*; 1992;42(4):385-8; Blunting by chronic phosphatidylserine administration of the stress-induced activation of the hypothalamo-pituitary-adrenal axis in healthy men).

If high level of C-Reactive protein: (inflammation)

> In addition to SOS, add Tumeric–1 gram AM and PM
>
> Don't skip meals. Eat less food, but the right SOS foods more often.

To help prevent prostate cancer:

> Nettle Root Extract–240 milligrams (helps protect the prostate against excess estrogen). But also important for women. Its anti-inflammatory compounds reduce tumor necrosis factor (TNF). TNF inflames tissues throughout the body, moderating rheumatoid arthritis and other age related diseases. Use has also been shown to lower blood sugar and stimulate urinary flow.
>
> Pygeum Extract–100 milligrams (suppresses high levels of prostaglandin). Take both the above to help prevent prostate cancer. If you already have it, consult a physician.
>
> Zinc–30 milligrams PM.
>
> Note: Copper–An important element required for our development and growth, not necessarily for prostate health, but mentioned here since it's often mistakenly taken along with zinc. Never take copper at the same time as zinc. While both are important minerals required by many of the enzymes our body requires, one decreases the level of the other. Take at different times, at least two hours or more apart. 9 milligrams daily.

4. THE PROGRAM—PART 2: THE SOS FOODS

Highest Quality Carbohydrates:

Eat as many colors of the right foods at one time as you can. It's that simple. Get familiar with the list of foods we've identified that follows. They'll lengthen your life, and the quality of each day, if you'll permit them to. Fortunately, the list of great foods to choose from is large. The more you become familiar with these foods, the easier it is to think of them and plan to eat them. In Chapter 7, my wife, Kelly, will share some of my favorite recipes featuring many of these foods. Just mix them up. While getting healthy fat is a challenge for some, I eat avocados often. A slice for breakfast, or on top of a synergy salad for dinner. It's easier than you think! That salad is generally topped with a sprinkling of almonds or pine nuts, some EVOO and a good dose of fresh lemon. Again, achieving synergy is worth the effort. And you'll find like we have, that your body gravitates toward healthy eating. No matter what you're used to!

1) Best Characteristics: Choose from the incredibly healthy foods that are listed below, grown as close to home as possible. Fresh, organic and if available, pesticide free.

The Key: The greater the number of combined SOS food group colors (Synergy), the greater their collective power to protect and heal you. Like the Legion of Super Heroes™ of comic book fame, the whole gang, each boasting their own special skill set, is greater than the sum of their parts.

How much: 5–7 servings of healthy fruits or vegetable carbohydrates daily.

What's a serving: Enough to fit in the palm of your hand. It's easier to accomplish this than you think. And if you use a blender, it's a cinch. I throw in enough healthful foods to produce a synergy drink that I keep refrigerated and draw from for days. Pour it in a smaller bottle, and take to work or school.

2) How often: The more often you eat the right foods the less your body experiences hunger, providing a gradual and consistent flow of nutrients from your drip system to your blood stream. Eat *small* meals of the recommended foods as *often* as you can. Since your blood sugar typically plunges every four hours, eat often enough to insure you reduce that consequence. You'll find the more you eat the balanced meals of SOS foods the more energy you'll feel and the more rapidly you'll lose weight. It's just as easy to get full on nutrient rich foods as it is on junk. You just won't stay full for as long a time. That means you get to eat delicious foods more often. Plate composite - 65 percent SOS Carbohydrates - 25 percent SOS proteins - and 10 percent SOS fats such as 1 teaspoon of EVOO (or 1 teaspoon of SOS nuts, or one 1/4 to 1/2 of avocado) and 1 teaspoon of EVCO. If EVCO is not available, double up on any of the later. Only if no EVCO is available, replace with one handful of SOS nuts to achieve the desired ration of Carbohydrate - Protein - Fat.

It's important to recognize how little protein we require. We've learned a bad habit and need to learn a better one. Share an entree when you go out dining. Your stomach is not capable of digesting any more protein at a given time than the amount you can fit in the palm of your hand. The rest will partially putrefy in your intestines. Give your brain time to feel that its cravings are satisfied. Allow 10 minutes for it to receive the signal from your stomach that it's full.

3) How much: For meals: 65 percent of a plate size should consist of all five color groups from the foods listed below if possible. If not possible, simply think "mixed colors" and combine as many as you can. The remainder of the plate

should contain no more than 25 percent protein and 10 percent healthy fat. The smaller the plate size, the easier it is to lose weight. As discussed, the less food we eat (often referred to as calorie restriction) the healthier we are, and according to animal studies, the longer we'll live. Leaving a table satisfied, but slightly hungry, produces great results in a short period of time.

If you chose to take the program to the next level, keep the food ratios the same, but cut the amount of food (or plate size using same amount of food) down by a quarter to one-third. Eat just as often, but eat smaller meals. Calorie deprivation has been shown to consistently lengthen the life in animal studies. Though more studies are required in human populations, I find that it works to energize me and keep me more clear and alert. Dr. John O. Holloszy, MD of the Department of Medicine, Washington University School of Medicine, St. Louis, Missouri observed that while it will take many more years of observation to be conclusive, persons that have undergone calorie restriction for 3–14 years were shown to have a great deal of protection against many secondary causes of aging and other disease, such as "type 2 diabetes, atherosclerosis and hypertension." According to Dr. Holloszy, "The caloric restricted (CR) individuals have very low serum triglyceride, total cholesterol and LDL cholesterol, insulin and glucose levels and extremely low blood pressure." They also were shown to have very low levels of inflammation.

On the shorter term, Dr. Phillip Miller recounts the effects of calorie deprivation on adults who were forced to restrict calories for 21 months when they discovered they lacked enough food to sustain themselves, after sealed in the famed Biosphere experiment. After reducing calories by 30 percent, but maintaining a balanced food ratio, women lost an average of 15 pounds, while men lost on average 27 pounds and experienced similar results to those reported by Dr. Holioszy—with substantial reduction in fasting blood sugar and blood pressure (which dropped by a whopping 25 percent, cholesterol and more).

And the downside? Holioszy found those practicing CR had reduced sex drive (which I suspect correlates with a reduction in blood pressure), and were sensitive to cold temperatures. I will address how to remain sexually aroused in my next work. On another note, while conjecture on my part, I'm of the belief that we receive far too much stimuli in the normal course of our lives. Some, far more than others. And, that the extent to which we reduce that revitalizes us. It's as true cognitively—born out of the proven results of meditation—as it is physiologically, by the reduction in the amount of food we eat. Again, this is only a theory that merits further research. (Note: since proteins become glycated, it stands to reason that the less we consume, the less we will glycate—though again, I believe that small portions of healthy SOS proteins are far more healthful, when eaten as part of a balanced meal, than a strict vegetarian diet.)

If you're an athlete, or wish to eat more healthful carbohydrates, grab a second plate and help yourself. No need to add additional protein. My recommended ratio for meals of carbohydrates-protein-fat (65-25-10) is not too dissimilar to the program suggested by The American Heart Association (they suggest 50/30 - 35/20-15). Other major health groups such as the American Cancer Society and the American Diabetes Association recommend a similar ratio of foods. They're based on solid research and they work! SOS snacks, as suggested below, need to be added and eaten in between and in addition to these balanced meals. The ratios above are approximate.

Easiest way to get there: support the following 8 simple habits.

1. Just blend!

Vita-Mix 5200® class juicer, the best pulverizing juicer I could find, is a great way to get there. You would have to chow down on a whole bunch of different vegetables, and several pieces of each, to eat the nutrients in just one serving from the right juicer. But which one is right? The Vita-Mix 5200® retains important fiber. I believe that makes it the best juicer for *prevention*. But if you're a victim of cancer or have autoimmune disease, my recommendation differs.[8]

2. Make more salad!

Enough to last from one night until the next, combining each of the color groups. Enjoy a portion of that salad for breakfast (yes, it's the best time), and another portion for dinner. Just two palmfuls for both meals is 4 servings! But since the objective is to eat at least 5 portions 5 times a day, don't forget the healthful snacks. Other research suggests it's not just the number of servings, but the number of times throughout the day they're eaten. Also a cinch …

3. Just pack your bags!

That's right. For those of you that work, or leave home for several hours at a time, pack! Just throw a few small items in your attaché case, purse or your child's backpack the night before you charge out the door (it's even easier for kids; their palms are smaller). Just throw one 6 ounce bottle of vegetable juice (low sodium version) or better still your own fresh blend, a bag of snack carrots, and a plum for example, in your attaché or carry bag. Now, you'll easily accomplish eating seven servings.

4. Improvise if you must!

Easier than you thought? Want more? Skip the salad for lunch if you wish and have a cup of mixed vegetables. Now you're up to 8! Or, have some pasta. That's right, pasta. 100 percent whole grain or live grain pasta. You can do this once a week. Since it may be difficult to find either type when you're eating out, just ask your server to cook it al dente, then ad EVOO, a squirt of lemon, cooked tomato, and if you like, garlic, roasted red and green peppers and onions. Now top with vegetables from the list below.

You can do the same thing with pizza. 100 percent whole wheat or sourdough crust when possible. If not, you'll be fine. Just be sure to top it with healthy fat (olive oil) and other ingredients above that will turn it into a very healthy, low glycemic *meal*. Once a week, pizza is fine as well.

A team of scientists led by Dr. Mario Negri of the Institute for Pharmaceutical Research in Milan studied the eating habits of 8,300 people and found that those that ate pizza at least once a week were 59 percent less likely to contract cancer of the esophagus, and 26 percent less likely to be stricken with cancer of the colon. Of course, this may have more to do with the power of just one ingredient, such as the tomato sauce, or the combination of them all. But in my opinion, it's due to the synergy of the food.

And I'm not alone. As study researcher Silvano Gallus said in a 2003 interview (Nutra Ingredients): "We knew that tomato sauce was protective against certain tumors, but we certainly didn't expect that pizza as a whole would provide such strong protection."

Remember, this is an easy to follow, incredibly healthful program, simply based on the synergy and interaction of nutrients. But if you do eat pasta or pizza, please make sure you add the recommended protein and a dash of healthy SOS fats (as previously discussed). For those travelers who will find themselves at the end of a road in a greasy diner, think SOS. Order healthful side dishes of steamed vegetables (with no margarine added) and mix them together in your salad. Ask the restaurant to top this with grilled chicken or a hard-boiled egg. You'll be amazed how accommodating short order cooks can be when you give them a challenge. Tell them you are on a special diet and need their help. I've enjoyed some excellent meals with the help of a creative cook in more than one greasy spoon. Remember, SOS is flexible.

5. Steaming!

I take other simple approaches to get my 5-7 serving fix, especially if I'm on the run. Steaming a meal is a wonderful way to enjoy the delicious taste and synergy of its nutrients. If you don't own a steamer, it's money well spent. Kale, purple cabbage, yellow and red peppers and almonds are among my favorites. And steaming is a no brainer. Just top with EVOO, pepper, and a hint of chili powder if you wish. It's a fast way to prepare a healthy meal, especially for those on the go. Just fill the base with water and set the timer to 10 or 15 minutes. Remember, we're only talking 5-7, some of which are healthy snacks (we call them hacks).

Grocery shopping should always include the snacks you need readily available each day. It's much easier to do when they're already on hand. When we were kids our parents packed our lunch bags. As adults, we eat junk food on the run. Why not adapt these simple healthy habits. Make more salad and pack your bag the night before. The latter is at least as important as watching TV. And it can easily be done during a simple commercial break. A small price to pay to live a longer life. It's just as easy to eat right on the run as it is to eat wrong. In fact, it's easier. You won't have to search for vending machines or airport food. It's in the bag!

6. Eat more often!

In addition to three meals a day (which most of us eat anyway) and three hacks, add one last meal. A mini meal. Just a couple of hours before bedtime. That meal should be the left over salad from the dinner I suggested you make more of the night before. That's all.

7. Keep it Simple!

You'll be surprised how easy this is. The key—it's those leftovers! The term has a negative connotation. But preparing enough healthy foods to draw from as needed, that retain their fresh flavor, is actually a positive approach to good eating. Make enough great salad to last for about a day and a half. Juice (masticate) enough to last for swigging periodically over the next couple of days, the enzymes do breakdown quickly (in minutes) but the nutrient value (though they too degrade over time), remains powerful. Prepare a large amount of seed and nut mix. Store in a jar and draw from whenever you want a hack. Pack them in baggies for travel or send off with your child to eat as part of their lunch at school. Make up a granola mix like the one suggested in the chapter that follows, and draw from as desired. Prepare enough delicious soup to last for days. Consider more variety in your breakfast—my wife Kelly's suggestions follow. Some of that same food can be enjoyed later that day and still retains its texture, flavor, and value. Pack hacks in advance. Keep it simple. We've made it easy to make healthy foods conveniently available. It's just a matter of preparing more SOS foods than you may need for a single meal. And spending a few moments a week preparing your hacks.

8. Supplement—as discussed in Chapter 5!

Supplement at breakfast and at dinner or at one mini meal a couple of hours before bed. Remember, this program is based on science not hype. And the SOS Supplements that follow are just as important as the SOS Foods. Collectively, they represent miracle Super-Nutrients that will extend and improve your life. Combine that with calorie restriction, leave each meal *slightly* hungry (something you'll get used to in short order), and you'll further empower yourself. So that's it! The carbohydrate portion of SOS is that simple, yet that powerful. Stay the course, incorporate it into your life, and become among the healthiest people in the world.

Rationale:

Eating foods synergistically empowers them. The *more often* you eat the *right* foods *the less you crave* the wrong ones. You'll avert the ravages that cause you to jump off the low blood sugar cliff. The more often you eat the right foods the less likely you'll binge eat.

The recommended carbohydrate foods provide the important fiber you need to regulate blood sugar, and balance the activity of your hormones. Eating the right ratio of foods improves your body's ability to regulate and, properly and efficiently use its powerful hormones. In the end, weight gain or loss is about caloric intake from the *right* (SOS) foods. But if you derive calories from this *mix,* your intake will be optimal. Remember, I've asked you to add three carbohydrates *hacks* to your intake daily, without additional protein or fat. This along with the proper balancing of these foods at mealtime will help insure that your caloric intake is moderate. Remember, there are 9 calories in a gram of fat and only 4 in a protein or carbohydrate. Those added snacks are like adding high octane to your fuel tank. In combination with balanced meals and the supplements that are summarized in the following section, your defense system and metabolism are both efficient and effective. Along with regular weight resistance and aerobic exercise, as well as meditation, yoga (or other relaxation technique) will put you over the top. Throwing in a dose of other fascinating anti-aging solutions (the subject of my next book) nails it.

In summary:

Eat three meals a day at normal mealtimes. Always select foods from the recommended food list below. The more colored food groups combined per

meal the better. Juice whenever possible with a machine like the Vita-Mix®
masticating machine that allows you to benefit from all of the fruit/vegetable's
precious contents, including skin, seeds and fiber (don't forget the juice bar you
drive by on your way to work). Pack a hack. Improvise when necessary. Steaming
is another great alternative. Eat more often with smaller but well-balanced meals.
Make and eat salads. They're a great way to help you get the full spectrum of
hues. So are a few slices of pizza occasionally, depending on how you top it.
Even an occasional dish of the right kind of pasta is fine if you top it properly.
Make more salad than you'll eat for dinner. *Three times as much.*

That way you are able to:

- Eat a normal size bowl or plateful of this same salad for your mini meal a
  couple of hours later before bedtime.
- Fill half your breakfast plate with salad the next morning.

1) Primary Foods Recommended. The bolded are better:

A. Carbohydrates:

Black, Blue and Purple	Red	Green	Yellow/ Orange	White/ Tan/ Brown
Group 1	Group 2	Group3	Group 4	Group 5
Black Bean	Cranberry	Artichoke Leaf	Cantaloupe	Coconut
Black Currant	Red Currant	Asparagus	Carrot	Garlic
Black Horse-Radish [1]	Red Guava	Avocado	Lemon	Kohlrabi (Purple, Green Too)
Black Plum	Red Pome-Granate	Broccoli	Pumpkin	Leek
Black Raspberry	Red Watermelon	Broccoli Sprout	Yellow Onion	Lentil
Blackberry	Ruby Red Grapefruit	Brussels Sprout	Yellow Pepper	Shallot
Blueberry (Low Bush)	Straw-Berry [2]	Collard Green	Yellow Grapefruit	Cauliflower

Black, Blue and Purple	Red	Green	Yellow/ Orange	White/ Tan/ Brown
Purple Cabbage	**Tomato**	**Kale**	Mango	Jicama
Black Mulberry	**Red Grape**	**Kiwi**		Parsnip
Purple Pepper	**Red Tart Cherry**	**Lime**		Pinto Bean
Purple Plum	Red Blood Orange	**Mustard Green**		White Horse-Radish[5]
	Red Pepper	**Parsley**		White Onion
	Red Radicchio	**Spinach**		Barley
	Red Pear	**Swiss Chard**[3]		
	Red Hot Chili Pepper	**Turnip Green**		
		Watercress		
		Green Apple[4]		
		Green Bean		
		Green Cabbage		
		Green Grape		
		Green Pear		
		Green Pea		
		Romaine Lettuce		
		Hot Peppers		

Table Footnotes:

1—Can promote blood thinning. Do not eat if you are taking aspirin, or after an injury. Avoid if taking antiplatelet or anticoagulant drugs. Strong diuretic. Those with kidney problems should avoid. 2—Only eat if labeled pesticide free. 3—High in oxalates. Those with kidney or gallbladder problems should avoid, though many, including professionals, feel they don't pose any real danger for those so effected. 4—Select Granny Smith or Fuji. 5—Same as 1.

Occasional Options:

For Group 1: substitute organic freeze dried blueberry powder and/or (and is better) organic freeze dried black raspberry powder.

For Group 2: Unsweetened pomegranate juice and unsweetened cranberry juice.

Super Option—*mix* powders from Option Group 1 juices from Option Group 2.

Other once a week meal suggestions to mix many color groups:

Once a week: Homemade pizza (with 100 percent whole wheat crust or sourdough bread crust (if possible). Mix it up. EVOO brushed on evenly. Lots of the above color groups, a sprinkle of lemon, garlic, spices and if you like, our recommended protein. Add spices to everything you can!!

Once a week: Pasta! Informed Living's 100 percent durum wheat pasta, infused with EVOO, herbs and spices. Mix and match all color groups, and recommended protein.

Once a week- Home-assembled Pizza.

More often:

Home made vegetable soup. Add garlic, protein from below such as pasteurized chicken if desired.

Plain yogurt with mixed berries (blueberries, strawberries), nuts (almonds, pistachios, macadamia) and fruit (kiwi or cantaloupe) and on occasion small amounts of mashed banana. Top with cinnamon and sesame seeds.

Special salads mixing fruits *and* vegetables *and* seeds *and* nuts, EVOO and spices, like Randy's salad in Chapter 7.

Select proteins below, stuffed with vegetables and fats. i.e., chicken with spinach, alpine cheese, almonds, and spices served with olive oil and black horseradish.

Whey shakes (no more than 1 a day as fourth meal) with above freeze dried fruit powders, cinnamon, and sprinkle of psyllium.

HIGHEST QUALITY PROTEIN

1. Best Characteristics:

Seek beef that's grass-fed and free range. Not just grass finished; pesticide and antibiotic free. Poultry should be free range pastured, pesticide and hormone free, allowed to scratch for insects, and fed purslane and other organic material. Fish should be from unpolluted, uncontaminated pristine water and not caged/farmed. While no fish can claim to be free of all mercury and contaminants, studies should show they are well below hazard levels. Alaskan fish from pristine rivers is under the wire. Yogurt should be *plain* with live cultures. Of course, you may add SOS fruits, nuts, cinnamon and even psyllium powder if you choose to (next section). Occasional eating of wild game, such as bison, is healthful.

- Organic Omega-3 Eggs
- Free Range Pasteurized Chicken
- Free Range Pasteurized Turkey
- Grass-fed Steak
- Grass-fed Steak Ground Sirloin
- Alaskan Sardines in EVOO
- Wild Alaskan Salmon Sausage
- Wild Alaskan Salmon
- Wild Alaskan Halibut
- Oregon Pink Shrimp
- Yogurt—Organic Plain unsweetened, comes with no fruit (fruit, nuts, spices such as cinnamon, seeds, can all be added)
- Alaskan Peppered Sable
- Arctic Char. The right char is one of the finest fish available, with *even more* Omega-3s than Wild Alaskan Salmon! And char fishing is sustainable. The problem is the wrong char is just as bad as the right char is good. Stay away from char unless you know the source (for a complete list of quality resources for this and all recommended foods in this book, go to our web site at RKInformedLiving.com). By all means, stay away from farmed *and* Scottish char (for an interesting read, go to http://en.wikipedia.org/wiki/Arctic_char, and scroll down to Scotland).

Occasional Option: To substitute or supplement (must still total no more than 20 percent of plate) above:

- Free Range Bison

- Grass-fed Beef Bacon
- Grass-fed Beef Bratwurst

*Option: To replace the above no more than twice a week:

- Grass-fed Bison
- Whey Isolate in water-Whey is one of the few foods that builds important Glutathione. Oral intake of glutathione itself doesn't appear to be effective. While taking a mouth full of foods high in anthocyanin might help it from being destroyed by enzymes, it's not yet been proven to do so. Two scoops full of isolated whey. It's easily digested and should be considered an option as part of your Good Night Sweep. It lacks the fiber and other important nutrients that some of the above protein do, but may be counted as a protein periodically. If you do so at nighttime, count it as your last meal and drink it while eating the extra salad from dinner.

2. How much?

Select 1 or more from the primary proteins list above. At each meal, this protein should be not larger than 1/2 deck of playing cards. Collectively, protein should make up no more than 25 percent of your plate.

3. The Key

The typical American is eating *far* more protein than we need and considerably more than we can properly digest. The hardest lesson to learn here: eat far less. If you go out for dinner, share an entree. More is not better. Keep protein to only 25 percent of that plate. The highest quality protein. Get used to lots of healthy fats and carbs. *Retrain* your brain. Remember 65 percent carbs, 25 percent protein, 10 percent healthy fats. Portion control. *Don't let the restaurant or the grocer dictate yours.* The restaurant will divide that entree any way you request they do. Start there. Or with your butcher. And by all means, at home.

Option: To replace above, you can substitute for 1 protein every other day for:

- Small bowl 40 percent filled with organic steel cut oat meal or organic full grain barley

To this you add approximately:

- 30 percent of at least two recommended fruits from different color groups
- 30 percent of primary nuts and seeds.
- Even better? Sprinkle ample amounts of *mixed* nuts *and mixed* seed mix.
- Make up a bowl full each week of your favorite mix of seeds add nuts based on those recommended here, and sprinkle them generously.

*Options: To top off above
- Small amount of coconut oil or organic butter
- Cinnamon and or other recommended spices
- Add a generous portion of berries, kiwi or other recommended fruits. And don't be afraid to add vegetables like parsley. Remember, the goal here is to mix it up!

Healthiest Fats:

In addition to the above, the following should be added to a full plate or bowl. All but the nuts and seeds should be added in moderation.

Recommended healthy fats:
- Extra Virgin Olive Oil
- Extra Virgin Coconut Oil
- Lightly roasted Organically Grown Almonds, no salt
- Organic Butter
- Ghee
- Pistachios Organically grown (Add other recommended nuts)
- Organically grown macadamia nuts
- Seeds Organically grown (Add other recommended seeds)

Spices:

I'm a big believer in spicing up food and mixing it up. Choose Organic spices from our recommended list. They're worth the extra cost:

Cloves, Cinnamon, Oregano, Turmeric, Parsley, Basil, Curry powder, Mustard Seed, Ginger, Pepper (ground or whole peppercorn), Chile Powder (it often contains cumin as an ingredient, not to be confused with curcumin, see below). Nor should cumin be confused with caraway, another spice as it often is. Cumin color is different (lighter) and its seeds are larger. It owes its aromatic fragrance to a high content of essential oil, Garlic (clove or powder), Onion, Turmeric (and curcumin, an extract of turmeric), and finally, Poppy Seed.

Sprinkle them generously, based on your preference. They allow you to add an important dimension to all SOS foods.

Healthy Extras:

Dessert: Choose one of the following for lunch or dinner (not at both)

2 Organic Extra Virgin Coconut Cookies

or

1 Cup Plain, Organic Yogurt with fruit, nuts and cinnamon

or

One handful of recommended seed and nut mix
Choose one of the following for a third meal if you choose none of the above:
Mixed Berrys and nuts and seeds in organic yogurt once a day.
Or
EVOO on Wasa Crackers (2) topped with Alpine Cheese and Daikon or
Broccoli Sprouts

Again, the above is what I do (other than AGE which I'm allergic to). Morning supplement program, and one teaspoon of fish oil. More often than not, I chase the oil with isolated blueberry whey powder.

Always take supplements with SOS foods to improve their absorption. For the same reason, I generally wait a while if time permits, before taking and chasing the teaspoon of fish oil with whey or my sweep—allowing my food and nutrients a head start, before I drown them with liquid and hinder their absorption. I also have a couple of tablespoons of cottage cheese whenever I take fish oil. It stabilizes the fat, and helps it absorb. Then I chase it. Evening supplement program, and 1 teaspoon of fish oil. I generally follow that with a dash of pomegranate juice in an 8 ounce glass of water, and sprinkle of lemon, and a teaspoon or more of psyllium as needed (what I call my "Good Night Sweep").

You've now received the most powerful program of its kind. Eating the right foods that you may select from the large menu provided (a lot easier and far more healthful than focusing on a list of top 10 super-foods!), mixing the color groups as often as you can, eating balanced meals in the right proportion, approximately 65-25-10 (SOS Carbohydrates-Protein-Fat) will change your life! As you'll quickly discover, the power of Super-Nutrients is extraordinary! You're only one meal away from a new way of living—for life ...

END NOTES

1. *Antioxidants and Redox Signaling*; 2005 Jan-Feb;7(1-2):32-41. Biswas et al.; Curcumin induces glutathione biosynthesis and inhibits NF-kappaB activation and interleukin-8 release in alveolar epithelial cells: mechanism of free radical scavenging activity
2. Mayo Clinic Staff: Mayo Clinic.com:March 28, 2008, Niacin to boost your HDL 'good' cholesterol
3. *Cornell Chronicle: www.news.cornell.edu/chronicle* Higher levels of resveratrol found among N.Y. red wines; Blaine P. Friedlander Jr.
4. *Science.* 1997 Jan 10;275(5297):218-20; Jang et al.

5. Vitaculture and Enology Research Center; Cryolite in Grapes/Flouride in Wine- A guide for Growers and Vintners to determine the optimum cryolite applications on grapevines; California Agricultural and Technology institute; Research Publication; Gwynn Sawyer Ostrom.

6. As recommended by Dr. Phillip Miller in his excellent book, *The Life Extension Revolution*

7. *Nutritional Neuroscience*; 2008 Aug;11(4):172-82

8. The Gerson Institute and others have demonstrated the importance of maximizing enzymatic activity for cancer victims above all other considerations relating to juicing. While again, a balance along with important fiber is most important for the *prevention* of many other diseases, the highest content of nutrients and enzymatic action appears to be the most important consideration of juicing for cancer victims. Enzymes and nutrients are their highest in the absence of fiber (fiber absorbs a portion of them). Studies by Michael Donaldson PhD. (Comparison of Juice Extractors: Enzymes) and others support the use of the more expensive two step (triturator/press combination). The Norwalk juicer (over $2,100) appears to be the very best for those persons. Donaldson's study also supports Max Gerson's claims (Gerson Institute for Alternative Cancer Treatment) that centrifugal juicers do the most damage to enzymes by deactivating them in the juicing process itself.

CHAPTER 7

RECIPES

My husband asked me to share with you a handful of his favorite recipes. I am neither a chef nor a dietician; I simply love to cook and love to see that smile on his face when he is eating something he loves that is actually good for him (which is a requirement in our household).

With every ingredient in the next few pages, try to use the *local, organic version* wherever possible ... the eggs, the butter, the meat, the vegetables, the canned products—*everything*. Don't forget to remove all pesticides from your fruits and vegetables, using your Tersano cleaning bowl. (www.RKInformedLiving.com)

1. LEMONY BRUSSELS SPROUTS

Believe it or not, this one will make you a believer in brussels sprouts...ask my neighbors, ask me. My husband loves brussels sprouts so I was on a mission to find a way that I could learn to love them too. Here it is...and very simple.

1.5   pounds brussels sprouts, core removed, cut into shreds
3   tablespoons butter
3   tablespoons EVOO
1   tablespoon poppy seeds
1-2   tablespoons fresh lemon juice
      kosher salt, fresh ground black pepper

Over low heat, cook the brussels sprouts in the butter/EVOO for about 5 minutes. Add poppy seeds and continue to cook until the sprouts are very wilted (about 10 more minutes). Turn heat off. Stir in fresh lemon juice, salt and pepper. Serves 6.

2. COCONUT CHICKEN FINGERS

12   free range chicken tenders, or 4 chicken breasts
½   cup hot sauce (I usually combine Louisiana with Tabasco)
½   cup coconut flour

¼   cup flaked unsweetened coconut (if you are not a coconut fan, you
      may leave this out)
1   teaspoon kosher salt
1   tablespoon cajun seasoning
      EVCO
      Dipping Sauce

Put the chicken in a baggie, cover with hot sauce and refrigerate for at least one hour. To a pie tin add the flour, flaked coconut, salt and cajun seasoning. Remove chicken from baggie, shake off excess liquid and dredge chicken in the flour mixture. Heat EVCO in skillet over medium heat. Brown chicken on both sides, approximately 3 minutes per side. Remove, drain on paper towels. Serve with a ramekin of either a blue cheese dipping sauce (you can make it or buy it) or a sauce made of diced onion, tomato and balsamic vinegar—or both. Serves 4.

3. RANDY'S KITCHEN SINK SALAD

This one we eat regularly for breakfast, lunch, or dinner to get our live veggie/greens fix. Use whatever you have in the fridge; this is just an example. Everything should be chopped into bite sized pieces ... so it all fits in a bite.

3-5   romaine lettuce leaves, chopped
      handful of arugula, chopped
      handful of radicchio, chopped
      handful of grape tomatoes
1   red bell pepper (or whatever color you have), chopped
3-4   artichoke hearts (from the jar) chopped
4   sun-dried tomatoes, chopped
      flat leaf parsley, or cilantro, or both, chopped
      handful of broccoli sprouts
      large handful almonds (chopped, whole, sliced—whatever seeds/nuts
      you have)
      fresh avocado cut in half, peeled, seeded, chopped
      jicama cut into sticks (great for crunch)
2   kiwi, chopped
6   pesticide-free strawberries, hulled, chopped (skip if your store does
      not have these)
      squeeze ½ fresh lemon over all for freshness
      kosher salt and black pepper to taste

Place all on a beautiful salad platter. Drizzle with your favorite EVOO dressing (when I do not have time to make a dressing, I like to use Paul Newman's Olive Oil and Spices). Toss. Serves 6–8.

4. PIZZA

The best part about pizza is you can put just about anything you like on it as long as it is an SOS food—vary the ingredients and make more than one at a time—and it is all wonderful. Below you will find a typical, throw it together pizza we eat for a quick meal after a round of golf on a Sunday afternoon … again, play with your food…add and remove any ingredients you like but keep the EVOO as the first layer, regardless.

1	organic pizza crust (I did not specify organic in each ingredient in this chapter, like I am doing with the crust; I am doing this here to make sure everyone knows they can buy Organic Pizza Crust)
2	tablespoons EVOO
	large handful grape tomatoes (sliced in half longwise)
	handful of fresh spinach
	handful of artichoke hearts
½	cup red bell pepper, diced
	large handful sliced fresh mushrooms
1	cup shredded mozzarella cheese
	handful basil leaves
1	teaspoon red pepper flake

Preheat oven to 400 degrees. Evenly brush EVOO over entire pizza crust. Sprinkle bell pepper, mushrooms, spinach, artichoke hearts and tomato evenly over pizza. Top with mozzarella cheese and torn basil leaves (to release their flavors)…sprinkle with red pepper flake. Bake for 14 minutes. Remove, cool for two minutes and serve.

I would like to mention a simple spicy version … also, if you cannot get the Organic Crust at your local store, I buy the Ultra Thin Margarita Version … and add the following in only minutes:

- diced bell pepper
- diced peppadeau (a spicy little red pepper found in many Deli sections, where they serve the specialty olives, etc.)
- handful of fresh spinach
- handful of artichoke hearts

- red pepper flake
- handful of mozzarella sprinkled over the top.

5. SEARED STEAK WITH MERLOT-MUSHROOM SAUCE

1	8-ounce grass-fed rib-eye or filet steaks
1	clove garlic, cut in half
2	teaspoons coarsely ground pepper
1½	tablespoons EVCO
3	tablespoons chilled unsalted butter
6	ounces fresh shiitake mushrooms, or any wild mushrooms with lots of flavor, stemmed, cut into 1/2-inch pieces
1	shallot, thinly sliced
1	cup Merlot (or any good red wine-must be one you would like to drink)
1	tablespoon chopped fresh thyme

Pat steak with paper towel to remove moisture. Rub garlic clove on both sides of each steak. Sprinkle steaks on both sides with salt and 2 teaspoons pepper; press to adhere. Heat oil in heavy medium skillet over medium-high heat. Add steaks; cook to desired doneness, about 3 minutes per side for medium. Transfer steaks to 2 plates (do not clean skillet). Add 1 tablespoon butter to pan. Add mushrooms and shallot; sauté about 4 minutes, be careful not to burn. Add wine and thyme and boil until wine is reduced by half, about 4 minutes. Remove from heat. Whisk in 2 tablespoons butter, 1 tablespoon at a time. Taste the sauce and then season with salt and pepper if needed. Pour over steaks. This is fabulous with cauliflower or roasted asparagus... please try and resist the mashed potato temptation. Serves 2.

6. STEAK, GRASS-FED BACON AND GINGERED EGGS— WE ARE TALKING WATERMELON STEAK FOR BREAKFAST!

For Watermelon Steak: Cut regular serving sized wedges of watermelon, at least 1 per person. Brush both sides with EVOO. Put on grill and cook for about 3 minutes on each side.

For Grass-fed Bacon:

Cook on grill until desired crispness, 2 slices per person.

For Gingered Eggs:

  1 omega-3 egg per person

  sliced ginger (can buy it in a jar)

Break open eggs into a skillet on the grill. Top with sliced ginger and black pepper. Cook until done and serve. We prefer to cook these on the grill but you could cook in the kitchen too.

7. EGG SALAD

7	omega-3 eggs
¼	cup real mayonnaise* or substitute with plain yogurt
1	teaspoon Dijon mustard
½	lime, juiced
	kosher salt and ground black pepper to taste
6	slices sourdough bread, toasted or grilled, with EVCO slathered
1	avocado, halved, peeled, seeded and sliced lengthwise
¼	cup fresh cilantro, chopped

Cover the eggs in water, bring to a medium boil, turn off heat and cover pot. Let eggs sit for about 10 additional minutes in the covered pot. Drain, rinse with cold water, and peel, when cool enough to handle. Roughly mash the eggs in a bowl with the mayonnaise, mustard and lime juice (don't over-mash—you want nice chunky texture). Season with salt/pepper. On each piece of toast, layer a few avocado slices, then spread with egg salad and arrange cilantro on top. Serve open faced. Serves 6.

*For a recipe for Corn-free, Sulfite-free and Soy-free Mayonnaise go to: http://foodallergies.about.com

8. WILD ALASKAN SALMON

1	(6-ounce) Wild Alaskan Salmon fillet per two persons (share one to leave room for more veggies)
	chili powder (enough to thinly cover one side of each salmon you are cooking)
	kosher salt
1	tablespoon EVCO
1	tablespoon EVOO

Rub your skillet with a nonstick oil, such as Dr. Fifes Cooking Oil (www.coconutresearchcenter.org) Heat a skillet over medium heat. Add the EVCO/EVOO. Rub the fillets with chili powder in a thin, but solid "crust." Sprinkle kosher salt and gently pat to hold the salt in. Gently lay the fish in the skillet (chili side down) and cook for about 3 minutes (do not disturb)…carefully turn over and cook for about 3 more minutes. Tent with foil for about 5 minutes and you are good to go. I like to serve this with the cabbage recipe…

9. BEAN SAUCE

½   onion, chopped
1   red bell pepper, cut into strips
1   yellow bell pepper, cut into strips
1   package fresh mushrooms, any kind, sliced
2   tablespoons EVOO
1   (16-ounce) can chopped tomatoes, undrained
1   (15-ounce) can dark red kidney beans, undrained
1   (15-ounce) can black beans, drained and rinsed
1   (15-ounce) can pinto beans, drained and rinsed
1   (3-ounce) jar capers
1   fresh jalapeno pepper diced, seeds removed (optional)
1   teaspoon cumin
      freshly ground black pepper to taste (I do not add salt to this recipe at all)
      fresh parsley for garnish
½   lemon, squeeze for garnish

Cook the onion, bell peppers and mushrooms in olive oil, over low heat just until starting to get tender. Add the rest of the ingredients, reduce heat and simmer for about 30 minutes stirring occasionally. While this is simmering, cook whatever wheat noodles you have according to package direction, drain well. Plate your noodles, ladle on a nice portion of Bean Sauce…and garnish with fresh parsley and a squeeze of fresh lemon! We sometimes eat this with our scrumptious Informed Living hard durum pasta, (RKInformedLiving.com), and at other times, with nothing at all. Serves 6. (Try to resist the mashed potato urge.)

10. HOT TOMATO HACK

      Several cut tomatoes
1   minced fresh garlic clove
      fresh chopped cilantro or flat leaf parsley

1   tablespoon EVCO
1   tablespoon EVOO

Heat over low EVCO/EVOO in skillet. Throw garlic in and cook for about 30 seconds. Add tomato and cook until softened, about 10 minutes. Add cilantro and cook a few more minutes. Serve as a side dish with anything!

11. VEGETABLE FRITTATA

1   large red or purple bell pepper, diced
16   ounces sliced fresh mushrooms (I prefer the flavor of portobello)
1½   cups shredded swiss cheese
¼   pound fresh asparagus, cut into 1 inch pieces (break off the bottom "tough" end first, cut into 1 inch pieces, weigh out the ¼ pound)
7   large Omega-3 eggs, lightly beaten
*½   cup mayonnaise substitute (see p.373)
¼   teaspoon kosher salt
3   tablespoons fresh basil, chopped

Layer the bell pepper, mushrooms and ½ swiss cheese in lightly greased 9.5" deep dish pie plate. Top with asparagus and remaining cheese. Combine the eggs and remaining 3 ingredients; pour evenly over cheese. Bake at 375 degrees for 40 minutes, or until a knife inserted in center comes out clean. Let stand 5 minutes. Serve warm. 6 Servings.

12. CAULIFLOWER GRATIN

Believe me, I love broccoli but I do have a hard time eating cauliflower. This is one of the few ways that I will eat cauliflower … sometimes, I mix both broccoli and cauliflower in this recipe. Randy, who will not eat potatoes, says he doesn't miss them at all when I serve this.

1   (10 ounce) package frozen cauliflower florets
½   cup coconut milk
½   teaspoon cayenne pepper
¼   teaspoon salt
½   cup shredded cheese (whichever you like, I use Mexican)
2   tablespoons Panko Italian-Style breadcrumbs
1   teaspoon EVOO

In a microwave-safe dish, stir to combine the cauliflower, milk, cayenne pepper, salt and shredded cheese. Lay a wet paper towel on top of ingredients and microwave on high for about 6 minutes.

In small ramekin combine the Panko and EVOO with a fork. Spoon over cauliflower and broil about 3 minutes, or until top is golden brown. Serves 4.

Option: if you have a few extra minutes, sauté 1 bunch of kale, large stems stripped and discarded, leaves chopped—in EVOO for 2 minutes or so. Before you top with breadcrumbs and broil, top with kale, then breadcrumbs, then broil.

13. GUACAMOLE

Almost everyone has a guacamole recipe, but in case you do not, here is a basic one to make that is ready in a snap:

3	ripe avocados
1	cup black beans, drained and rinsed
2	tablespoons Pine Nuts
1	lime, juiced
¼	cup diced sweet white onion
1	garlic clove, minced
1	serrano chile, minced
1	handful of fresh cilantro, chopped
1	teaspoon EVOO
½	teaspoon cumin
	kosher salt and ground black pepper to taste

Scoop the flesh of the avocados with a spoon, into a mixing bowl. Gently mash with a fork, leaving some large chunks. Fold in the rest of the ingredients. Cover with plastic wrap (make sure it is touching the avocado) and chill at least an hour before serving. We serve with eggs, fresh vegetables, or a large spoonful as a hack...but you can serve with anything you like. 3 Servings.

14. GREEN CHILI AND ONION CHEESE BUFFALO BURGER

2.25	pounds grass-fed ground buffalo meat
2	tablespoons worcestershire sauce
1	tablespoons minced garlic
1	teaspoon cajun seasoning
1	vidalia sweet onion
3	poblano chiles
6	slices swiss cheese
6	hamburger bun
	salt and pepper

½   cup hickory smoked BBQ sauce

Gently mix the ground meat, salt, pepper worcestershire sauce, garlic and cajun seasoning, form 6 patties, cover. Let stand at room temperature for 30 minutes before grilling. Cut the onion into ½" thick slices. Rub the cut onion slices and the whole poblano chiles with EVOO on all sides and grill until soft and brown. Char the peppers. Remove from grill and peel, seed and chop the peppers, along with chopping the onion. Put both together in a small bowl with a pinch of salt and pepper. Grill burgers; during last two minutes top with a slice of swiss cheese. Assemble: spoon onion/pepper mixture on bottom bun, hamburger, spread BBQ sauce mixture on top bun. Enjoy. Makes 6 Hamburgers.

15. ROASTED VEGGIES

Use any veggies you have but the below is one that I make frequently— sometimes I only do tomatoes, sometimes just asparagus. Your Mom was wrong by the way, you should definitely play with your food—play with this recipe.

2   large bell peppers, varying colors, seeded and cut into 1 inch pieces

3   baby eggplant, quartered lengthwise

4   baby zucchini, quartered lengthwise

4   plum tomatoes, seeded (squish the seeds out over the sink) quartered lengthwise

1   handful fresh mushrooms, sliced in large chunks

2   shallots, peeled and sliced
     EVOO
     kosher salt and fresh black pepper to taste
     Preheat oven to 500 degrees.

Combine all veggies on a large cookie sheet. Drizzle well with EVOO and season with salt and pepper. Roast about 15 minutes, or until just tender. Serves 6-8.

16. ARTICHOKE CHICKEN

1   chicken breast (free range) per person (or use several chicken tenderloins)

4   tablespoons coconut flour

3   tablespoons EVOO

14½ oz. chicken stock

3   tablespoons capers
1   tablespoon diced jalepeno (I use from the jar)
      freshly ground black pepper
1   14 oz. can artichoke hearts, quartered

Dredge chicken in flour. Heat EVOO in skillet over low heat. Cook until lightly brown, about 3 minutes on each side. Add the next 4 ingredients, bring to a boil, reduce heat and simmer for about 20 minutes or until sauce starts to thicken. Stir in the artichoke hearts and just heat through. Serve with freshly steamed asparagus. Note on the "stock," I don't have time to make stock so I buy the boxed organic versions from the grocery store and they keep in the fridge for some time.

17. ASPARAGUS HACK

¾   pound asparagus
      balsamic vinegar
      shredded cheese—whatever you like—I use mozzarella

Cook asparagus in steamer (or small amount of boiling water) for about 4 minutes. Dump into bowl of ice water to stop the cooking. Drain the water, pat the asparagus dry. Arrange on little plate … drizzle with Balsamic vinegar and sprinkle with shredded cheese. Serves 4.

18. PILE HIGH FRUIT

My favorite quick, sweet, dish to throw together for a snack, a side dish or breakfast. Onto a flat salad plate, place one triangle-shaped watermelon wedge in center. Pile a small handful each of the following freshly washed (remove pesticides) fruit items, on top of the watermelon wedge: red raspberries, black-berries, blueberries, strawberries (hulled, quartered), kiwi (cut into quarters), and chunks of cantaloupe. GORGEOUS AND FRESH!

19. LENTIL AND LEEK SOUP

½   onion, diced
1   carrot, sliced
1   large leek, sliced
½   tablespoon tomato paste
⅓   cup lentils, washed

2 ½   cups vegetable stock
2   cloves
       bay leaf
       salt and pepper to taste
       freshly chopped flat leaf parsley

In a large saucepan sauté the onion, carrot, and leek until soft. Add the tomato paste, lentils, vegetable stock, cloves and bay leaf. Bring to a boil. Lower heat and simmer, partially covered about 20 minutes, until the lentils are tender. Remove bay leaf. Puree in a processor or blender until smooth. Season to taste. Pour into bowls and sprinkle fresh parsley over top.

20. NUTTY GREENS

Use whatever greens you have but use an assortment for interest and health—remember, play with your food.

1   tablespoon olive oil
1   clove garlic, minced
1   small onion, halved and sliced thin
1   small can water chestnuts, drained and thinly sliced
3   shiitake mushrooms, sliced (if using dried, soak, discard the stems and slice)
⅓   pound kale, washed and cut into large pieces
⅓   pound spinach, washed and cut into large pieces
⅓   pound mustard greens, washed and cut into large pieces
½   cup watercress
2   teaspoon balsamic vinegar
½   cup walnuts (or whatever nuts you have)
       freshly ground black pepper, to taste

Heat the oil in a large skillet over low heat. Add the garlic and onions and sauté until onions are translucent. Be careful not to brown the garlic or it will give a bitter taste. Add the water chestnuts and shiitake mushrooms. Sauté for 3 minutes. Add the greens and sauté for 1 minute. Add the balsamic vinegar, walnuts, and pepper and sauté until the greens are tender. Serves 4–6.

21. ARUGULA BEANS

3 cups pinto beans or white cannellini beans, drained, rinsed (or mix them both)

1 bag arugula

1 teaspoon cumin seeds

1 tablespoon EVOO

1 sliced clove garlic

Heat EVOO and garlic in skillet, add the cumin seeds. When the seeds start sizzling, add in the beans. Cook until the beans are heated through then dump in the arugula. Cook a few minutes, until it wilts. Turn off the heat and you are ready to serve. Serves 4-6.

22. MEAT LOAF (THIS MAKES ONE LOAF, DOUBLE FOR TWO LOAVES)

1	omega-3 egg, lightly beaten
½	cup oats (raw)
¼	cup coconut milk
½	teaspoon salt
¼	teaspoon fresh black pepper
1	pound grass-fed ground sirloin
¾	cup shredded jalapeno cheddar cheese (use whatever cheese you like)
⅓	cup shredded carrot
⅓	cup diced sweet onion
¼	cup brown sugar
¼	cup ketchup
1	tablespoon mustard

Preheat oven to 350 degrees. In a large bowl, combine the egg, oats, milk, salt and pepper. Add to this the ground sirloin, cheese, carrot and onion. Mix this gently with clean, jewelry-free hands. In a lightly greased meatloaf pan, bake in oven for about 30 minutes. Option: do not put in loaf pan, place on lightly greased cookie sheet which will give a textured crust. While this is baking, combine the brown sugar, ketchup and mustard (for glaze). After the 30 minutes, pull the loaf out of the oven (keep oven temp ON), spoon glaze over the top and cook for an additional 15 minutes. Serves 6.

23. BASIC CABBAGE

1   small head red cabbage
1   tablespoon EVCO
1   tablespoon EVOO
     kosher salt and black pepper to taste

Cut the cabbage in half and, with the cut-side down, slice it very thinly around the core. Discard the core. Melt the EVCO/EVOO in skillet over medium heat. Add the cabbage, salt and pepper and sauté for about 15 minutes, stirring occasionally. The cabbage needs to get a bit brown in color. Serves 6. There are many variations of this—throw in some fresh tomato for lycopene, throw in some cashews, almonds etc. Don't buy the cabbage that the produce manager has already cut in half (loss of nutrients). Please buy it whole.

24. STEAMER BASKET

If you have no time, this is the answer. I highly recommend you purchase a steamer, I have several of the Black and Decker steamers ... you put water in the bottom, cut up your veggies, throw them in the basket, put the lid on, plug it in and set the timer...the timer rings when it is done. That simple. You can throw just about anything in the steamer, but the following is a list of the typical items that I regularly steam, plate, drizzle with EVOO and/or balsamic vinegar, dust with salt and pepper and you are good to go. And yes, there are many mornings that I serve Randy a plate of piping hot steamed veggies for breakfast—fill the bowl full, mix up the colors. Most veggies take about 10 minutes (broccoli and carrots a few minutes longer) while asparagus only takes about 4 minutes. Typical steamed veggies at our house: broccoli, spinach, cabbage, carrot, kale, asparagus, bell pepper.

25. FAVORITE VEGETABLE PLATE (FOR ANY MEAL)

In a large skillet, I cook on low heat every veggie we have in the fridge ... start out on low in EVOO, add some balsamic vinegar and cover. Cook for about 12 minutes or until the veggies are just starting to get tender. Top with pine nuts for a fantastic meal. A typical vegetable plate at our house would consist of:

Brussels sprouts, broccoli, red cabbage, carrot, asparagus, bell pepper all piled high on a dinner plate, topped with pine nuts and black pepper.

26. HIGH SPEED BLENDS

While we use the Vita-Mix® for all of our fruits and vegetable drinks, I realize not every household has one. If you don't, you will need something comparable ... and again, this is worth every penny. Throw in the whole fruit if your blender can handle it. Remember to sprinkle a small amount of Psyllium occasionally. We blend all kinds of things (we make enough to last for Randy's hacks as well) but a typical blender breakfast might look as follows:

	cantaloupe, a small piece (remove skin, keep seeds)
	kiwi, one half (remove skin or leave on)
	handful of grapes
1–2	scoops of blueberry whey
1	small carrot (just cut the two ends off, leave skin)
¼	apple (keep skin, stem, and core)
	A piece of red bell pepper (remove nothing)
	1 small slice jalapeno (if you like spice)
	1 teaspoon fish oil
	ground nutmeg and ginger
	ice, water

Blend until smooth.

Another example:

¼	cup watercress
2	broccoli florets
1	tablespoon pine nuts
1	small carrot
¼	apple
1	teaspoon fish oil
	cinnamon
	ice, water

And a third example (possibilities are endless):

1	cup spinach
½	apple
1	small carrot
½	cup watercress
½	scoops of whey
2	broccoli florets

1   teaspoon fish oil
     pinch red pepper flakes
     ice, water

27. TIPS: I HOPE SOME OF THESE YOU WILL FIND HELPFUL

Get rid of the cookie jar that is sitting on your countertop and replace it with seed/nut jars. I keep two jars out at all times for hacks. I typically mix seeds and nuts. When I am making Randy's Kitchen Sink salad I just grab that handful from this jar that is already good to go.

Make sure your produce is pesticide-free. For the sanitizing bowl that we use, go to www.RKInformedLiving.com.

Incorporate cherries into your snack regime…just wash them well and watch out for the pit. These really do help me with my sweet tooth—I hope they help you too.

Slice an apple and spread natural chunky peanut butter all over it.

We all know we are supposed to snack on carrots, red bell peppers, etc… please, start doing this…how about dipping into some Roasted Red Pepper or Asparagus/Artichoke Dip (make it or buy it). Avoid the crackers, use the fresh veggies dippers.

Do not buy chips—then you will not eat them. I am addicted to Tostitos® type chips…so I have compromised…I no longer buy them for the house, however, when I do go out for an occasional Mexican dinner, I am allowed to eat them.

I was raised on potatoes…mashed, baked, scalloped, au gratin—you name it—every night we had some form of potato. I now rarely buy potatoes for the house … but if I am out to dinner and wish to order a baked potato, that is my treat…but keep them out of your kitchen.

Do not buy soft drinks for the house. Again, an occasional soft drink at a restaurant is OK (Randy would not agree with this but this is my section!).

Bread—I just flat "SAY NO." Ignore it at the restaurants. And of course we know there are breads that are better choices … so when you must, select one of those.

Make it easy on yourself. We plan for leftovers. A great salad made for dinner carries over nicely for tomorrow's breakfast, lunch or hack. We make enough blended breakfast to last a day. We're only a handful away from our favorite nut and seed mix for an easy hack. We also make our own version of trail mix. We take our nut and seed mix, add shredded coconut, carob or cacao chips, and a small amount of granola.

The above are great examples of SOS foods that you can mix and match to make delicious SOS meals. Again, the combinations are endless. In addition to suggesting the salmon with the cabbage above as a complete meal, a couple of typical days might look as follows:

Day 1:
   B: Nutty Greens or Alaskan Salmon
   H: Nut/Seed mix
   L: Salad
   H: Apple or #18 Fruit or Blended Juice
   D: Alaskan Salmon or Pizza or Egg Salad
   H: Banana with Peanut Butter
   H: Nut/Seed Mix

Day 2:
   B: Gingered Eggs or Blended Juice
   H: Salad
   L: Basic Cabbage or Yogurt/Nut/Seed
   H: Black Plum or Carrots
   D: Seared Steak in EVOO
   H: Boiled Egg or Sliced Avocado or cup of Soup
   H Nut/Seed Mix

Remember, if you make a batch of soup on a Sunday, you will have it all week to hack on. Eating this way is easy, fun and healthful! One final suggestion, use organic fish, poultry or beef stock whenever possible when making soup. It helps to naturally produce hydrochloric acid, which diminishes as we grow older (more on this in our next book on anti-aging). If you have any recipe suggestions you'd like to share with others, please visit Randy and I on our web site at www.RKInformedLiving.com.

BIBLIOGRAPHY

PREFACE

Alemayehu, B. & Warner, K. E. (June 2004). The Lifetime Distribution of Health Care Costs. *Health Services Resource, 39*(3), 627-42. Retrieved June 14, 2008, from http://www.blackwell synergy.com/doi/abs/10.1111/j.1475-6773.2004.00248.x

Sahadi, J. Retiring couples need $215K for health costs. New research from Fidelity finds health care costs could eat up a bigger portion of Social Security benefits. *CNNMoney.com.* Retrieved June 15, 2008, from http://money.cnn.com/2007/03/27/pf/retirement/health_costs/index.htm

CHAPTER 1 PROTEIN

Abrams, S.A., Griffin, I.J., Hawthorne, K.M., Liang, L. et al. (2005) A combination of prebiotic short- and long-chain inulin-type fructans enhances calcium absorption and bone mineralization in young adolescents. Am J Clin Nutr. (2005, Aug:82(2):471-6. Related Articles, Links

Akagi, H., Malm, O., Branches, F.L.P., et al. (1995, February) Human exposure to mercury due goldmining in the Tapajos River basin, Amazon, Brazil: speciation of mercury in human hair, blood and urine. Water-air-soil-pollut. Dordrecht : Kluwer AcademicPublishers. v. 80 (1/4) pp. 85-94. Environ Health Perspect. 2003, April; 111(4): 604–608. PMCID: PMC1241452

Anderson, L. D., Remington, P., Trentham-Dietz, A., et al. (June 2002). Assessing a Decade of Progress in Cancer Control. The Oncologist, 7(3), 200-204

Barzel, U.S., & Massey, L.K. Excess Dietary Protein Can Adversely Affect Bone. The Journal of Nutrition Vol. 128 No. 6 June 1998, pp. 1051-1053. American Society for Nutritional Sciences

Black, R., Saul, M., & Bryce, J. (2003, June 28) Where and Why Are 10 Million Children Dying Every Year?"The Lancet Vol. 361, pp. 2226-2234. Retrieved from http://www.cfwshops.org/download/child_survival.pdf. PMID: 12842379 [PubMed - indexed for MEDLINE]

Bread for the World Institute (2004) Are We On Track To End Hunger? Hunger Report

Brenner, B. Dr. (2004 December) Daring to Dream. Your Medicine Online. Retrieved from http//:www.brighamandwomens.org/dom_newsletter/December_04

Brooks, N., Layne, J.E., Gordon, P.L., et al. (2006, December 18) Strength training improves muscle quality and insulin sensitivity in Hispanic older adults with type 2 diabetes. Int J Med Sci. 2007; 4(1): pp. 19–27. PMCID: PMC1752232

Calabrese, J. R., et al. (1999). Fish Oils and bipolar disease. Archives of General Psychiatry, (56), 413-414.

Campbell, T.C., Campbell, T.M., Robbins, J., and Lyman, H. (2006) The China Study: The Most Comprehensive Study of Nutrition Ever Conducted and the Startling Implications for Diet, Weight Loss and Long-term Health. Dallas, TX.: Benbella Books

Cane, M.D., Enzymes: The Difference between Raw and Cooked Foods. Retrieved April 14, 2008, from http://www.living-foods.com/articles/rawvscooked.html

CBS News Early Show, February 6, 2004: New York

Cohen, R. (1997) MILK: The Deadly Poison by Robert Cohen. Englewood Cliffs, NJ.: Argus Publishing

Cumming, R.G., and Klineberg, R. (1994) Case-Control Study of Risk Factors for Hip Fractures in the Elderly. American Journal of Epidemiology Vol. 139, No. 5: 493 503. The Johns Hopkins University School of Hygiene and Public Health

Daily mercury intake in fish-eating populations in the Brazilian Amazon. Journal of Exposure Science and Environmental Epidemiology (2008). (2008). Nature Publishing Group, 18., pp. 76-87

Davis, A. (1970) Lets Eat Right to Keep Fit, New York: Harcourt, Brace & Jovanovich

Department of Health and Human Services (Centers for Disease Control and Prevention) Get Smart: Know When Antibiotics Work, About Antibiotic Resistance Accessed. Retrieved March 12, 2008 from http://www.cdc.gov/drugresistance/community/anitbiotic resistance.htm

Department of Nutrition, School of Public Health, School of Medicine, University of North Carolina at Chapel Hill, North Carolina

Descalzo, A.M., Insani, E.M., Biolatto, A., et al. (2005). Influence of pasture or grain based diets supplemented with vitamin E on antioxidant/oxidative balance of Argentine beef. Meat Science; 70:35-44

Dourson, M. L., Wullenweber, A. E. & Poirier, K. A. (October 2001). Uncertainties in the Reference Dose for Methylmercury. NeuroToxicology (Elsevier Science, Inc.), 22(5), 677 689

Dwyer, J., Navab, M., Dwyer, K. M., Hassan, K., Sun, P., Shircore, A., et al. (in press). Oxygenated Carotenoid Lutein and Progression of Early Atherosclerosis. The Los AngelesAtherosclerosis Study

Eades, M.R. & Eades, M.D. (1996). Protein Power, New York: Warner Books

Fallon, S. (2002). Tragedy and Hype. (Electronic Version) The Third International Soy Symposium. Retrieved from Nexus Magazine, Vol. 7, No. 3

Feskanich, D., Willet, W. C. & Colditz, G. A. (1997). Milk: dietary calcium, and bone fractures on women: a 12 year prospective study. American Journal of Public Health, (87), 992-997

Food and Agriculture Organization of the United Nations (2006) Viale delle Terme di Caracalla, 00153 Rome, Italy. Retrieved from http://www.unicef.org

For cooking tips, try this Food Safety web site: http://www.ehso.com/ehshome/FoodSafety/foodsturkeyfaqs.php.

Food and Nutrition Board, Institute of Medicine. Dietary Reference Intakes for Energy, Carbohydrate, Fiber, Fat, Fatty Acids, Cholesterol, Protein, and Amino Acid. Washington, DC: National Academy Press, 2002

From "Protein Content of Common Foods", First Databank.Inc. San Bruno, CA.

From Wikipedia, from http://en.wikipedia.org/wiki/Amino_acid

Green P., Gispan-Herman I. & Yadid G. Laboratory for the Study of Fatty Acids –Increased arachidonic acid concentration in the brain of Flinders Sensitive Line rats, an animal model of depression. Felsenstein Medical Research Center, Petah Tiqva, Israel. PMID: 15805551 [PubMed - indexed for MEDLINE]

Grandjean, P., White, R. F., Nielsen, A., et al. (July 1999). Methylmercury neurotoxicity in Amazonian children downstream from gold mining. Environ Health Perspect (PMCID: PMC1566671), 7(107), 587-591

Hall, J.B. & Silver, S. (2001). Nutrition and Feeding of the Cow-Calf Herd: Digestive System of the Cow. Publication Number 400-010, Posted June 2001 from Virginia Tech http://www.ext.vt.edu/pubs/beef/400-010/400-010.html

Harada, M., Nakanishi, J., Yosada, E., et al. (October 2001). Mercury pollution in the Tapajos River basin, Amazon: mercury level of head hair and health effects. PMID: 11686639 (PubMed - indexed for MEDLINE), 4(27), 285-290

Health Resources and Services Administration. National Vaccine Injury Compensation Statistics Report. Retrieved January 8, 2008, from http://www.hrsa.gov/vaccinecompensation/statistics_report.htm

Hightower, J. & Moore, D. "Environmental Health Perpsective." Mercury levels in high end consumers of fish. 4. PMCID: PMC1241452. 111th ed. San Francisco, CA. California Pacific Medical Center, April 2003. 604-608

Hightower, J.M., O'Hare, A., and Hernandez, G.T. (2006, February) Blood Mercury Reporting in NHANES: Identifying Asian, Pacific Islander, Native American, and Multiracial Groups. Environ Health Perspect. 114(2): 173–175. Published online 2005 September 21. doi: 10.1289/ehp.8464. Veterans Administration, San Francisco, CA. PMCID: PMC1367827

Howell, E. Dr. and Murray, M. (1985) Enzyme Nutrition - The Food Enzyme Concept. Wayne, NJ: Avery Publishing Group, Inc.

Human Society of the Unites States (n.d.) Welfare Issues with Selective Breeding for Rapid Growth in Broiler Chickens and Turkeys. Retrieved 2/1/2002 from www.hsus.org/web-files

Hunger Report: Are We On Track To End Hunger? Hunger Report 2004. (2004) Bread for the World Institute. 2004. Retrieved from http://www.bread.org/learn/hunger reports/are we-on-track-to-end.html

Hyman, M. & Liponic, M. (2005) Ultrprevention: The 6-Week Plan That Will Make You Healthy For Life. New York, NY. : Atria Books

Johnson, C.J., Peterson, D.R., & Smith, E.K. Myocardial tissue concentrations of magnesium and potassium in men dying suddenly from ischemic heart disease agnesium and sudden death. S. AFR. MED., 64/18 (697-698) ORIGINAL RESEARCH COMMUNICATIONS (1983)

Journal of the College of Nutrition (2000) Nutritional Contribution of Eggs to American Diets, Vol. 19, No. 90005, 556S-562S. Abstract from Song,

W.O. & Kerver, J.M., Michigan State University, from http://www.jacn. org/cgi/gca?sendit=Get+All+Checked+Abstract%28s%29&SEA CHI D=1&FULLTEXT=Nutritional+Contribution+of+eggs+to+american +diets&VO ME=19&FIRSTPAGE=556&FIRSTINDEX=0&hits=10 &RESULTFORMAT=&gca=jamc utr%3B19%2Fsuppl_5%2F556S

J Lipid Res. (2005, Jun); 46(6):1093-6. Epub 2005, Apr 1

Katz, S.L. (2008, February). All-night roast: Slow cooking is great way to intensify meat's flavor: The Washington Post

Kane, E, N.D., (2002). Enzymes: The Difference Between Raw And Cooked Foods. The Oncologist, Vol. 7, No. 3, 200-204, Assessing a Decade of Progress in Cancer Control. Retrieved from American Association of Naturopathic Physicians database

Lemon, P.W., Tarnopolsky, M.A., MacDougall, J.D., & Atkinson, S.A. Protein requirements and muscle mass/strength changes during intensive training in novice bodybuilders. J Appl Physiol. 1992 Aug;73(2):767-75

Leena Isac , The Truth about Protein and Calcium. American Journal of Clinical Nutrition, Vol. 32, 967-970 (1979)

Lund, E., Engeset, D., Alsaker, E., Skeie, G., Hjårtaker, A., Lundebye, A-K., et al. (2004) Cancer Risk and Salmon Intake. Science Magazine, Vol. 305, no. 5683, 477 – 478

MacArthur, J. D. The Eagle, Ben Franklin and the Turkey. GreatSeal.com. Retrieved March 1, 2008, from http//www.greatseal.com

Macpherson, G. (Ed.), (1992) Black's Medical Dictionary by C.W.H. Harvard, London: A & C Books

Macarulla, et al. (2001). The Effects of the Whole Seed and a Protein Isolate of Faba Bean. British Journal of Nutrition, 85(5), 607-14.

Mangels, R. Ph.d., (2006 April, 26) Protein in the Vegan Diet. The Vegetarian Resource Group. Retrieved from http//:www.vrg.org/nutrition/protein

McKibben, B. Taking the Pulse of the Planet. Audubon Magazine. Retrieved January 1, 2008, from www.audubonmagazine.org/population

MedicineNet.com (2000, October 6) Milk for Your Bones? Is Milk Best? Retrieved from www.medicinenet.com

MedicineNet.Com (2008, March 9),WebMD Weight Loss Clinic - Expert Column Slow but

Sure Recipes. Take the heat off with these 3 simple slow-cooker suppers. Retrieved February 1, 2002, from http://www.hsus.org/web-files.

Retrieved from FarmAnimalWelfare.org. An HSUS Report: Welfare Issues with Selective Breeding for Rapid Growth in Broiler Chickens and Turkeys

Minden, J. Transcript Interview with Jon Minden. Science NetLinks. Retrieved May 9, 2008, from http://www.sciencenetlinks.com/sci_update.cfm?DocID=117

Mori, M., Kawada, T., Ono, T., & Torii, K. Taste preference and protein nutrition and L amino acid homeostasis in male Sprague-Dawley rats. Physiol Behav. 1991 May;49(5):987-95. Ajinomoto Co., Inc., Life Sciences Laboratories, Central Research Laboratories, Yokohama, Japan. PMID: 1653438 [PubMed indexed for MEDLINE]

Most contaminants in state's fish are low, but mercury remains a concern Minnesota Department of Health releases annual fish consumption advisor. (2003, April 22). Minnesota Department of Health from http://www.health.state.mn.us/news/pressrel/fishad

Mulvad, G., Pedersen, H. S., Hansen, J. C., et al. The Inuit diet. Fatty Acids and Antioxidants, their role in Ischemic Heart disease, and Exposure to Organochlorines and Heavy Metals. An International study. Arct. Med. Res., 55(Suppl): 20-24, 1996.

Munro, H. (1989). Protein Nutriture and Requirements of the Elderly. In: Munro, H. & Danford, D. (Eds.), Human Nutrition a Comprehensive Treatise. Nutrition, Aging, and the Elderly. Vol. 6 (pp. 153-181). New York: Plenum Press

National Vaccine Injury Compensation statistics reports (n.a.). Health Resources and Services Administration. Retrieved 2008, January 8 from http://www.hrsa.gov/vaccinecompesation/statistics_report.htm

Nutrition and Austism. Retrieved June 14, 2008, from http://www.nutritionandautism.com/step1.asp

Ohio Fishing Information from http://www.geaugalink.com/recreatn/fishing.html

Olejnik, B. (2003, September) Dwindling Spent Hen Disposal Outlets Causes Concerns. Poultry Times

Omega-6 Fatty Acids Cause Prostrate Tumor Cell Growth In Culture. University of California, San Francisco, CA. Science Daily, August 2, 2005

Park, M. MD., Ross, G.W. MD., Petrovitch, H. MD., et al. (2005) Consumption of milk and calcium in midlife and the future risk of Parkinson disease. American Academy of Neurology: Vol. 64, pp. 1047-1051

Parracho, H., Bingham, M. O., Gibson, G. R., et al. (July 4, 2005). Differences between the gut microflora of children with autistic spectrum disorders and that of healthy children. The Journal of Medical Microbiology, 54, 987-991.

Pedersen, M. G., Hansen, J. C., Dewailly, E., et al. (1996). The Inuit diet. Fatty Acids and Antioxidents, their role in Ischemic Heart Disease, and Exposure to Organochlorinnes and Heavy Metals. An International Study. Arct. Med. Res., 55., pp. 20-24

Pollan, M. (2002, 10 March) Power Steer. The New York Times Magazine

Price, W. A., D.D.S. "Nutrition and Physical Degeneration" Copyright, 1997 (6th ed.) by

Keats Publishing, Inc., Connecticut ISBN 0-87983-816-7, 524. La Mesa, CA, USA. Price-Pottenger Nutrition Foundation, 2000. Price- Pottenger Nutrition Foundation L MESA, CA 91943-3614

Protein: Moving Closer to Center Stage. Harvard School of Public Health USDA National Nutrient Database for Standard Reference (2004). Release 17. U.S. Department of Agriculture, Agricultural Research Service. Retrieved April 24, 2008, from http://www.hsph.harvard.edu/nutritionsource/what-should-you-eat/protein full story/index.html

Reddy, S.T., Wang, C.Y., Sakhaee, K., et al. Effect of low-carbohydrate high-protein diets on acid base balance, stone-forming propensity, and calcium metabolism. Am J Kidney Dis. 2002 Aug;40(2):265-74. Department of Internal Medicine, The University of Chicago, IL. [PubMed - indexed for MEDLINE]

Reeves, M., Remington, P. M.D., M.P.H & Anderson, L. D. Assessing a Decade of Progress in Cancer Control. The Oncologist, 200-204, 2002 June (Vol. 7), No. 3, PMID

Robinson, J. (2000) Why Grassfed Is Best!: The Surprising Benefits of Grassfed Meats, Eggs, and Dairy Products. Seattle, WA.: Vashon Island Press

Rylander, R., Remer, T., & Berkemeyer, S. Acid-Base Status Affects Renal Magnesium Losses in Healthy, Elderly Persons. Journal of Nutrition, September 1, 2006; 136(9): 2374 – 2377

Rylander, R. Drinking Water Constituents and Disease. The Journal of Nutrition: February 2008, 138:423S-425S

Schwalfenbery, MD. (2006, 10 June) Omega-3 fatty acids, their beneficial role in cardiovascular health. Retrieved from Can Fam Physician. 2006 June 10; 52(6): 734-740. PMCID: PMC1780156

ScienceDaily. (2005, August 2). Omega-6 Fatty Acids Cause Prostate Tumor Cell Growth In Culture. Omega-6 Fatty Acids Cause Prostate Tumor Cell Growth In Culture. University of California - San Francisco. Retrieved from: http://www.sciencedaily.com/releases/2005/08/050802123505.htm

Sears, B., Dr., (2003) THE OMEGA RX ZONE: THE MIRACLE OF THE NEW HIGH-DOSE FISH OIL. New York, NY: Regan Books

Smith, M. (2000, October 6) Milk for Your Bones? Is Milk Best? WebMD Feature. Retrieved from http://www.medicinenet.com

Smriga, M., Kameishi, M,, Uneyama, H., & Torii, K. Dietary L-lysine deficiency increases stress induced anxiety and fecal excretion in rats. J Nutr. 2002 Dec;132(12):3744-6. Ajinomoto Company Incorporated, Institute of Life Sciences, 210-8681, Kawasaki, Japan. PMID: 12468617 [PubMed - indexed for MEDLINE]

Sousa Passos, C. J., Da Silva., D. S., Lemire, M. F., et al. (2008). Daily mercury intake in fish-eating populations in the Brazilian Amazon. Retrieved from http//:www.nature.com/jes. Journal of Exposure Science and Environmental Epidemiology. Vol. 18, pp. 76-87

Spencer, H., Kramer, L. & Osis, D. (1998) Do Protein and Phosphorus Cause Calcium Loss? Journal of Nutrition Vol. 118 No. 6 June 1988, pp. 657-660

Stone, N. J. (1996). Fish Consupmtion, Fish Oil, Lipids, and Coronary Heart Disease. Nutrition Committee of the American Heart Association, (94), 2337-2340

The Lancelot (2003) Where and Why Are 10 Million Children Dying Every Year (Vol. 361, pp.2226-2234) Black, R., Morris, S. & Bryce, J, from http://www.cfwshops.org/download/child_survival.pdf

Thiomersal controversy. (2008, March 11). Wikipedia. Retrieved March 11, 2008, from http://en.wikipedia.org/w/index.php?title=Thiomersal_controversy&oldid=197 67543

Thimerosal in vaccines. Center for Biologics Evaluation and Research (n.a.) U.S. Food and Drug Administration. Retrieved on 2007 October 1

USDA National Nutrient Database for Standard Reference. "Release 17." [Book] US Department of Agricultural Research Service, 2004

U.S. National Library of Medicine and the National Institutes of Health. (1998). Diet, lifestyle, and the etiology of coronary artery disease: The Cornell China study, November 1998 (10B, 18T–21T). Division of Nutritional Sciences, Cornell University,Ithaca, New York

Watson, D. Mercury in Dental Filling Disclosure and Prohibition Act. MercuryPolicy. org. Retrieved November 5, 2001, from http://www.mercurypolicy.org

Weber, M.L., SeaWeb Aquaculture Clearinghouse (2003) What Price Farmed Fish, A review of the environmental & social costs of farming carnivorous fish. From http://www.seaweb.org/resources/reports.php#wpff

Weil, A., MD., (2001). Eating Well For Optimum Health, New York: Random House

Whitaker, J.W. (1975) Feedlot Empire: beef cattle feeding in Illinois and Iowa, 1840-1900. The Iowa State University Press

www.unicef.org

Young, V.R., and Pellett, P.L. (1994) Plant proteins in relation to human protein and amino acid nutrition. Am J Clinical Nutrtion Vol. 59: pp. 1203S-1212S

Zeisel, MD., Phd. (n.d.) Choline: Needed for Normal Development of Memory. Vol. 19, No. 90005, 528S-531S (2000). Retrieved (n.d.) http://www.jacn. org/misc/terms.shtml

CHAPTER 1 ADDITIONAL RESOURCE

Chopra Dr., D. (Audio Cassette) Magical Mind, Magical Body, Mastering the Mind/Body Connection for Perfect Health and Total Well Being. Nigthingale-Conant Production, (n.d.)

Humane Society of the United States. (Photo) The Human Society of the United States Factory Farming Campaign. (2008) http://www.hsus.org/ farm/multimedia/gallery/layers/space.html

http://www.farmsanctuary.org/issues/factoryfarming/photos/downers.html. [Photo] New York: Farm Sanctuary, 2008

Iron Content in Common Foods. (Chart) USDA Nutrient Database for Standard Reference, November 1, 1997.

NCBA Zinc in Human Nutrition. (Chart) Ohio: National Cattlemen's Beef Association, 1997.

Medeiro, L. C. (Chart). "Nutritional content of game meat". B-920R. Wyoming: College of Agriculture, University of Wyoming., 2002

Prectel, B. (Photo) Retrieved from http://www.ars.usda.gov/is/graphics/ photos/k5643-20.htm. Feeding Cattle Regularly. USDA's Image Gallery, May 23, 2006.

CHAPTER 2 FATS

Aberg, F., et al. (1992). Coenzyme Q10. *Archives of Biochemistry and Biophysics*, (295), 230-234. Retrieved June 25, 2008, from http://en.wikipedia.org/wiki/Coenzyme_Q10

Alemayehu, B. & Warner, K. E. (2004). The Lifetime Distribution of Health Care Cost. *Health Services Research*, *39*(3), 627-42 doi:10.1111/j.1475-6773.2004.00248x.

Ali, M. (December 2005). Mechanisms by which garlic (Allium sativum) inhibits cyclooxygenase activity. Effects of raw versus boiled garlic extract on the synthesis of prostanoids. *Prostaglandins, Leukotrienes and Essential Fatty Acids*, *53*(6), 397-400.

Alpha-Linolenic acid metabolism in men and women: nutritional and biological implications. Lipid metabolism and therapy. *Delicious Living*. Retrieved February 3, 2008, from http://healthnotes.deliciouslivingmag.com/healthnotes.cfm?lang=EN&org=nh& ContentID=2845003

Ames, B. N. (2004). A Role for Supplements in Optimizing Health: The Metabolic Tune-Up. *Archives of Biochemistry and Biophysics*, *423*(1), 227-34.

Bang, H.O., Dyerberg, J.: Plasma lipids and lipoproteins in Greenlandic west coast Eskimos. Acta Med Scand 192:85-94, 1972

Beauchamp, G. K., Keast, R. S., Morel, D., et al. (September 1, 2005). Phytochemistry: ibuprofen-like activity in extra-virgin olive oil. *Nature*, 437, 45-46.

Behar, S., et al. (1997). Low total cholesterol is associated with high total mortality in patients with coronary heart disease. *European Heart Journal*, *18*, 52-9.

Belch, J. F. & Hill, A. (January 2000). Evening primrose oil and borage oil in rheumatologic conditions. *American Journal of Clinical Nutrition*, *71*(1), 352S-356S.

Berschauer, F., et al. (1984). Nutritional-physiological effects of dietary fats in rations for growing pigs. *Arch. Tieremahr*, *34*(1), 19-33.

Best, B. Fats You Need — Essential Fatty Acids. Retrieved February 2, 2008, from http://www.benbest.com/health/essfat.html

Bhatt, D. L. & Topol, E. J. "Current Perspective." Need to Test the Arterial Inflammation Hypothesis. Cleveland Clinic Foundation, Cleveland, OH. Dept. of Cardiovascular Medicine.

Blankson, H., Stakkestad, J. A., Fagertun, H., et al. (December 2000). Conjugated linoleic acid reduces body fat mass in overweight and obese humans. *Journal of Nutrition*, *130*(12), 2943-8.

Bio Alternatives. Oxford Universities' Dr. RA Newsholme was the first to conclude that polyunsaturated fats actually cause cancer. Retrieved March 12, 2008, from www.bio-alternatives.net

Biology Daily. Nitric Oxide. Retrieved March 6, 2008, from http://biosphere. biologydaily.com/biology/Nitrogen_monoxide

Bioriginal's Borage Oil Free From PAs. (2007). *Allergy Research Group*. Retrieved March 3, 2008, from http://www.allergyresearchgroup.com/ _search.php?q=broken+Borage+Oil+Free+form+pbs

Bonettia, P. O., Lermanc, L. O., Napolid, C. & Lermana, A. (February 2003). Statin effects beyond lipid lowering - are they clinically relevant? *European Heart Journal*, *24*(3), 225-248.

Braly MD., J. & Holford, P. (2003). *Homocysteine: The H Factor Solution*. Bergen, NJ. Basic Health Publications.

Brazil Nuts. (July 3, 1990). *Federal Register*, *55*(128), 27522.

Brazil Nuts. (October 17, 2007). Brazil Nuts. *Oak Ridge Associated Universities*. Retrieved March 8, 2008, from www.orau.org/ptp/collection/ consumer%20products/consumer.htm

Britannica Concise Encyclopedia. (2006). Glutamic acid. Encyclopedia Britannica, Inc. Retrieved January 28, 2008, from http:www.answers.com/topic/ glutamic-acid

Bryant, D. (March 29, 2009). Grower gaps programs urged for almond food safety. *Western Farm Press*.

Burdge & Graham. (March 2004). Current Opinion in Clinical & Metabolic Care. *7*(2).

Canola—a new oilseed from Canada. (September 1981). *Journal of the American Oil Chemists' Society*, 723A-729A.

Casas, E. M., Albadalejo, M. F., Planells, M. I., et al. (2001). Tyrosol Bioavailability in Humans after Ingestion of Virgin Olive Oil. *Clinical Chemistry*, (47), 341-243.

Casper, R. (1987, Sep.). *2nd International Symposium on PMS*. A double blind trial of evening primrose oil in premenstrual syndrome. Kiawah Island.

Change in diets of cattle might control E. coli. (October 1998). *Infectious Disease News.* Retrieved February 2, 2008, from http://www.infectiousdiseasenews.com/199810/frameset.asp?article=diet.asp

Cholesterol-Lowering Effect of a Teaflavin-Enriched Green Tea Extract: A Randomized Controlled Trial. (June 2003). *Original Investigation, 163*(12).

Chung-Yen, C., Milbury, P. E., Lapsley, K. & Blumberg, J. B. (June 2005). Flavonoids from Almond Skins Are Bioavaolable and Act Synergistically with Vitamins C and E to Enhance Hamster and Human LDL Resistance to Oxidation 1.2. *The American Society for Nutritional Sciences, J. Nutr., 135*, 1366-73.

CNN. Health Study: A third of kids eat fast food daily. Retrieved June 29, 2008, from http://www.cnn.com/2004/HEALTH/parenting/01/05/fast.food.ap/index.html

Comas, H. & Nahkla, A. (September 1997). The Potential of Seal Oil as Omega 3 Polyunsaturated Fatty Acid (Omega 3 PUFA) Supplements. *The Benefits of Omega 3 Fatty Acids found.* Retrieved February 3, 2008, from http://www.omega3sealoil.com/Chapter4_3c.html

Covas, M. I., de la Torre, K., Farre-Albaladejo, M., et al. (February 15, 2006). Postprandial LDL phenolic content and LDL oxidation are modulated by olive oil phenolic compounds in humans. *Free Radic Biol Med. PMID: 16458191, 40(4)*, 608-16.

Covas, M. I., Nyyssonen, K., Poulsen, H. E., Kaikkonen, J., et al. (September 5, 2006). The effect of polyphenols in olive oil on heart disease risk factors: a randomized trial. *Annals of Internal Medicine, PMID:16954359, 145*(5), 333-41.

Cox, C. (September 2005). Fats and Oils: The Good, the Bad, and the Downright Slippery. *NutritionAdvocate.com, 3*(9).

Debe Dr., J. A. DHEA - The Real Story. *drdrebe.com.* Retrieved March 11, 2008, from http://www.drdebe.com/dhea.html

de Lorgeril, M., Salen, P., Martin, J. L., et al. (1999). Mediterranian diet, traditional risk factors, and the rate of cardiovascular complications after myocardial infarction: the final report of the Lyon Diet Heart Study. *American Heart Association, 99*, 779-785.

DeSmet, P. (1991). Safety of borage seed oil. *Can. Pharm Journal, 124*, 5.

Dietary Reference Intakes for Water, Potassium, Sodium, Chloride, and Sulfate. (February 11, 2004). *Institute of Medicine of the National Academies.*

Dietary Reference Index: Energy, Carbohydrate, Fiber, Fat, Acids, Cholesterol, Protein, and Amino Acids (Macronutrients). (2002). *National Academies Press*, 11-7.

Diez-Gonzalez, F., Callaway, T. R., Kizoulis, M. G. & Russell, J. B. (September 11, 1998). Grain Feeding and the Dissemination of Acid-Resistant Escherichia coli from Cattle. *Science, 281*(5383), 1666-8.

Doeser, L. (1981). *The Little Green Avocado Book.* New York, NY. St. Martin's Press.

Downey, R. K. (1964). Genetic Control of Fatty Acid Biosynthesis in Rapeseed. *Journal of the American Oil Chemists' Society,* (41), 475-478

Earth Save Canada. Ethical Considerations. Retrieved July 2, 2008, from http://www.earthsave.ca

Enig PhD., M. & Fallon, S. (1999). *Nourishing Traditions: The Cookbook that Challenges Politically Correct Nutrition and the Diet Dictocrats* (2nd ed.). New Trends Publishing.

Enig PhD., M. G. & Fallon, S. W. The Oiling of America. *Nexus,* 6, 1 & 2. Retrieved January 29, 2008, from http://www.westonaprice.org.oiling.htm

Erasmus, U. Why I Use Evening Primrose Oil, Not Borage Oil In Udo's Choice Oil Blend. Retrieved March 4, 2008, from http://www.udoerasmus.com

Erasmus Dr., U. Pyrrolizidine Measurements and Limits of Detection. Evening Primrose Oil versus Borage Oil. *udoerasmus.com.* Retrieved March 6, 2008, from http://www.udoerasmus.com

Fallon, S. & Enig PhD., M. G. (2001). *Nourishing Traditions* (2nd ed.). Washington, DC. New Trends Publishing, Inc.

Fallon, S. & Enig PhD, M. G. (August 1993). Dangers of Statin Drugs: What You Haven't Been Told About Popular Statin Lowering Drugs, Wise Traditions in Food Farming and The Healing Arts. *The Weston A. Price Foundation, 71S,* 134-136,145-149.

Fallon, S. & Enig PhD., M. G. Comments on the Report of the 2005 Dietary Guidelines Advisory Committee. Washington, DC. Weston A. Price Foundation, September 27, 2004.

Fallon, S. & Enig PhD., M. G. (June 14, 2004). Dangers of Statin Drugs: What You Haven't Been Told About Popular Cholesterol-Lowering Medicines. *The Weston A. Price Foundation.*

Fallon, S. & Enig, PhD, M. G. (1999). *Nourishing Traditions: The Cookbook that Challenges Politically Correct Nutrition and the Diet Dictocrats* (Second). New trend Publishing, Inc.

Fallon, S. & Enig PhD, M. G. (July 28, 2002). The Great Can-ola. *The Weston A. Price Foundation.* Retrieved March 19, 2008, from http:www.weston-price.opg

Fallon, S. & Enig PhD, M. G. (1999). Tripping Lightly Down the Prostaglandin Pathways. *Price-Pottenger Nutrition Foundation Health Journal, 20*(3).

FDA Authorizes New Coronary Heart Disease Health Claim for Plant Sterol and plant Stanol Esters. (September 5, 2000). *U.S. Department of Health and Human Services, 4144,* 202-205.

Fielding, J. M., Rowley, K. G., Cooper, P. & O'Dea, K. (2005). Increases in plasma lycopene concentration after consumption of tomatoes cooked with olive oil. *Asia Pacific Journal of Clinical Nutrition, PMID: 15927929. 14*(2), 131-6.

Fife, B. (2004). *The Healing Miracles of Cocnut Oil* (3rd ed.). Healthwise.

Flesch, M., Schwarz, A. & Bohn, A. (September 1998). Effects of red and white wine on endothelium dependent vasorelaxation of rat aorta and human coronary arteries. *Am J Physiol Heart Circ Physiol, 275,* H1183-H1190.

Fraser, Sabate, J., Beeson, W. L. & Strahan, T. M. (July 1, 1992). A possible protective effect of nut consumption on risk of coronary heart disease. The Adventist Health Study. *Archives of Internal Medicine, 152*(7).

Garg, Rekha, et al. (December 1999). Niacin treatment increases plasma homocysteine levels. *American Heart Journal, 138,* 1082-87.

Gaullier, J., et al. (2004). Conjugated Linoleic Acid (CLA) supplementation for one year reduces body mass in healthy overweight humans. *American Journal of Clinical Nutrition, 79*(6), 1118-25.

Giessen, C. (2001). *Diets and why most don't work.* Chula Vista, CA: New Century Press.

Goldacre, M. J., Seagroatt, V., Yeates, D. & Acheson, E. D. (2004). *Skin cancer in people with multiple sclerosis: a r, 58,* 142-144.

Goldberg, A. C., Ostlund, R. E., Bateman, J. H., et al. (February 2006). Effect of plant stanol tablets on low-density lipoprotein cholesterol lowering in patients on statin drugs. *American Journal of Cardiology, 97*(3), 376-9.

Grodstein, F., Levine, R., Troy, L., et al. (1996). Three-year follow-up of participants in a commercial weight loss program: can you keep it off? *Archives of Internal Medicine, 156*(12), 1302-6 Pubmed: 8651838.

Govens, P. L., Spilker, M. E., Zock, P. L., et al. (July 1, 2005). Compartmental modeling to quantify alpha linolenic acid conversion after longer term intake of multiple tracer boluses. *Journal of Lipid Resources, 46*(7), 1474-1483.

Hall, E. R., Townsend, G. L., Linthicum, D. D. & Frasier-Scott, K. F. (January 1991). Substrate inactivation of lung thromboxane sythase preferentially decreases thromboxane A2 production. *Prostaglandins Leukotrienes Essential Fatty Acids. PMID:2011609, 42*(1), 31-7.

Halvorsen, B. L., et al. "A systematic screening of the total antioxidants in dietary plants." J Nutr. 132. (2002): 461-71.

Hancock, Jr., A. B. (1984). Unsaturated Pyrrolizidines from Borage. *Journal of Natural Products, 47*(4), 747-8.

Henning, PhD, RD, FACN, B., Toborek, MD, PhD, FACN, M. & McLain, MD, FACN, C. J. (2001). High-Energy Diets, Fatty Acids and Endothelial Cell Function: Implications for Atherosclerosis. *Journal of the American College of Nutrition, 20*(2), 97-105.

Hollis, B. W. (February 2005). Circulating 25-hydroxyvitamin D levels indicative of vitamin D sufficiency: Implications for establishing a new effective dietary intake recommendation for vitamin D. *Journal of Nutrition*, (135), 317-322.

Ho, M., Maple, C., Bancroft, A., et al. (July 1999). The benficial effects of omega-3 and omega-6 essential fatty acid supplementation on red blood cell rheology. Prostaglandins, Leukotrienes and Essential Fatty Acids, *61*(1), 13-17. Retrieved July 15, 2008, from http://www.sciencedirect.com/science?_ob=ArticleURL&_udi=B6WPH-45FCRX4 1M&_user=10&_rdoc=1&_fmt=&_orig=search&_sort=d&view=c&_ acct=C000050221&_version=1&_urlVersion=0&_userid=10&md5=4facf816e1500a ebf13a42998d6de1b3

Honey, K. (2007). Drug designed to raise HDL levels falls down. *Journal of Clinical Investigation, 117*(2), 282-2.

Horrobin, K. (1997). Calcium metabolism, osteoporosis and essential fatty acids: a review. *Prog Lipid Res, 36*(2-3), 131-151.

Hornstra, G. (May 2000). Essential fatty acids in mothers and their neonates. *American Journal of Clinical Nutritional, 71* (Supplement), 1262S-1269S.

Hu, F. B., Stampfer, M. J., Manson, J. E., et al. (November 14, 1998). Frequent nut consumption and risk of coronary heart disease in women: prospective cohort study. *British Medical Journal, 317*(7169), 1341-5.

Hu, F. B., Manson, J. E. & Willet, W. C. (2001). Types of Dietary Fat and Risk of Coronary Heart Disease: A Critical Review. *J. Am. Coll. Nutr.,* *20*(1), 5-19.

Hudson, T. (January 1, 2001). Premenstrual Syndrome. *Townsend Letter for Doctors and Patients,* (203), 176-179. Retrieved March 2, 2008, from http://www.tldp.com/

Immune Attack Teacher Guide. (2007). *Federation of American Scientists, 2007.* Retrieved June 26, 2008, from http://fas.org/immuneattack/technical-support/ia-database/blood-vessel-network

IP, C., Banni, S., Angioni, E., et al. (1999). Conjugated Linoleic Acid–Enriched Butter Fat Alters Mammary Gland Morphogenesis and Reduces Cancer Risk in Rats. *Journal of Nutrition,* (129), 2135-2142.

Jia, X., Li, N., Zhang, W., et al. (2006). A pilot study on the effects of almond consumption on DNA damage and oxidative stress in smokers. *Nutr Cancer. PMID: 16898862, 54*(2), 179-83

Johnson, M. M., Swan, D. D., Surette, M. E., et al. (August 1997). Dietary Supplementation with Linolenic Acid Alters Fatty Acid Content and Eico-sanoid Production in Healthy Humans. *The Journal of Nutrition, 127*(8), 1435-1444.

Journal of the American Oil Chemists' Society. (December 1986). *46*(12), 1510.

J Lipid Res. (July 2005). *7*(46), 1474-83.

Journal Watch. Multidrug-Resistant Salmonella on the Rise. *Journal Watch.* Retrieved July 1, 2008, from http://emergency-medicine.jwatch.org/cgi/content/full/1998/601/1

Kabara, J. (Ed.). "Life Science." Symposium on the Pharmacological Effect of Lipids 27. Champaign, IL. American Oil Chemists Society, 1980. 1351-1358.

Kelloff, G. J., Hawk, E. & Sigman, C. (2004). Cancer Chemoprevention, Vol. 1. *The Annals of Pharmacotherapy, 38,* 2182-3. Retrieved June 10, 2008, from http://www.theannals.com/cgi/content/full/38/12/21

Kinosian, B., Glick, H. & Garland, G. (November 1, 1994). Cholesterol and Coronary Heart Disease: Predicting. *Annals of Internal Medicine, 121*(9), 641-647.

Kris-Etherton, P., Eckel, R. H. & Howard, B. V. (April 3, 2001). AHA Science Advisory: Lyon Diet Heart Study. Benefits of a Mediterranian-style,

National Cholesterol Education Program/American Heart Association Step 1 Dietary Pattern on Cardiovascular Disease. *American Heart Association*, *103*(13), 1823-5, PMID: 11282918.

Krumholz, et al. (1990). Lack of association between cholesterol and coronary heart disease mortality and morbidity and all-cause mortality in persons older than 70 years. *Journal of American Medical Association*, *272*, 1335-40.

Lau, V. W., Journoud, M. & Jones, P. (June 2005). Plant sterols are efficacious in lowering plasma LDL and non-HDL cholesterol in hypercholesterolemic type 2 diabetic and nondiabetic persons. *American Journal of Clinical Nutrition*, *18*(6), 1351-8.

Leaf, A. (1999). Dietary prevention of coronary heart disease: the Lyon Diet Heart Study. *American Heart Association*, *99*(6), 733-5.

Leitzmann, M. F., Stampfer, M. J., Michaud, D. S., et al. (July 2004). Dietary intake of n-3 and n-6 fatty acids and the risk of prostate cancer. *American Journal of Clinical Nutrition*, *80*(1), 204-16.

Levine, L. (2003). Statins stimulate arachidonic acid release and prostaglandin I2 production in rat liver cells. Lipid World. Retrieved March 3, 2008, from http://www.Lipidworld.com/content/2/1/1

Lifescript. Evening Primrose Oil Supplement, A Closer Look @ Suppliments. Retrieved March 4, 2008, from http://www.lifescript.com/channels/food_nutrition/supplements/evening+primr ose_oil.asp

Lu, Q. Y., Artega, J. R., Zhang, Q., et al. (January 2005). Inhibition of prostate cancer cell growth by an avocado extract role of lipid-soluble bioactive substances. *The Journal of Nutritional Biochemistry*, *16*(1), 23-30.

Mann, G. V., et al. (1964). Cardiovascular disease in Masai. *Journal of Atherosclerosis Research*, *4*, 289 312.

Mann, G. V., et al. (December 25, 1965). Physical fitness and immunity to heart-disease in Masai. *Lancet*, *2*(7426), 1308-1310.

Mann, G. V., et al. (January 1975). Atherosclerosis in the Masai. *American Journal of Epdemiology* (1) 26-37.

Marnett, L. J. (December 27, 2002). Oxy Radicals, lipid peroxidation and DNA damage. *Toxicology*, 181 2:219-22.

Mason, M. (2006, October 10). A Dangerous Fat and Its Risky Alternatives. *The New York Times*. Retrieved March 4, 2008, from http://www.nytimes.com

Mateos, R., Dominguez, M. M., Esparteo, J. L. & Cert, A. (November 19, 2003). Antioxidant effect of phenolic compounds, apha-tocopheral, and other minor components in virgin olive oil. *J Agric Food Chem.*, *51*(24), 7170-5.

McCully, K. S. (1997). *The Homocysteine Revolution* Keats.

McCully, K. S., and McCully, M. Homocysteine, Cuts Your Risk of Heart Disease, and Protects Your Health. 1st ed. New York: Harper Collins, 1999.

Mensick, R. P., Zock, P. I., Kester, A. D. & Katan, M. B. (2003). Effects of dietary fatty acids and carbohydrates on the ration of serum to total HDL. *Journal of Clinical Nutrition*, *77*, 1146-55.

Mensick, R. P. (2005). Effects of stearic acid on plasma lipi and lipoproteins in human. *Lipid*, *40*, 1201-5.

Mierendorff, H. J. (1995). Determination of pyrrolizidine alkaloids by thin-layer chromatography in the oil of seeds of Borago officinalis. *Fett Wissenschaft Technologie*, *97*(1), 33-7.

Miller, C., Bryce, G. R. & Conlee, R. K. (1984). Adaptations to a high-fat diet that increase exercise endurances in male rats. *Journal of Applied Physiology*, *56*(1), 78-83.

Miller, MD, P. L. (2006). *Life Extension Revolution, the New Science of Growing Older Without Aging.* Bantam Dell.

Mirsky, S. & Heilman, J. (2006). *Diabetes Survival Guide.* New York: Ballentine Books.

Mozaffarian, D., Rimm, E. B. & Herrington, D. M. (November 2004). Dietary fats, carbohydrates, and progression of coronary atherosclerosis in postmenopausal women. *American Journal of Clinical Nutrition*, *80*, 1175-84.

Muller, H., Lindman, A. S., Blomfeldt, A., et al. (November 2003). A diet rich in coconut oil reduces diurnal postprandial variations in circulating tissue plasminogen activator antigen and fasting lipoprotein (a) compared with a diet rich in unsaturated fat in women. *Journal of Nutrition*, *133*(11), 3422-3427.

Mozaffarian, D., Rimm, E. B. & Herrington, D. M. (November 2004). Dietary fats, carbohydrate, and progression of coronary atherosclerosis in postmenopausal women1,2,3. *American Journal of Clinical Nutrition*, *80*(5), 1175-1184. Retrieved February 2, 2008, from http://www.ajcn.org/cgi/content/abstract/80/5/1175

National Report on Human Exposure to Environmental Chemicals. (March 2001). *Center for Disease Control and Prevention.* Retrieved June 26, 2008, from http://www.cdc.gov/exposurereport/

Newell, C. A., Anderson, L. A. & Phillipson, J. D. (1996). *Herbal Medicines: a guide ofr health care professionals* London: The Pharmaceutical Press.

Newsholme, E. A. (1977). Mechanism for starvation suppression and refeeding activity of infection. *Lancelot, i,* 654.

Nordstrom, D. C., Honkanen, V. E., Nasu, Y., et al. (1996). Alpha-linolenic acid in the treatment of rheumatoid arthritis. A double blind, placebo-controlled and randomized study: flaxseed vs. safflower seed. *Rheumatol Int,* 14, 231-4.

Ocerman, P., et al. (1986). Evening primrose oil as a treatment of the premenstrual syndrome. *Rec Adv Lin Nutr,* 2, 404-5.

O'Dowd, Y., Driss, F., Dang, P. M., et al. (November 15, 2004). Antioxidant effect of hydroxytyrosol, a polyphenol from olive oil: scavenging of hydrogen peroxide but not superoxide anion produced by human neutrophils. *Biochem Pharmacol,* 68(10), 2003-8.

Okamoto, M., Mitsunobu, F., Ashida, K., et al. (2000). Effects of Perilla Seed Oil Supplementation on Leukoptriene Generation by Leucocytes in Patients with Asthma Associated with Lipometabolism. *International Archives of Allergy and Immunology,* 122(2).

Okamoto, T., et al. (1989). Coenzyme Q10. *J.Vit.Nutr.Res.,* (59), 288-292. Retrieved June 25, 2008, from http:en.wikipedia.org/wiki/Coenzyme_Q10 - 71k

Olive oil's benefits left on the shelf. (2005, August 27). *New Scientist.* Retrieved February 1, 2008, from http:www.newscientist.com/article/mg18725145.300.html

Olive Oil Council. Retrieved February 1, 2008, from http://www.internationaloliveoil.org/

Olive Oil Quotation. Retrieved January 31, 2008, from http://oliveoilquotation.com/

Omega 3 Fatty Acids, II: Fish or Flax? (1996). *The Prostate Cancer Forum,* 8(7). Retrieved July 12, 2008, from http://www.prostateforum.com/backissues.htm

Outbreak of Salmonella serotype Enteritidis infections associated with raw almonds—United States and Canada, 2003-3004. (June 11, 2004). *Morb Mortal Wkly Rep.,* 53(22), 484-7.

Oxy radicals, lipid peroxidation and DNA damage. (December 27, 2002). *Toxicology*, 181-2-219-22.

Pandav, R., Belle, S. H. & DeKosky, S. T. (2000). Apolipoprotein E polymorphism and Alzheimer's disease. The Indo-US Cross-National Dementia Study. *Archives of Neurology*, *57*, 824-30.

Papendorp, D., Coetzer, H. & Kruger, M. (1995). Biochemical profile of osteoporotic patients on essential fatty acid supplementation. *Nutrition Research*, *15*(3), 323-4.

Pariza, M. W., Park, Y. & Cook, M. E. (2000). Mechanisms of Action of Conjugated Linoleic Acid: Evidence and Speculation. *Proceedings of the Society for Experimental Biology and Medicine*, *223*, 8-13. Retrieved June 14, 2008, from http://www.ebmonline.org/cgi/gca?sendit=Get+All+Checked+Abstract%28s%2 9&SEARCHID=1&FULLTEXT=Mechanisms+of+action &VOLUME=223&FIRST PAGE=8&FIRSTINDEX=0&hits=10&RE SULTFORMAT=&gca=psebm%3B223%2F1%2F8

Parsell, D. (2004, November 27). Saturated Fat Shows Unexpected Benefit. *Science News Online*, *166*, 22.

Parvais, O. B., et al. (1004). TLC detection of pyrrolizidine alkaloids in oil extracted from the seeds of Borago officinalis. *Journal of Plant Chromatographt Modern TLC*, *7*(1), 80-2.

Patrick, ND, L. (August 2000). The Importance of Redox Homeostasis in HIV. *Alternative Medicine Review*, *5*(4), 290-305.

Peat, R. Coconut Oil. *raypeat.com*. Retrieved January 29, 2008, from http://raypeat.com/articles/articles.coconut-oil.shtml

Peat, R. (1996). Pathogen Reduction/HACCP & HACCP Implementation. *From PMS to Menopause*. Eugene, WA.

Pendergast, EdD, FACN, D. R., Leddy, MD, J. L. & Venkatraman, PhD, J. T. (2000). Review: A perspective on Fat Intake in Athletes. *Journal of American College of Nutrition*, *19*(3), 345-50.

Plotnick, G. D., Corretti, M. C. & Vogel, R. A. (1997). Effect of antioxidant vitamins on the transient impairment of endothelial dependent brachial artery vasoactivity following a single high fat meal. *JAMA*, *278*(26), 1682.

Prostaglandins, Leukotrienes and Essential Fatty Acids. (July 1999). Prostaglandins, Leukotrienes and Essential Fatty Acids. *61*(1), 13-17. Retrieved July 13, 2008, from http://www.ncbi.nlm.nih.gov/sites/entrez

Prostate Cancer Forum: Omega 3 Fatty Acids, II: Fish or Flax?(n.d.). Retrieved May 10, 2008, from http://www.prostateforum.com

Puolakka, J., et al. (1985). Biochemical and clinical effects of treating the premenstrual syndrome with prostaglandin synthesis precursors. *J Rep Med, 30*(3), 149-153.

Pristin, T. (1997, July 23). Counterfeit Olive Oil. *The New York Times.* Retrieved January 30, 2008, from http://www.usdoj.gov/usao/nj/press/files/pdffiles/oliveoilseizurewarrant.pdf

Rao, G. N., Glascow, W. C., Eling, T. E. & Runge, M. S. (November 1, 1996). Role of Hydroperoxyeicosatetraenoic Acids in Oxidative Stress-induced Activating Protein 1 (AP-1). *The American Society for Biochemistry and Molecular Biology, Inc., 271*(44), 27760-4.

Rasyslami. "Image of several fatty acid molecules created by me with POV-ray. Originally in Lojban for a nuzban article, later translated." [Image] Retrieved January 29, 2008, from Image:Rasyslami.jpg Wikipedia.

Ravnskov, MD, PhD, U. (June 2004). The Benefits of high Cholesterol. *The Weston Price Foundation.*

Raw Foods. Retrieved March 4, 2004, from http://www.rawfoods.com/articles/oliveoil.html

Related Articles, Links. (2005). *Epub.*

Rehm, DPM, K. What You Need To Know About Depression and Diabetes. *Podiatry Today.* Retrieved June 25, 2008, from http://www.podiatrytoday.com

Reinforcing the mucus: a new therapeutic approach for ulcerative colitis? *BMJ Publishing Group Ltd. & British Society of Gastroenteroly.* Retrieved June 30, 2008, from http://gut.bmj.com/cgi/citemap?id=gutjnl;54/7/900

Report Sets Dietary Intake Levels for Water, Salt. (February 11, 2004). Report Sets Dietary Intake Levels for Water, Salt, and Potassium To Maintain Health and Reduce Chronic Disease Risk. *National Academies of Science.* Retrieved January 28, 2008, from http://www.canadafreepress.com/2005/health020105.htm Mindfully.orgnote.

Resources.ebd.gov.hk. Keeping Fit. Retrieved June 29, 2008, from http://resources.edb.gov.hk/biology/english/health/definition_health/keeping_fit.html

Reuter, B. (August 2000). Dietary Fat and Carbohydrates in Endurance Activities. *Strength and Conditioning Journal, 22*(4), 62-63.

Ridker Dr., P. M., Hennekens Dr., C. H., Buring, J. E., et al. C-Reative Protein and Other Makers of Inflammation in the Prediction of Cardiovascular Disease in Women. Cleveland Clinic Foundation, Cleveland, OH. Dept. of Cardiovascular Medicine.

Robinson, J. (2000). *Why Grassfed is Best.* US Department of Agriculture: Food Safety and Inspection Service.

Robinson, J. (2004). *Pasture Perfect: The Far-Reaching Benefits of Choosing Meats, Eggs, and Dairy Products from Grass-Fed Animals.* Washington: Vashon Island Press.

Romero, C., Brenes, M., Yousfi, K., et al. (February 2004). Effect of cultivar and processing method on the contents of polyphenols in table oil. *Journal of Agriculture and Food Chemistry, 52*(3), 479-84.

Rose, D. P., Connolly, J. M., et al. (1995). Influence of Diets Containing Eicosapentaenoic or Docasahexaenoic Acid on Growth and Metastasis. *Journal of Nutrition.*

Rosedale MD., R. (1999, Aug.). *Insulin and its Metabolic Effects.* Designs for Health Institute. Boulder Fest.

Sapkota, A. R., et al. "What Do We Feed to Food-Production Animals? A Review of Animal Feed Ingredients and Their Potential Impacts on Human Health." Environ Health Perspect. 115.5 (May 2007): 663-70 PMCID: PMC1867957.

Science, Society, and America's Nuclear Waste. (July 3, 1990). *Federal Register, 55128,* 27522. Retrieved May 9, 2008, from http://www.osti.gov/bridge/

Scimeca, J. A. & Miller, G. D. (2000). Potential Health Benefits of Conjugated Linolec Acid. *Journal of the American College of Nutrition, 19*(4), 470S-471S.

Sears Dr., B. (2005). *The Anti - Inflammation Zone.* NY, NY. Harper Collins.

Sears Dr., B. (2002). *The Omega Rx Zone: The Miracle of the New High-Dose Fish Oil.* NY: Harper Collins.

Schafer, K. Nowhere to Hide:Persistent Toxic Chemicals in the U.S. Food Supply. *Pesticide Action Network North America, 2000.* Retrieved June 25, 2008, from http://www.panna.org

Shindo, Y., Witt, E., Han, D., et al. (1994). Enzymic and non-enzymic anti-oxidants in epidermis and dermis of human skin. *Journal of Investigative Dermatology*, (102), 122-124. Retrieved June 26, 2008, from http://www.nature.com/jid/journal/v102/n1/abs/5611404a.html

Simeoui, S., Hoffmann, B. R., Winkemann, B. R., et al. (September 2, 2004). Association between the A 2518G polymorphism in the monocyte chemoat-tractant protein-1 gene and insulin resistance and Type 2 diabetes mellitus. *Epub, 47*(9), 1574-80.

Simopoulos, A. P. "Nutrition and Health." Diets Including Walnuts Can Reduce the Risk of Heart Disease. Docket # 02P-0292. College Park, MD. Food and Drug Admin., August 14, 2002.

Smith, C. (2004). Retail Prescription Drug Spending In the National Health Accounts. *Health Affairs, 23*(1), 160-167. Retrieved July 10, 2008, from http://content.healthaffairs.org/cgi/content/full/23/1/160

Smith, J. S., Goldweber, M., Tyson, R., et al. (1983). Utilization potential for semi-tropical and tropical fruits and vegetables in therapeutic and family diets. *Proc. Fla. State Hort. Soc., 96*, 241-3.

Spiller PhD, G. A., Miller, A., Olivera, K., Reynolds, J., et al. (2003). Effects of Plant-Based Diets High in Raw or Roasted Almonds, or Roasted Almond Butter on Serum Lipoproteins in Humans. *Journal of the American College of Nutrition, 22*(3), 195-200.

Stampfer, M. J., Malinow, R., Willet, W. C., et al. (1992). A prospective study of plasma homocysteine and risk of myocardial infarction in US physicians. *Journal of American Medical Association, 268*, 877-81.

Steinhart, C. E., Doyle, M. E. & Cochrane, B. A. (1994). *Food Safety 1994* (1st ed.). Research Institute.

Steinhart, C. E., Doyle, M. E. & Cochrane. (1995). *Food Safety 1995*. Research Institute.

Steinhart, C. (December 1996). Chemistry behind the news. *Conjugated Lioleic Acid The Good News About Animal Fat, 73*(12), A302. Retrieved February 1, 2008, from http://jchemed.chem.wisc.edu/journal/issues/1996/Dec/absA302.html

Stenmark, P., Grunler, J., Mattsson, J., et al. (June 21, 2001). A New Member of the Family of Di-iron Carboxylate Proteins A Membrane-Bound Hydroxylase Involved In Ubiquinone Biosynthesis. *J. Biol. Chem., 276*(36), 33297-33300. Retrieved June 29, 2008, from http://www.jbc.org/cgi/

content/abstract/276/36/33297?maxtoshow=&HITS=10& hits=10&RE
SULTFORMAT=&fulltext=new+member+of+the+family+of+di-iron +ca
rboxylate+proteins&searchid=1114091714873_4085&stored_search=&F
IRSTINDEX=0&volume=276&issue=36&journalcode=jbc

Stoney, C. M. & Engebretson, T. O. (2000). Plasma homocysteine concentrations are positively associated with hostility and anger. *Life Science, 66,*
2267-75.

Taheri, F., Ochoa, J. B., Faghiri, Z., et al. (March 7, 2001). L-Arginine regulates
the expression of the T-cell receptor zata chain (CD3zeta) in Jurkat cells.
Clin Cancer Res., 7(3 Suppl), 958s-965s.

Tarantino, PhD, L. M. Qualified Health Claims: Letter of Enforcement
Discretion—Walnuts and Coronary Heart Disease. Center For Food Safety
and Applied Nutrition: FDA, March 9, 2004.

Tayyem, R. F., Health, D. D., Al-Delaimy, W. K., et al. (July 2006). Curcumin
Content of Turmeric and Curry Powders. *Nutrition and Cancer, 52*(2),
126-31.

*The Dangers of Statin Drugs: What You Haven't Been Told About Cholesterol-
Lowering Medicine, Part 1.* [Book] July 21, 2004. Retrieved March 8, 2008,
from http://www.mercola.com/2004/jul/21/statin_drugs.htm

The Organic Trade Association. Health of the Planet and It's Inhabitants.
Retrieved June 26, 2008, from http://www.ota.com

The unique benefits of Perillo Oil. (1998, November) *LE Magazine.*

The Worlds Healthiest Foods. Retrieved January 28, 2008, from http://www.
whfoods.com

thinkquest.org. Computer vs. brain: a thinquest project. Retrieved September
20, 2008, from http:www.library.thinquest.org

Tulloch, I., Smellie, W. & Buck, A. (1994). Evening primrose oil reduces
urinary calcium excretion on both normal and hypercalciuric rats. *Urol
Res, 22,* 227-230.

Turner, R. C., Radley, J. M. & Mayneord, V. W. (1958). The Naturally Occurring Alpha Ray Activity of Foods. *Health Physics,* 268-75.

Unit I: Cellular Communication. *4CelluarComm.* Retrieved June 26, 2008,
from http://www.bio.davidson.edu/courses/Bio111/wordfiles/study%20
guide/4CellularComm.DOC

University of Maryland. Feature Stories: Trans Fats 101. Retrieved June 28,
2008, from http://www.umm.edu/features/transfats.htm

Unlu, N. Z., Bohn, T., Clinton, S. K. & Schwartz, S. J. (March 2005). Cartenoid Absorption from Salad and Salsa by Humans Is Enhanced by the Addition of Avocado or Avocado Oil. *Journal of Nutrition*, *135*, 431-6.

Whelton, P. K., He, J., Cutler, F. L., et al. (May 28, 1997). Effects of oral potassium on blood pressure. Meta-analysis of randomized controlled clinical trials. *JAMA*, *277*(20), 1624-1632.

Whigham, L. D., Watras, A. C. & Schoeller, D. A. (May 2007). Efficiacy of Conjugated Limoleic Acid for Reducing Fat Mass: A Meta-Analysis in Humans. *American Journal of Clinical Nutrition*, *85*(5), 1203-11.

Whole Foods. Retrieved March 4, 2008, from http://www.whfoods.com/genpage.php?tname=foodspice&dbid=132

Wikipedia, The Free Encyclopedia. Coenzyme Q10. Retrieved June 29, 2008, from http://en.wikipedia.org/w/index.php?title=Coenzyme_Q10&oldid=221854594

Wikipedia, The Free Encyclopedia. Insulin resistance. Retrieved July 26, 2008, from http://en.wikipedia.org/w/index.php?title=Insulin_resistance&oldid=219913725

Wikipedia. The Free Encyclopedia, Olive oil. Retrieved January 28, 2008, from http://en.wikipedia.org/wiki/Olive_oil

Winfried MD., M., Scharnagal PhD., H., Winkler Dr., K., et al. (2004). Low-Density Lipoprotein Triglycerides Associated With Low-Grade Systemic Inflammation, Adhersion Molecules, and Angiographic Coronary Heart Disease. *American Heart Association*, *110*, 3068-74.

Wolk PhD., A., Reinhold PhD., B., Hunter, Dr., D., et al. (1998). A prospective study of association of monounsaturated fat and other types of fat with risk of breast cancer. *Archives of Internal medicine*, 41-5.

Wong, C. Statin Drugs May Lower CoQ10 Levels. *Alternative Medicine.* Retrieved March 8, 2008, from http://altmedicine.about.com/od/consumerreviewsalerts/a/statins_coq10.htm

CHAPTER 3 LOVE STORY

Agricultural Baseline Projections: U.S. Crops, 2008-2017. (February 12, 2008). *USDA, Economic Research Service.* Retrieved May 11, 2008, from http://www.ers.usda.gov/briefing/Baseline/crops.htm

Agricultural Research Center, U.S. Department of Agriculture. Retrieved July 23, 2008, from http://www.ars.usda.gov

American Society of Agricultural and Biological Engineer. Retrieved April 16, 2008, from http://www.asabe.org/

Ames, B., et al. (February 19, 2002). Proceedings of the National Academy of Sciences. *99*(4): 2356-61, 99(4): 1876-81, 99(4): 1870-5.

Anderson, J. W., Story, L., Sieling, B., et al. (1984). Hypocholesterolemic Effects of Oat-Bran or Bean Intake for Hypocholesterolemic Men. *American Journal of Clinical Nutrition, 40,* 1146-55.

Anderson, MD, M. (n.d.). Guide to Sulfited Foods. *Center for Science in the Public Interest.*

Answers.com. Milton Hershey. Retrieved June 9, 2008, from http://www.answers.com/milton+hershey?cat=biz-fin

Arias, R., Lee, T. C., Logendra, L. & Janes, H. (May 2000). Correlation of lycopene measured by HPLC with the L, a, b color readings of a hydroponic tomato and the relationship of maturity with color and lycopene content. *Journal of Agricultural Food Chemistry, 48*(5), 1697-1702. PMID: 1082008 [PubMed - indexed for MEDLINE

Avery, A. (2002). Organic Food Marketers Make False Health Claims Organic pesticides may cause cancer and liver damage. *Center for Global Food Issues, 540,* 337-363.

Bach Knudseni, K. E., Wisker, E., Daniel, M., et al. (1994). Digestibility of energy, protein, fat and non starch polysaccharides in mixed diets: comparative studies between man and the rat. *British Journal of Nutrition, 71*(1Y94), 471-487. Retrieved May 13, 2008, from http://journals.cambridge.org/download.php?file=%2FBJN%2FBJN71_04%2F S0007114594000553a.pdf&code=7aac3fabb63c732f5367dab8427fc72d

Balzer MD., J., Rassaf MD., T. & Heiss MD., C., et al. (2008). Sustained Benefits in Vascular Function Through Flavanol-Containing Cocoa in Medicated Diabetic Patients. *The Journal of the American College of Cardiology, 51,* 2141-49. Retrieved June 9, 2008, from http://content.onlinejacc.org/cgi/content/abstract/51/22/2141

Bao, S. L. The effect of lycium barbarum polysaccharide on vasculr tension in two-kidney, one clip model of hypertension *50.* 3. June 1998. 309-314. PMID: 11324572 [PubMed - indexed for MEDLINE

Bauer, S. (June 2002). Watermelon Packs a Powerful Lycopene Punch. *USDA, Agricultural research service.* Retrieved April 27, 2008, from http://www.nps.ars.usda.gov

Bednar, G. E., Patil, A. R., Murray, S. M., et al. (2001). Starch and Fiber Fractions in Selected Food and Feed Ingredients Affect Their Small Intestinal Digestibility and Fermantability and Their Large Bowel Fermantability In Vitro in a Canine Model. *Journal of Nutrition, 131,* 276-86.

Beecher, C. (1994). Cancer preventive properties of varieties of Brassica oleracea: a review. *Am. J. Clin. Nutr., 59 (Suppl),* 1166S-1170S.

Beekwilder, J., Hall, R. D. & Ric de Vos, C. H. (2005). Identification and dietary relevance of antioxidants from raspberry. Biofactors, 23(4), 197-205. Retrieved May 24, 2008, from http://www.ncbi.nlm.nih.gov/pubmed/16498206. PMID: 16498206 [PubMed - indexed for MEDLINE

Beiseigel, J. M., Hunt, J. R., Glahn, R. P., et al. (August 2007). Iron bioavailability from maize and beans: a comparison of human measurements with Caco-2 cell and algorithm predictions. American Journal of Clinical Nutrition, 86(2), 388-96.

Better Health Channel. Antioxidants. Retrieved April 3, 2008, from http://www.betterhealth.vic.gov.au/bhcv2/bhcarticles.nsf/pages/Antioxidants

BMJ USA: Minerva. (September 17, 2005). *BMJ Medical Publication of the Year, 331*(E382), 7517. Retrieved July 22, 2008, from http://bmj.com/cgi/content/full/331/7517/E382

Borek, C. (2001). Journal of Nutrition. *Supplement: Recent Advances on the Nutritional Effects Associated with the Use of Garlic as a Supplement, 131,* 1010S-1015S.

Brazilian berry destroys cancer cells in lab, UF study shows. (January 12, 2006). *Research, Health, Sciences, Agriculture (University of Florida News).*

Britannica Online Encyclopedia. Nutrition. Retrieved July 21, 2008, from http://www.britannica.com

Broccoli Protects Eye Health. *The World's Healthiest Foods, George Mateljian Foundation,* (Broccoli Protects Eye Health). Retrieved May 5, 2008, from http://www.whfoods.com/genpage.php?tname=news&dbid=37

Brown, M. J., Ferruzzi, M. G., Nguyen, M. L., et al. (2004). Carotenoid bioavailability is higher from salads ingested with full-fat than fat-reduced salad dressings as measured with electrochemical detection. *American Journal of Clinical Nutrition, 80,* 396-403.

Brunswick Labs. Antioxidants Today: Similarities and Differences. Retrieved May 8, 2008, from http://brunswicklabs.com/compare.shtml

Canene-Adams, K., Lindshield, B., Jeffrey, E., et al. (January 9, 2007). Combinations of Tomato and Broccoli Enhance Antitumor Activity in Dunning R3327-H Prostate Adenocarcinomas. *Cancer research, 67*(2), 836-843. Retrieved April 21, 2008, from http://cancerres.aacrjournals.org/content/vol67/issue2/

Carter, C. A., Chalfant, J. A. & Goodhue, R. E. (2002). Agricultural and Resource Economics Update. *Giannini Foundation of Agricultural Economics, 5*(4).

Carter, C. A., Chalfant, J. A. & Goodhue, R. E. (2005). China's Strawberry Industry: An Emerging Competitor for California? *Agricultural and Resource Economics Update, 9*(1), Update V9N1.

Casiari, J. J., et al. (June 1, 2001). Cytotoxicity of ascorbate, lipoic acid, and other antioxidants in hollow fiber in vitro tumors. *British Journal of Cancer, 84*(11), 1544-50.

CBS News. Ethanol Pollution Surprise: EPA Finds Worrisome Levels Of Toxic Air Pollutants At Ethanol Plants. Retrieved July 22, 2008, from http://www.cbsnews.com/stories/2002/05/03/tech/main508006.shtml

Center for Disease Control and Prevention Report. (November 17, 2007). Retrieved July 18, 2008, from http://www.cdc.gov/flu/weekly/weeklyarchives2007-2008/weekly46.htm

Certified Organic Associations of British Columbia. Sustainable Food Systems, Corporate-ownership Horizon Organic. Retrieved April 16, 2008, from http://www.certifiedorganic.bc.ca/sitesearch.php?query=Corporate-ownership&search=1

Choudhary, R., Bowser, T. J., Weckler, P. R., et al. Rapid Estimation of Lycopene Concentration in Watermelon and tomato puree by Visible Reflective Spectroscpoy. *American Society of Agricultural and Biological Engineers.* Retrieved April 19, 2008, from http://asae.frymulti.com/abstract.asp?aid=17968&t=1

Choung, M. G., Choi, B. R., Yn, A., et al. (November 19, 2003). Anthocyanin profile of Korean cultivated kidney beans (Phaseolus vulgaris L.) *Journal of Agricultural Food Chemistry, 51*(24), 7040-3.

Commodity Boom: How Long Will It Last? (2008, March). *Finance and Development, 45,* 1. Retrieved May 24, 2008, from http://www.imf.org/external/pubs/ft/fandd/2008/03/index.htm

"ConAgra Foods Stops Adding Diacetyl to Popcorn Butter Flavoring." Occupational Health & Safety. (December 19, 2007). 22 July 2008 http://www.ohsonline.com/articles/56934/

Consumer Reports. Greener Choices Eco-Labels Center, "Natural" Retrieved July 22, 2008, from http://www.greenerchoices.org/eco-labels

Cooper, S. (March 2003). Reappraisal of serum starvation, the restriction point, G0, and G1 phase arrest points. *The FASEB, 17.*

Coudray, C., Demigne, C. & Rayssiguier, Y. (January 2003). Effects of dietary fibers on magnesium absorption in animals and humans. *Journal of Nutrition, 133*(1), 1-4.

Cox, S. I Say Tomayto, You Say Tomahto. Retrieved April 21, 2008, from http://lamar.colostate.edu/~samcox/Tomato.html

Curl, C. L., Fenske, R. A. & Elgethum, K. (March 2003). Organophosphorous pesticide exposure of urban and suburban preschool children with organic and conventional diets. *Environmental Health Perspectives, 111*(3), 377-82.

Davis PhD, D. R., Epp PhD, M. E. & Riordan, MD, H. D. (2004). Changes in USDA Food Composition Data for 43 Garden Crops, 1950 to 1999. *Journal of the American College of Nutrition, 23*(6), 669-682.

DeNoon, D. J. Dark Chocolate Is Healthy Chocolate. Dark Chocolate Has Health Benefits Not Seen in Other Varieties. *WebMD Health News.* Retrieved June 8, 2008, from http://www.webmd.com/diet/news/20030827/dark-chocolate-is-healthy-chocolate

Domfield, A., Domfield, M. & Domfield, L. (2001). Pomegranate juice consumption inhibits serum angiotensin converting enzyme activity and reduces systolic pressure. *Atherosclerosis, 158*, 195-8.

Dreosti PhD, I. E. (October 2000). Recommended dietary intake levels for phytochemicals: Feasible or fanciful? *Asia Pacific Journal of Clinical Nutrition, 9*(s1), S119-S122.

Diamond Organics. Organic foods delivered to your door. Retrieved May 10, 2008, from http://www.diamondorganics.com

Drachman MD, D. A. (2005). Do we have brain to spare? *Department of Neuology, University of Massachusetts Medical School, Worcester, MA., 64,* 2004-2005. Retrieved July 22, 2008, from http://www.neurology.org/cgi/content/full/64/12/2004

Duarte, S., Gregory, S., Singh, A. P., et al. Inhibitory effects of cranberry poly-phenols on formation and acidogenenicity of Streptococcus mutans biofilms *257*. 1. FEMS microbiology letter, 2006. 50-6.

Duttary, A. K. & Jorgensen, A. (August 2004). Effects of kiwi fruit consumption on platelet aggregation and plasma lipids in healthy human volunteers. *Plasma*, *15*(5), 287-97.

Edward, A. J. & Clevidence, B. A. (June 2002). Watermelon Packs a Powerful Lycopene Punch. *Agricultural Research*.

Environmental Protection Agency Office of Air and Radiation. Global Warming and Our Changing Climate - FAQ. Retrieved March 15, 2005, from http://yosemite.epa.gov/oar/globalwarming.nsf/UniqueKeyLookup/ SHSU5BUN 59/$File/gw_faq.pdf

Erick MS, R. D., et al. (May 2, 2003). Vitamin B-6 and Ginger in Morning Sickness. *Journal of Nutrition*, *95*(4), 416.

Extoxnet: Extension Toxicology Network, Cornell University. Copper Sulfate. Retrieved March 16, 2008, from http://pmep.cce.cornell.edu/profiles/ extoxnet/carbaryl-dicrotophos/copper-sulfat

Fink, B. N., Steck, S. E., Wolff, M. S., et al. (March 27, 2001). Dietary flavonoid intake and breast cancer risk among women on Long Island. *America Journal of Epidemiology*, *165*(5), 514-23. PMID: 17158855 [PubMed indexed for MEDLINE

Fintelmann, V. (1996). Antidyspeptic and lipid-lowering effect of artichoke leaf extract. *Zeitschrift fur Allegemeinmed*, *72*, 1-19.

Fixed Obstructive Lung Disease in Workers at a Microwave Popcorn Factory — Missouri, 2000–2002. (2002, April 26). *Morbidity and Mortality Weekly Report*, *51*, 16., pp. 345-7.

Fleet, J. C. (May 1994). New Support for a folk remedy: cranberry juice releases bacteriuria and pyuria in elderly women. *Nutrition Review*, *52*(5), 168-70. PMID: 8052456 [PubMed - indexed for MEDLINE

Flegal, K. M., Carroll, M. D., Kuczmarski, R. J. & Johnson, C. L. (January 1998). Overweight and Obesity in the United States: prevalence and trends, 1960-1994. *International Journal of Obesity*, *22*(1), 39–47.

Food Quality News.com. (October 5, 2004). Nobel prize for pioneers in smell. *Food Quality News.com*. Retrieved July 21, 2008, from http://www. foodqualitynews.com/news

Forastiere, F., Pistelli, R., Sestini, P., et al. (April 2000). Consumption of fresh fruit rich in vitamin C and wheezing symptoms in children. *Italian Studies on Respiratory Disorders in Children and the Environment*, 55(4), 283-8.

Fromartz, S. (2007). *Organic Inc. Natural Foods and How They Grow*. Harvest Books.

Galeone, C., et al. (November 2006). Onion and garlic use and human cancer. *American Journal of Clinical Nutrition*, 84(5), 1027-32.

Galli, R. I., Bielinski, D. F. & Szprengiel, A. (February 1, 2006). Blueberry Supplemented Diet Reverses Age-Related Decline in Hippocampal HSP70 Neuroprotection. *Neurobiol Aging, USDA*, 2, 344-350. Retrieved May 12, 2008, from http://www.ars.usda.gov/research/publications/publications.htm?SEQ_NO_115=139924

Gau, G. W., Yang, W. G. & Du, P. Observation of the Effects of Lycium Barbarum Polysaccharides (LBP) In Combination with LAK/IK-2 Therapy In The Treatment of 75 Cancer Patients. *Rich Nature*. Retrieved May 13, 2008, from http://www.richnature.com

Gaziano MD, J. M., Hennekens MD, C. H., O'Donnel MD, C. J., et al. (1997). Fasting Triglycerides, High Density Lipoprotein, and Risk of Myocardial Infarction. *American Heart Association*, 96, 2520-25. Retrieved July 18, 2008, from http://www.circ.ahajournals.org/cgi/content/full/96/8/2520

Gelinas, B. & Seguin, P. (May 19, 2007). Oxalate in Grain Amaranth. *Journal of Agriculture and Food Chemistry*, 55(12), 4789-94.

Gille, J. J., Pasman, P., von Berkel, C. G., et al. (1991). Effect of antioxidants on hyperoxia-induced chromosomal breakage in Chinese hamster ovary cells: protection by carnosine. *Mutagenesis*, 6(4), 313-8.

Giovannucci, E., Ascherio, A., Rimm, E. B., et al. (December 6, 1995). Intake of carotenoids and retinol in relation to risk of prostate cancer. J Natl Cancer Inst., 87(23), 1767-76. Retrieved April 20, 2008, from http://www.ncbi.nlm.nih.gov/pubmed/7473833 e-ext.html

Giovannucci, E., E. B. Rimm, and Y. Liu. "A Prospective Study of Tomato Products, Lycopene, and Prostate Cancer Risk." Journal of the National Cancer Institute. 94.5 (March 06 2002): 391-8.

Gojiberry.com. Gogi office of tietan goji berry company. Retrieved May 18, 2008, from http://www.gojiberry.com

Goldstein, D. (2006). "Miracle Or False Hope In A Bottle?" Los Angeles: CBS.

Greenpeace. Retrieved March 20, 2008, from http://archive.greenpeace.org/geneng/reports/food/record_harvestembargo.pdf

Greenwell, I. "The Antioxidant Network." Life Extension Magazine Aug. 1999. 16 May. 2008 http://www.lef.org/magazine/mag99/aug99-report5.html

Grieve, M. Cacao. *Botanical.com*. Retrieved June 8, 2008, from http://www.botanical.com/botanical/mgmh/c/cacao-02.html

Guthman, J. (2004). *Agrarian Dreams: The Paradox of Organic Farming in California*. California: University of California Press.

Hagelin DR, J. Food Fight (June 17, 1999) *Newsweek.com*. Retrieved July 23, 2008, from http://www.newsweek.com

Harborne, J. B. (1964). *Biochemistry of phenolic compounds*. London: Academic Press.

Halliday, J. New process pits watermelon against tomato as lycopene source. *FoodNavigator.com/Europe*. Retrieved April 15, 2008, from http://www.foodnavigator.com/news/ng.asp?id=70632

Harris DR, E. & Patil DR, B. (2004, Dec, 1). "Science Daily." *Science Daily*. Texas Agricultural Experiment Station.

Hecht, S. S. (August-November 2000). Chemoprevention of cancer by isothio-cyanates, modifiers of carcinogen metabolism. *Drug Metabolism Review*.

Hecht, S. S., Huang, C., Stoner, G. D., et al. (March 7, 2006). Identification of cyanidin glycosides as constituents of freeze-dried black raspberries which inhibit anti-benzo[a]pyrene-7,8-diol-9, 10 epoxide induced NFkB and AP-1 activity. *Carcinogenisis, Oxford Journals, 27*(8), 1617-26.

Henry, S. Diabetes and Fiber. *A Healthy Me*. Retrieved March 15, 2008, from http://www.ahealthyme.com/topic/fiberdiabetes

Heo, H. J. & Lee, C. Y. (May 2006). Phenolic phytochemicals in cabbage inhibit amyloid B protein-induced neurotoxicity. *Food Science and Technology, 39*(4), 331-7.

Holt, C. "Why Milk Has the White Stuff for Children." Earth Friendly, Farm Friendly™. February 08 2006. 13 May 2008 http://www.earthfarmfriendly.com/News/2_08_06_white_stuff.html

Holtmann, G., Adam, B., Haag, S., et al. Efficacy of artichoke leaf extract in the treatment of patients with functional dyspepsia: a six-week placebo-controlled, double blind, multicentre trial. (December 2003). *Aliment Pharmacology Therapy, 18*(11-12), 1099-105. PMID: 14653829 [PubMed – indexed for MEDLINE

Howard, L. A., et al. (October 2003). Kinetic modeling of vitamin C loss in frozen green vegetables under variable storage conditions. *Journal of Food Science, Food Chemistry, 83*(1), 33-41.

Howard, L. A., Wong, A. D., Perry, A. K. & Klein, B. P. (1999). B-carotene and ascorbic acid retention in fresh and processed vegetables. *Journal of Food Science, 64*, 929-936.

Hunt, J. R. (December 2003). High-, but not low-bioavailability diets enable substantial control of women's iron absorption in relation to body iron stores, with minimal adaptation within several weeks. *Amer. Journal of Clin. Nutr., 78*(6), 1168-77.

Ignarro, L. J., Byrns, R. E., Sumi, D., et al. (September 2006). Pomegranate juice protects nitric oxide against oxidative destruction and enhances the biological actions of nitric oxide. *Nitric Oxide, 15*(2), 93-102.

Integrated Environmental Management, Inc. Microwave Radiation. Retrieved July 22, 2008, from http://www.iem-inc.com

Intergovernmental Panel on Climate Change. Greenhouse Gas Inventory Reference Manual, 1996. Retrieved March 15, 2008, from http://www.ipcc-nggip.iges.or.jp/public/gl/invs1.html

International Sprout Growers Association. Sprouts. Retrieved May 7, 2008, from http://www.isga sprouts.org

Jacobs, D. R., Steffen, L. M. & Steffen, J. (September 2003). Supplements —Nutrients, foods, and dietary patterns as exposures in research: a framework for food synergy. *American Journal of Clinical Nutrition, 78*(3), 508S-513S.

Jacobson PhD, M. F. (June 5, 2002). Liquid Candy, How Soft Drinks Are Harming Americans' Health. *Center for Science in the Public Interest.* Retrieved July 22, 2008, from http://www.cspinet.org/new/pdf/liquid_candy_final_w_suppliment.pdf

Jiang He, M. D., et al. (September 15, 2005). Majors causes of death among men and women in China. *The New England Journal of Medicine, 353*(11), 1124-34.

Johansen, R. (March 13, 2008). The health food product Noni--does marketing harmonize with the current status of research? *Tidsskr Nor Laegeforen, 128*(6), 694-7. PMID: 18337850 [PubMed indexed for MEDLINE

Johnson, C. J., Peterson, D. R. & Smith, E. K. (May 1979). Myocardial tissue concentrations of magnesium and potassium in men dying suddenly from ischemic heart disease. *American Journal of Clinical Nutrition, 32*, 967-70.

Johnson, I. T. (January 2002). Gluconsinolates: bioavailability and importance to health. *International Journal for Vitamin Nutritional Research, 72*(1), 26-31.

Join Together: China Tries to Cope with Smoking Epidemic. (January 12, 2007). *Join Together.* Retrieved July 18, 2008, from http://www.jointogether.org/news/headlines/inthenews/2007/china-tries to-cope-with.html

Josef, H. H. Delay Sought in Climate Talks. *Lycos News.* Retrieved March 15, 2008, from http://news.lycos.com/head.article.asp?docid= APVO695&date=20010124

Joseph, J. A., Shukitt-Hale, B., Denisova, N. A., et al. (October 1, 1998). Long-term dietary strawberry, spinach, or vitamin E supplementation retards the onset of age-related neuronal signal transduction and cognitive behavioral deficits. *Journal of Neuroscience, 18*(19), 8047-8055; PMID: 9742171 [PubMed – indexed for MEDLINE

Kabagambe, E. K. & Campos, H. (July 2005). Decreased consumption dried mature beans is positively associated with urbanization acute myocardial infarction. *Journal of Nutrition, 135*, 1770-75. Retrieved May 9, 2008, from http://www.nutirion.org/cgi/content/abstract/135/7/1770

Kalt, W., Ryan, D. A., Duy, J. C., et al. (September 11, 2001). Interspective Variation in Anthocyanins, Phenolics, and Antioxident Capacity among Genotypes of Highbush and Lowbush Blueberries (Vaccinium Section cyanoccus spp.) *Journal of Agriculture and Food Chemistry, 49*(10), 4761-7.

Kelishadi MD., R. Cacao to Cocoa to Chocolate: Healthy Food? *ARYA Journal.* Retrieved June 9, 2008, from http://crc.mui.ac.ir/arya/arya/display.aspx?id=1614

Kittredge, J. Pesticides in Food. *NOFany.org.* Retrieved May 6, 2008, from http://nofany.org/hottopics/pesticidesinfood.html

Koschinsky, T., He, C., Mitsuhashi, T., et al. (June 10, 1997). Orally absorbed reactive glycation products (glycotoxins): An environmental risk factor in diabetic nephropathy. *PNAS, 94*(12), 6474-9.

Kreft, S., Knapp, M. & Kreft, I. (November 1999). Extraction of rutin from buckwheat (Fagopyrum esculentum Moench) seeds and determination by capillary electrophoresis. *Journal of Food Chemistry, 47*(11), 4649-52.

Kresty, L. A., Morse, M. A., Carlton, P. S., et al. (August 15, 2001). Chemoprevention of esophageal tumorigenesis by dietary administration of lyophilized black raspberries. *Cancer research, 61*(16), 6112-9.

Kulze Dr., A. (2004). *Dr. Ann's 10 Step diet.* South Carolina: Just Wellness, LLC.

Layrisse, M. & Martinez-Torres Marcel Roche, C. (October 21, 1968). Effect of Interaction of various foods on iron absorption. *American Journal of Clinical Nutrition, 21*, 1175-1183. Retrieved May 10, 2008, from http:// www.ajcn.org/cgi/content/abstract/21/10/1175

Lecos, C. W. (1986, October). SULFITES: FDA Limits Uses, Broadens Labeling. *FDA Consumer, 20.*

Leu, A. Organic Food Is Better for You! *International Institute for Ecological Agriculture.* Retrieved April 16, 2008, from http://www.permaculture. com/drupal/node/144

Lichtenthaler, R., Rodrigues, R. B., Maia, J. G., et al. (February 2005). Total oxidant scavenging capacities of Euterpe oleracea Mart. (Acai) fruits. *International Journal of Food Sciences and Nutrition, 56*(1), 53-64. PMID: 16019315 [PubMed – indexed for MEDLINE

Lipophilic and Hydrophilic Antioxidant Capacities of Common Foods in the United States. (2004). *J. Agric. Food Chem., 52*, 4026-4037.

London School of Hygeine and Tropical Medicine. Retrieved March 15, 2008, from http://www.lshtm.ac.uk

Lustig DR, R. H. (2006, Aug, 7). "Drinking juice is no better than drinking soda." *Obscenity Discussion.*

Magdoff, F., Foster, J. B. & Buttel, F. H. (Eds.). (2000). *HUNGRY FOR PROFIT.*

Martin, et al. Study Detects Protein In Human Milk Linked To Reduced Risk Of Obesity. Cincinnati Children's Hospital Medical Center, May 3, 2004.

McPherson, J. D., Shilton, B. H. & Walton, D. J. (1988). Role of fructose in glycation and cross-linking of proteins. *Biochemistry, 27*, 1901-7.

Meck Higgins PhD., M. L. (August 2004). Color Me Healthy: Enjoying Fruits and Vegetables. *Kansas State University.* Retrieved May 2, 2008, from http://www.oznet.ksu.edu/library/FNTR2/samplers/mf2649.asp

Mertens-Talcott, S. M., Rios, J., Jilma-Stohlawetz, P., et al. (2008). Acai Human Consuption Trail: Bioavailability of Anthocyannins Pharmacokinetics of Anthocyanins and Antioxidant Effects after the Consuption of Anthocyanin-Rich Acai Juice and Pulp (Euterpe oleracea Mart) in Human Healthy Volunteers. *Journal of Agricultural and Food Chemistry.*

Morris, K. L. & Zemel, M. B. (1999). Glycemic index, cardiovascular disease and obesity. *Nutrition Reviews, 57*(9), 273-6.

Motohashi, N., et al. (2002). Cancer prevention and therapy with kiwifruit in chinese folklore medicine: a study of kiwifruit extracts. *Journal of Ethnopharmacology, 81*(3), 357-64.

Murray, R. K., et al. (1994). *Harper's Biochemistry* (23rd ed.). New York: Appleton & Lange.

National Farm to School Online. Retrieved May 7, 2008, from http://www.farmtoschool.org

New-Chapter.com. Tumeric - High potency named turicforce. Retrieved May 11, 2008, from http://www.new-chapter.com

Nixon, D. (November 1999). Alternative and Complementary Therapies in Oncology Care. *Journal of Clinical Oncology, 117*(11S (November Supplement)), 35-7.

Northrup, C. (1994). *Women's Bodies, Women's Wisdom* New York: Bantam Books.

Novus Research, Gilbert, AZ. Phenolic Compounds in Plants. Retrieved May 12, 2008, from http://www.organicashitaba.com/pc.html

Nutrition Data. Selenium. Retrieved April 24, 2008, from http://www.nutritiondata.com/help/glossary

Nuutila, A. M., Puupponen-Pimia, R., Aami, M. & Oksman-Caldentey, K. (June 2003). Comparison of antioxidant activities of onion and garlic by inhibition of lipid peroxidation and radical scavenging activity. *Food Chemistry, 81*(3), 489-493. Retrieved July 23, 2008, from http://cat.inist.fr/?aModele=afficheN&cpsidt=14719486

Office of Dietary Supplements - National Institutes of Health. Magnesium. Retrieved May 6, 2008, from http://www.ods.od.nih.gov/factsheets/magnesium.asp

Oliveres MD., M. & Uauy PhD., MD., R. (August 2004). Comprehensive Overview Paper: Essential Nutrients in Drinking Water. *World Health Organization.* Retrieved March 15, 2008, from http://www.who.int/water_sanitation_health/dwq/nutoverview.pdf

Opinion of the Scientific Committee on Food on Tahitian Noni Juice. (December 11, 2002). *Health & Consumer Protection Directorate-General.*

Organic Food is More Nutritious than Conventional. (1993). Organic Food is More Nutritious than Conventional Food. *Journal of Applied Nutrition, 45,* 35-39.

Packer PhD., L. & Colman, C. (1999). *The Antioxidant Miracle.* New York: John Wiley & Sons.

Pantuck, A. J., Leppert, J. T., Zomorodian, N., et al. (July 2006). Phase II Study of Pomegranate Juice for Men with Rising Prostate-Specific Antigen following Surgery or Radiation for Prostate Cancer. *Clinical Cancer Research, 12,* 4018-26.

Parker, R. S. (January 1989). *Journal of Nutrition, 119,* 101-4.

Pear Bureau Northwest. Vitamins, nutrients and Phytonutrients - Oh my! Retrieved March 14, 2008, from http://www.usapears.com/healthy/nutrition.asp

Perricone M.D., N. (2006). *7 secrets to beauty, health and longevity* (1st ed.). New York: Ballantine Books.

Perkins-Veazie, P. & Collins, J, K. (February 2004). Flesh quality and lycopene stability of fresh-cut watermelon. *Postharvest Biology and Technology, 31*(2), 159-166. Retrieved April 20, 2008, from http://www.citeulike.org/article/16729

Philips, H. Instant Expert: The Human Brain (September 4, 2006) *NewScientist.com news service.* Retrieved July 18, 2008, from http://www.newscientist.com

Philpott, T. (April 26, 2007). How food processing got into the hands of few giant companies. *Grist: Environmental News and Commentary.* Retrieved April 16, 2008, from http://www.grist.org/comments/food/2007/04/26/giants/

Pittler MH, E. E. (March 2000). Efficacy of ginger for nausea and vomiting: a systematic review of randomized clinical trials. *British Journal Anesthesia, 84*(3), 367-71.

Pirog, R. Food, Fuel, and Freeways: An Iowa perspective on how far food travels, fuel usage, and greenhouse gas emissions. Retrieved March 15, 2008, from http://www.leopold.iastate.edu/pubs/staff/ppp/food_mil.pdf

Pirog, R. Checking the food odometer: Comparing food miles for local versus conventional produce sales to Iowa institutions. Retrieved March 15, 2008, from http://www.leopold.iastate.edu/pubs/staff/files/food_travel072103.pdf

Pirog, R. & Benjamin, A. (Spring 2002). How far do your fruit and vegetables travel? *Leopold Letter, 14*(1).

Pottoroff, L. P. (1999). Some Pesticides Permitted in Organic Gardening. *Colorado State University Extension.* Retrieved July 21, 2008, from http://www.colostate.edu/Depts/CoopExt/4DMG/VegFruit/organic.htm

Preventing prostate cancer and diet. Excerpted from Prostate Disease: Finding the Cause and Cure. (2003). *Harvard Health Publications.* Retrieved April 16, 2008, from http://www.health.harvard.edu/newsweek/Preventing_prostate_cancer_and_diet.htm

Prospective Study of Fruit and Vegetable Intake and Risk of Prostate Cancer Kirsh et al. *J. Natl. Cancer Inst..*2007; 99: 1200-1209

Putnam, J., Allshouse, J. & Kantor, L. S. (January 2003). U.S. Per Capita Food Supply Trends: More Calories, Refined Carbohydrates, and Fats. *Economic Research Service, USDA, 2*(5), 2-15. Retrieved April 20, 2008, from http://www.ers.usda.gov/publications/FoodReview/DEC2002/frvol25i3.pdf

Ramberg, J. & McAnalley, B. From Farm to the Kitchen Table: A Review of Nutrient Losses in Foods. *GlycoScience & Nutrition, 3*(5), 1-12. Retrieved March 16, 2008, from http://www.lightforyou.net/optimalhealthproducts.htm

Ramljak, D., Romamczyk, L. J., Metheny-Barlow, L. J., et al. (2005). Pentameric procyanidin from Theobroma cacao selectively inhibits growth of human breast cancer cells. *Molecular Cancer Therapeutics, 4*(4), 537-46.

Red Blossom Tea Company. Tea buds loaded with polyphenols. Retrieved May 11, 2008, from http://www.redblossontea.com

Reitveld, A. & Wiseman, S. (October 2003). Supplement: Proceedings of the Third International Scientific Sympoosium on Tea and Human Health Antioxidant Effects of Tea: Evidence from Human linical Trials. *The American Society for Nutritional Service J. Nutr. 133*, 3285S-3292S.

Research At Great Lakes Meeting Shows More Vitamin C In Organic Oranges Than Conventional Oranges. (2002, June 2). *Science Daily.* Retrieved May 18, 2008, from http://www.sciencedaily.com/releases/2002/06/020603071017.htm

Ribaya-Mercado, J. D. & Blumberg, PhD, J. B. (2004). Lutein and Zeaxanthin and Their Potential Roles in Disease Prevention. *Journal of the American College of Nutrition, 23*(90006), 567S-587S.

Roberts, M. (2007, March 27). Cocoa nutrient for 'lethal ills' *BBC News International Edition.* Retrieved June 9, 2008, from http://news.bbc.co.uk/2/hi/health/6430777.stm

Rosedale MD, R. (1999). Insulin and Its Metabolic Effects. Dr. Stanley S Bass ,Super Nutrition &Superior Health. Retrieved July 18, 2008, from http://drbass.com/rosedale.html

Sahlstrom, S. & Brathen, E. (1997). Effects of enzyme preparations for baking, mixing time and resting time on bread quality and bread staling. Food Chemistry, 58, 1, 75-80. Effects of wheat variety and processing conditions in experimental bread baking studied by univariate and multivariate analyses

Saito, M., Hirata-Koizumi, M., Matsumoto, M., et al. (2005). Undesirable effects of citrus juice on the pharmacokinetics of drugs: focus on recent studies. *Drug Safety, 28*(8), 677-94.

Sanchez-Moreno, C., Cao, G., Ou, B. & Prior, R. L. (August 13, 2003). Anthocyanin and proanthocyandin content in selected white and red wines. Oxygen radical absorbance capacity comparison with nontraditional wines obtained from highbush blueberry. *Journal of Agriculture and Food Chemistry, 51*(17), 4889-96. PMID: 12903941 [PubMed – indexed for MEDLINE

Sandberg, A. (2002). Bioavailability of minerals in legumes. *British Journal of Nutrition, 88*(Suppl 3), 8281-5.

Santa Ana, R. (June 30, 2008). Watermelon May Have Viagra-effect. *Science Daily.* Retrieved July 18, 2008, from http://www.sciencedaily.com/releases/2008/06/080630165707.htm

Sauser, B. (2007, February 13). Ethanol Demand Threatens Food Prices. *Technology Review.* Retrieved May 24, 2008, from http://www.technologyreview.com/read_article.aspx?ch=specialsections&sc=biofuels&id=181 3&a=

Schlosser, E. (Video DVD) Fast Food Nation. 2006.

Science Daily. (2007, March 12). Cocoa 'Vitamin' Health Benefits Could Outshine Penicillin. Retrieved June 5, 2008, from http://www.sciencedaily.com/releases/2007/03/070311202024.htm

Science Daily. (2007, November 20). Flavonoid-rich Diet Helps Women Decrease Risk of Ovarian Cancer. Retrieved July 18, 2008, from http://www.sciencedaily.com/releases/2007/11/07111918402.htm

Seddon, J. M., Ajani, U. A., Sperduto, R. D., et al. (November 9, 1994). Dietary carotenoids, vitamins A, C, and E, and advanced age-related macular degeneration. Eye Disease Case-Control Study Group. *JAMA, 272*(18), 1413-20.

Seeram, N. P., Adams, L. S., Zhang, Y., et al. (December 13, 2006). Blackberry, black raspberry, blueberry, cranberry, red raspberry, and strawberry extracts inhibit growth and stimulate apoptosis of human cancer cells in vitro. *J. Agric. Food Chem.*, (25), 9329-39. PMID: 17147415 [PubMed indexed for MEDLINE

Shapiro, T. A., Fahey, J. W., Wade, K. L., et al. (May 2001). Chemoprotective Glucosinolates and Isothiocyanates of Broccoli Prouts: Metabolism and Excretion in Humans. *Cancer Epidemiology, Biomarkers & Prevention, 10*, 501-508.

Schauss, A., Wu, X., Prior, R., et al. (November 15, 2006). Antioxidant capacity and other bioactivities of the freeze-dried Amazonian palm berry, Euterpe oleraceae mart. (acai). *Journal of Agricultural and Food Chemistry (USDA).*

Schroeter, H., Heiss, C., Balzer, J., et al. (January 24, 2006). Epicatechin mediates beneficial effects of flavonal-rich cocoa on vascular function in humans. *The National Academy of Sciences of the USA, 103*(4), 1024-29. Retrieved June 10, 2008, from http://www.pnas.org/cgi/reprint/103/4/1024.pdf

Shapiro DRPH, RD, L. R., Crawford MPH, RD, P., Clark BS,RD, M. J., et al. (September 1984). Obesity Prognosis: A Longitudinal Study of Children From the Age of 6 Months to 9 Years. *American Journal of Public Health, 74*(9), 968-72. PMCID: PMC1651774 [PubMed – indexed for MEDLINE

Sharp, D. (2003). Acrylmide in Food. *Lancet, 9355*(361), 361-2.

Singh, M., Krishanappa, R., Bagewadi, A. & Keluskar, V. (July 2004). Efficacy of oral lycopene in the treatment of oral leukoplakia. *Oral Oncology, 40*(6), 591-6.

Smith, M. A., Marley, K. A., Seigler, D., et al. (2000). Bioactive properties of wild blueberry fruits. *Journal of Food Science, 65*, 352-6.

Smith PhD., C., Crowther MD., C., Franzcog, et al. (April 2004). A Randomized Controlled Trial of Ginger to Treat Nausea and Vomiting in Pregnancy. *Obstetrics & Gynecology, 103*, 639-645. Retrieved May 16, 2008, from http://www.greenjournal.org/cgi/search?sortspec=relevance&author1=&fulltext =&pubdate_year=2004&volume=103&firstpage=639

Soy Infant Formula Could Be Harmful to Infants: Groups Want It Pulled. (December 10, 1999). *Nutrition Week, 29*(46), 1-2.

Spectrum Organic. Coconut Oil. Retrieved May 9, 2008, from http://www.spectrumorganics.org

Stapleton, L. (2006). Want Pesticides with your Orange Juice? *Terrain Magazine.* Retrieved May 5, 2008, from http://www.ecologycenter.org/terrain/article.php?id=13507

Stocker PhD, R. (November 2002). Possible Health Benefits of Coenzyme Q10. *Linus Pauling Institute at Oregon State University.* Retrieved July 23, 2008, from http://lpi.oregonstate.edu/f w02/coenzymeq10.html http://www.lpi.oregonstate.edu.

St-Onge, M., Sy, M., Heymsfield, S. B. & Hirsch, J. (May 2005). Human Cortical Specialization for Food: a Functional Magnetic Resonance Imaging Investigation. *The Journal of Nutrition – Nutritional Neurosciences, 135*, 1014-18.

Stonyfield Farms. Retrieved April 18, 2008, from http://www.stonyfield.com/Wellness/HealthandNutritionGuide.cfm

Stuerenburg, H. J. & Kunze, K. (1999). Concentrations of free carnosine (a putative membrane-protective antioxidant) in human muscle biopsies in rat muscles. *Archives of Gerontology and Geriatrics, 29*, 107-13.

Sumathi, R., et al. (May - June 1993). *Pharmacology Resources, 27*, 309-18.

Sun, J., Chu, Y. & Liu, R. H. (March 15, 2008). Antioxidant and antoproliferative activities of common fruit. *J Agric Food Chem, 50*, 7449-7454.

Talcott Dr., S. A Phytochemical-Rich Oil from Acai Fruit. College Station, TX. Texas A&M University, Dept. of Nutrition and Food Science. Retrieved May 12, 2008, from http://nfscfaculty.tamu.edu/talcott/Commidities/New%20Acai%20Oil.pdf

Taubert, D., Berkels, S., Roesen, R. & Klaus, W. (August 27, 2004). Chocolate and blood pressure in elderly individuals with isolated systolic hypertension. *The Journal of the American Medical Association, 290*, 1029-30. Retrieved June 10, 2008, from http://www.ncbi.nlm.nih.gov/pubmed/12941673

The Kyoto Global Accord Treaty calls for sharp reductions in heat-trapping green-house gases by the United States and 37 other industrialized nations. Retrieved March 15, 2008, from http://earthrenewal.org/global_warming.htm

The Organic Myth. (2006, October 16). *Business Week.* Retrieved April 16, 2008, from http://www.businessweek.com/magazine/content/06_42/b4005001.htm

The Worlds Healthiest Foods, George Mateljian Foundation. Black Beans. Retrieved May 8, 2008, from http://www.whfoods.org/genpage.php?tname=foodspice&dbid=2

The Worlds Healthiest Foods. The George Mateljian Foundation. Ginger. Retrieved March 12, 2008, from http://www.whfoods.com

The Worlds Healthiest Foods. The George Mateljan Foundation. Kiwi-fruit. Retrieved March 15, 2008, from http://www.whfoods.com/genpage.php?tname=foodspice%dbid=41

The Worlds Healthiest Food, The George Mateljian Foundation. Rasp-berries. Retrieved May 21, 2008, from http://www.whfoods.org/genpage.php?tname=foodspice&dbid=39

The Worlds Healthiest Foods, The George Mateljan Foundation. Turnip Greens. Retrieved March 13, 2008, from http://www.whfoods/com/genpage.php?tname=foodspice&dbid=144

The Worlds Healthiest Foods. The George Mateljian Foundation. Swiss Chard. Retrieved March 12, 2008, from http://www.whfoods.com

The *Worlds Healthiest Food The George Mateljian Foundation.* Water-melon. Retrieved April 19, 2008, from http://www.whfoods.org/genpage.php?tname=foodspice&dbid=31#healthbenefits

Tian, Q., Aziz, R. M., Stoner, G. D. & Schwartz, S. J. (January 2005). p53: Keeping Cancer in Check. *Journal of Food Science, 70*(1). Retrieved May 22, 2008, from http://www.rockefeller.edu/pubinfo/p53.html The Rockefeller University.

Ting, L. & Zhang, Y. (August 2004). Dietary Isothiocyanates Inhibit the Growth of Human Bladder Carcinoma Cells. *Journal of Nutrition, 134,* 2004-10.

Torrey PhD, G. Zeaxanthin May Decrease Your Risk. *American Macular Degeneration Foundation.* Retrieved May 21, 2008, from http://www.macular.org/nutrition/zeaxan.html

ToxFAQs™ for Polycyclic Aromatic Hydrocarbons (PAHs). (September 1999). *ATSDR*. Retrieved May 8, 2008, from http://www.atsdr.cdc.gov/tfacts69.html

University of Florida News. Brazilian berry destroys cancer cells in lab, UF study shows. Retrieved May 9, 2008, from http://news.ufl.edu/2006/01/12/berries

University of Maryland Medical Center. Ginger. Retrieved May 9, 2008, from http://www.umm.edu/altmed/articles/ginger

Unlu, N. Z., Bohn, T., Clinton, S. K. & Schwartz, S. J. (2005). Carotenoid absorption from salad and salsa by humans is enhanced by the addition of avocado or avocado oil. *Journal of Nutrition, 135*, 431 43.

USA.com. The 5 most important antioxidants. Retrieved May 10, 2008, from http://www.usaweekend.com/99_issues/990404eatsmart.html

U.S. Environmental Protection Agency. Children's Environmental Exposure Research Study. Retrieved May 2, 2008, from http://www.epa.gov/cheers/

U.S. Food and Drug Administration. Natural and Organic Foods. Retrieved July 22, 2008, from http://www.fda.gov

U.S. Highbush Blueberry Council. Retrieved May 5, 2008, from http://www.blueberry.org/faq.htm

Vaal Eden Nutriceudicals. Activated Lycopene. Retrieved April 5, 2008, from http://www.bodyandmind.co.za/merchant_nc.php?pid=978&step=4

Vallejo, F., Tomas-Barberan, F. A., Garcia-Viguera, C., et al. (October 15, 2003). Phenolic compound contents in edible parts of brocoli inflorescences after domestic cooking. *Journal of the Science of Food and Agriculture, 83*(14), 1511-16.

Wada, L. & Ou, B. (May 9, 2002). Antioxidant Activity and Phenolic Content of Oregon Cranberries. *J Agric. Food Chem., 50*, 3495-3500.

Wang, Y., Chang, C. F., Chen, H. L., et al. (May 2005). Dietary supplementation with blueberries, spinach, or spirulina reduces ischemic brain damage. *Exp. Neurol., 193*(1), 75-84; PMID: 15817266.

Washington Red Raspberry Commission. Phytochemicals in Red Raspberries. Retrieved July 23, 2008, from http://www.info@red-raspberry.org

Watermelons Are Healthier When Served Warm. HealthDay News. Retrieved April 20, 2008, from http:www/antioxidant-vitamins.info/Antioxidant-Chemistry.php

Wei, J., Wang, X., Shi, H., et al. (2007). A critical role of luteolin - induced reactive oxygen species in blockage of tumor necrosis factor - activated nuclear factor - B pathway and sensitization of apoptosis in lung cancer cells. *Molecular Pharmacology*, *71*, 1381-8. PMID: 17296806 [PubMed - indexed for MEDLINE

Weisell PhD, R. C. (1996). Trace elements in human nutrition. *World Health Organization.*

Which?. (March 31, 2004). Which? exposes the cereal offenders. *Europe.com.* Retrieved July 19, 2008, fromhttp://www.which.co.uk/press/press_topics/campaign_news/food/Which_exposes_the_c real_offenders_571_56095.jsp

Whitehouse.Gov. President's Remarks at Ask President Bush Event in Ohio. Retrieved May 2, 2008, from http://www.whitehouse.gov/omb/query.html?lk=1&charset=iso-8859-1&st=61& ct=1011860316&qt=url%3Awww.whitehouse.gov/news/releases/2004/09+% 7C%7C+url%3Awww.white-house.gov/news/releases/2004/09+%7C%7C+url %3Awww.whitehouse.gov/news/releases/2004+%7C%7C+Releasing+and+ Sharing+of+Data

WikiAnswers. Is the tomato a fruit or a vegetable? Retrieved April 23, 2008, from http://wiki.answers.com/Q/Is_the_tomato_a_fruit_or_a_vegetable

Wikipedia, The Free Encyclopedia. Acai Palm. Retrieved May 5, 2008, from http://en.wikipedia.org/w/index.php?title=A%C3%A7a%C3%AD_Palm&oldid=21045042

Wikipedia, The Free Encyclopedia. Blowing a raspberry. Retrieved May 1, 2008, from http://en.wikipedia.org/w/index.php?title=Blowing_a-Raspberry&oldid=151626

Wikipedia, The Free Encyclopedia. Catechin. Retrieved May 30, 2008 from http://en.wikipedia.org/w/index.php?title=Catechin&oldid=215947912

Wikipedia, The Free Encyclopedia. Herion. Retrieved May 4, 2008, from http://en.wikipedia.org/w/imdex.php?title=Herion&oldid=153713083

Wikipedia, The Free Encylopedia. Kyoto Protocol. Retrieved March 14, 2008, from http://en.wikipedia.org/wiki/Kyoto_Protocol

Wikipedia, The Free Encyclopedia. Mitosis. Retrieved May 23, 2008, from http://en.wikipedia.org/w/index.php?title=Mitosis&oldid=153077673

Wikipedia, The Free Encyclopedia. Noni. Retrieved May 9, 2008, from http://en.wikipedia.org/w/index.php?title=Noni&oldid=209920702

Wikipedia, The Free Encyclopedia. Oxygen radical absorbance capacity. Retrieved May 17, 2008, from http://en.wikipedia.org/wiki/Oxygen_Radical_Absorbance_Capacity

Wikipedia, The Free Encyclopedia. Superoxide. Retrieved May 5, 2008, from http://en.wikipedia.org/w/index.php?title=Superoxide&oldid=210261461

Wikipedia, The Free Encyclopedia. Vasodilator. Retrieved June 7, 2008, from http://en.wikipedia.org/w/index.php?title=Vasodilator&oldid=216751467

Wikipedia, The Free Encyclopedia. Wolfberry. Retrieved May 8, 2008, from http://en.wikipedia.org/wiki/Wolfberry

Wisner, R. Impacts of Iowa's Rapid Expansion in Corn-based Ethanol Production on Crop Acreage Needs, Grain Prices, Basis Behavior and Distillers Grain Supplies. Iowa State University, October 2006. Retrieved May 24, 2008, from http://www.extension.iastate.edu/ag/WisnerPresent.indd.pdf

Wong, C. What are goji berries? *About.com: Alternative Medicine.* Retrieved May 13, 2008, from http://altmedicine.about.com/od/completeazindex/a/goji.htm

Wood, A. W., Huang, M., Sayers, J., et al. (September 1982). Inhibition of the mutagenicity of bay-region diol epoxides of polycyclic aromatic hydrocarbons by naturally occurring plant phenols: Exceptional activity of ellagic acid (ultimate carcinogen/Ames' Salmonella typhimurium/Chinese hamster V79 cells/kinetics o. *Proceedings of the National Academy of Science, USA, 79,* 5513-17.

Worldwatch Institute News Release. The World Can't Wait for Another Climate Treaty. Retrieved March 15, 2004, from http://www.worldwatch.org/alerts/010328.html

Wu, H., et al. (2006). Effect of Lycium barbarum polysaccharide on the improvement of antioxidant ability and DNA damage in NIDDM rats. *USDA-Agricultural Research Service (Grand Forks), 126.5,* 365-71.

Xia, R., Huang, P. & Shao, G. (June 2007). Nourishing Yin and Promoting Blood Circulation of TCM to Treat Hemorheologic Disorder Induced by Diabetes Mellitus in Rats. *Evid Based Complement Alternative Medicine, 4*(2), 203-7.

Young PhD, R. O. (October 28, 2006). Are The Exotic Fruit Juices Like Noni and Goji Safe For Human Consumption. *Articles of Health*. Retrieved May 21, 2008, from http://articlesofhealth.blogspot.com/2006/10/are-exotic-fruit-juices-like-noni-and.html

Young PhD, R. O. (October 9, 2006). Mangosteen, Noni, Goji, Xango, Thai-Go, are ALL Acidic and detrimental to Health. *Articles of Health*. Retrieved May 21, 2008, from http://articlesofhealth.blogspot.com/2006/10/are-exotic-fruit-juices-like-noni-and.html

Young PhD., R. O. & Young, S. R. (2008). *The pH Miracle: Balance Your Diet, Reclaim Your Health*. Wellness Center.

Zhang, Y. (November 2, 2004). Cancer-preventative isothiocyanates: measurement of human exposure and mechanism of action. *Mutat Res.*, 555(1-2), 173-190.

Zimmerman C.N., M. Phytonutrients & Nutraceuticals: Nutrients Of The Future. *Phytonutrients & Nutraceuticals: Overview*. Retrieved July 22, 2008, from http://www.realtime.net/anr/phytonu.html#Lipoic

Zuckett, G. Paybacks: How the White House and Congress Are Neglecting Our Health Care Because of Their Corporate Contributors. *Common Dreams*. Retrieved July 22, 2008, from http://www.commondreams.org/cgi-bin/print.cgi?file=/news2004/0818-06.htm

CHAPTER 4 FRANKENFOODS

Barboza, D. (2000, May 16). AstraZeneca to Sell a Genetically Engineered Strain of Rice. *The New York Times*.

Bijman, J. "Advanta: Worldwide challenges." AgBioForum 4. 6.1 (2004): Article 6. 23 May 2008 http://library.wur.nl/WebQuery/wurpubs/lang/314972.

Brookes, G. & Barfoot, P. Global Impact of Biotech Crops: Socio-Economic and Environmental Effects in the First Ten Years of Commercial Use. *AgBioForum*, 9(3), Article 2. Retrieved May 27, 2008, from http://www.agbioforum.org/v9n3/v9n3a02-brookes.pdf

Farndon, J. (2006). *From DNA to GM Wheat: Discovering Genetic Modification of Food*. Library Binding.

Fumento, M. (2003). *Bioevolution: How Biotechnology Is Changing Our World*. Encounter Books.

Genetic Engineering and Biotechology News. Retrieved May 26, 2008, from http://www.genengnews.com/

Greenpeace International. Say No to Genetic Engineering. Retrieved May 26, 2008, from http://www.greenpeace.org/international/campaigns/genetic-engineering

Harlanger, S. & Roller, S. (Eds.). (1998). *Genetic Modification in the Food Industry: A Strategy for Food Quality Improvement.* Culinary and Hospitality Industry Publications Services.

Mercola Dr. The GMO Food Guide. Take Control of Your Health. *Mercola.com.* Retrieved May 23, 2008, from http://articles.mercola.com/sites/articles/archive/2007/09/18/the-gmo-food-guide-aspx

Mindfully.org. Genetically Modified Crops in the United States 2004. Retrieved May 24, 2008, from http://www.mindfully.org/GE/2004/US-GMO-Crops-Pewlaug04.htm

SourceWatch.org. Monsanto and the Roundup Ready Controversy. Retrieved May 26, 2008, from http://www.sourcewatch.org/index.php?title=Monsanto_and_the_Roundup_Ready_Controversy

Stringam, R., Ripley, V. L., Love, H. K. & Mitchell, A. (2003). Transgenic Herbicide Tolerant Canola – The Canadian Experience. *Crop Science Society of America, 43,* 1590-1593.

The Pew Charitable Trusts. Agricultural Biotechnology. Retrieved May 26, 2008, from http://www.pewtrusts.org/our_work_detail.aspx?id=442

USDA - National Agricultural Service. 2004 - 2005 Statistical Highlights of US Agriculture. *USDA –National Agricultural Service.* Retrieved May 18, 2008, from http://www.usda.gov/nass/pubs/stathigh/content.htm

U.S. Department of Agriculture – Environmental Research Service. Adoption of Genetically Engineering Crops in the U.S. Retrieved May 26, 2008, from http://www.ers.usda.gov/Data/BiotechCrops/

Wikipedia, The Free Encyclopedia. BioScience. Retrieved May 29, 2008, from http://en.wikipedia.org/w/index.php?title=BioScience&oldid=138738966

Wikipedia, The Free Encyclopedia. Canola. Retrieved May 27, 2008, from http://en.wikipedia.org/w/index.php?title=Canola&oldid=215272602

Wikipedia, The Free Encyclopedia. Monsanto Canada Inc v Schmeiser. Retrieved May 21, 2008, from http://en.wikipedia.org/w/index.php?title=Monsanto_Canada_Inc._v_Schmeise r&oldid=213904954

Wikipedia, The Free Encyclopedia. Phytoremediation. Retrieved May 3, 2008, from http://en.wikipedia.org/w/index.php?title=Phytoremediation&old id=209985231

CHAPTER 5 THE SOS SUPPLEMENTS

Tanaka, S., Haruma, K., Yoshihara, M., et al. (March 20006) Aged Garlic Extract Has Potential Suppressive Effect on Colorectal Adenomas in Humans. *The Journal of Nutrition, 136,* 821S-826S.

Baggio, E., Gandini, R., Plancher, A. C., et al. (1993). Italian multicenter study on the safety and efficacy of coenzyme Q10 as adjunctive therapy in heart failure (interim analysis). The CoQ10 Drug Surveillance Investigators. *The Journal of Clinical Investigation, 71*(8 Supplements), S145-9.

Bierenbaum, M. L. (1997). Palm oil antioxidant effects in patients with hyper-lipidemia and carotid stenosis - 2 year experience. *Asia Pacific Journal of Chinese Nutrition, 6*(1), 72-5.

Bierenbaum, M. L. (1995). Tocotrienol in patients with carotid stenosis. *Lipids, 30,* 1179-83.

Bodor, N., Farag, H. H. & Brewster 3rd, M. E. (December 1981). Site-specific, sustained release of drugs to the brain. *Science, 214*(4527), 1370-2.

Chen, T. C., Chimeh, F., Lu, Z., et al. (April 15, 2007). Factors that influence the coetaneous synthesis and dietary sources of vitamin D. *Archives of Biochemistry and Biophysics, 460*(2), 213-7.

Cooke, M., Iosia, M., Buford, T., et al. (2008). Effects of acute and 14-day coenzyme Q10 supplementation on exercise performance in both trained and untrained individuals. *Journal of the International Society of Sports Nutrition, 5,* 2783-5.

Curry Powder: For Health and Enjoyment. Retrieved May 27, 2008, from http://www.lionsgrip.com/curry.html

DrugDigest.com. Horseradish. Retrieved May 24, 2008, from http://www.drug digest.org/DD/DVH/HerbsWho/0,3923,4103%7CHorseradish,00.html

Durga, J., von Boxtel, M. P., Schouten, E. G., et al. (January 20, 2007). Effect of 3-year folic acid supplementation on cognitive function in older adults in the FACIT trial: a randomized, double blind, controlled trial. *Lancet, 369*(9557), 208-16.

Eating Pizza 'cuts cancer risk'. (2003,July). *BBC News.* Retrieved May 17, 2008, from http://news.bbc.co.uk/2/3086013.stm

Hasselwander, O., Kramer, K., Hoppe, P. P., et al. (2002). Effects of feeding various tocotrienol sources on plasma lipids and aortic atherosclerotic lesions in cholesterol-fed rabbits. *Food Research International, 35*(2-3), 245-51.

Heart Disease and Stroke Statistics. (2008). *American Heart Association, Update.*

Hickey, S. & Roberts, H. Ascorbate: The Science of Vitamin C. Retrieved August 29, 2008, from http://www.lulu.com/ascorbate

Hornero-Mendez, D. & Minguez-Mosquear, M. I. (February 2006). Bioaccessibility of carotenes from carrots: Effect of cooking and addition of oil. *Chemistry and Biochemistry of Pigments Group, Instituto de la Grasa.* Retrieved September 4, 2008, from http://www.ig.csic.es/Congresos/comco06.html

Jiang, Q., et al. (2001). Gamma tocopherol, the major form of vitamin E in the US diet, deserves more attention. *American Journal of Clinical Nutrition, 74*, 714-22.

Jolliet, P., Simon, B., Barre, J., et al. (1998). Plasma coenzyme Q10 concentrations in breast cancer prognosis and therapeutic consequence. *International Journal of Clinical Pharmacology, 36*(9), 506-9.

Kline, K. (2004). Review of cancer prevention by Vitamin E stated that gamma-tocopherol is the most potent form for preventing breast cancer. *Journal of Nutrition, 134*, 345S-346S, 15.

Kris-Etherton PhD, P. M., Harris PhD, W. S. & Appel MD, L. J. (2002). Fish Consumption, Fish Oil, Omega-3 Fatty Acids, and Cardiovascular Disease. *American Heart Association, 106*, 2747.

Lands, L. C., Grey, V. L. & Smountas, A. A. (October 1999). Effect of supplementation with a cysteine donor on muscular performance. *Journal of Applied Physiology, 87*(4), 1381-5.

Lang, C. A. (June 1, 2001). The Impact of Glutathione on Health and Longevity. *The Journal of Anti-Aging Medicine, 42*(2), 137-44.

Langsjoen, P. H., Folkers, K., Lyson, K., et al. (July 1998). effective and safe therapy with coenzyme Q10 for cardiomyopathy. *Department of Medicine, Scott and White Clinic, Temple, Texas, 66*(13), 583-90.

Lipid Acid Could Reduce Atherosclerosis, Weight Gain. (2008, January 17). *ScienceDaily.* Retrieved August 10, 2008, from http:///www.sciencedaily.com-/releases/2008/01/080114162506

Losonczy, K. G., Harris, T. B. & Havlik, R. J. (August 1996). Vitamin E and Vitamin C Supplement Use and Risk of All-cause and Coronary Heart Disease Mortality in Older Persons: The Established Populations for Epidemiologic Studies of the Elderly. *American Journal of Clinical Nutrition*, *64*(2), 190-6.

Montonen, J., Knekt, P., Jarvinen, R., et al. (2004). Dietary antioxidant intake and risk of type 2 diabetes. *Diabetes Care*, *27*(2), 326-66.

Mustad, V. A., Smith, C. A., Ruey, P. R., et al. (December 2002). Supplementation with 3 compositionally different tocotrienol supplements does not improve cardiovascular disease risk factors in men and women with hypercholesterolemia. *American Journal of Clinical Nutrition*, *76*(6), 1237-43.

Nutraingredients.com/Europe. Pizza, the latest functional food? Retrieved May 18, 2008, from http://www.nutraingredients.com/news/ng.asp?id=38274

Papucci, L., Schiavone, N., Witort, E., et al. (July 23, 2003). Coenzyme Q10 Prevents Apoptosis by Inhibiting Mitochondrial Depolarization Independently of Its Free Radical Scavenging Property. *Biol. Chem.*, *278*(30), 28220-8.

Qureshi, A. A., Qureshi, N., Wright, J. J., et al. (April 1991). Lowering of serum cholesterol in hypercholesterolemic humans by tocotrienols (palmvitee) *American Journal of Clinical Nutrition*, *53*(4 Supplement), 1021S-1026S.

Reynolds, E. H. (June 22, 2002). Education and debate, Folic acid, ageing, depression, and dementia. *British Medical Journal*, *324*, 1512-15.

Roum, J. H., Buhl, R., McElvaney, N. G., et al. (December 1993). Systemic deficiency of glutathione in cystic fibrosis. *Journal of Applied Physiology*, *75*(5), 2419-24.

Schreibelt, G., Musters, R. J., Reijerkerk, A., et al. (2006). Lipoic Acid Affects Cellular Migration into the Central Nervous System and Stabilizes Blood-Brain Barrier Integrity. *The Journal of Immunology*, *177*, 2630-7.

Singh, R. B., Neki, N. S., Kartikey, K., et al. (April 2003). Effect of coenzyme Q10 on risk of arthero sclerosis in patients with recent myocardial infarction. *Molecular Cell Biochemistry*, *246*(1-2), 75-82.

Solomon, PhD., P. R., Adams, BA, F., Silver, BA, A., et al. (2002). Ginkgo for Memory Enhancement A Randomized Controlled Trial. *JAMA*, *288*, 836-40.

Statistical yearbook. Retrieved August 28, 2008, from http://www.fao.org/statistics/yearbook/vol_1_2/pdf/United-States-of-America.pdf

The Effect of Ascorbic Acid Supplementation on the Blood Lead levels of Smokers. (1999). *Journal of American College of Nutrition*, *18*(2), 166-70.

Thomas, D. (2003). A study on the mineral depletion of the foods available to us as a nation over the period 1940 to 1991. *Nutrition and Health*, *17*(2), 85-115.

Trivedi, D. P., Doll, R. & Khaw, K. T. (2003). Effect of four monthly oral vitamin D3 (cholecalciferol) supplementation on fractures and mortality in men and women living in the community: randomized double blind controlled trial. *The British Medical Journal*, *326*, 469-75.

Tuohimaa, P., Pukkala, E., Scelo, G., et al. (July 2007). Does solar exposure, as indicated by the non melanoma skin cancers, protect from solid cancers: Vitamin D as a possible explanation. *European Journal of Cancer*, *43*(11).

Verhoef, P., Stampfer, M. J., Buring, J. E., et al. (May 1, 1996). Homocysteine metabolism and risk of myocardial infarction: vitamins B6, B12< and folate. *American Journal of Epidemiology*, *143*(9), 845-59.

Wikipedia, The Free Encyclopedia. Artic char. Retrieved May 24, 2008, from http://en.wikipedia.org/w/index.php?title=Artic_char&oldid=214090490

Wikipedia, The Free Encyclopedia. Cumin. Retrieved May 18, 2008, from http://en.wikipedia.org/w/index.php?title=Cumin&oldid=213270764

Wikipedia, The Free Encyclopedia. Vitamin D. Retrieved August 16, 2008, from http://en.wikipedia.org/w/index.php?title=Vitamin_D&oldid=232312605

Wortsman, J., Matsuoka, L. Y., Chen, T. C., et al. (September 2000). Decreased bioavailability of vitamin D in obesity. *American Journal of Clinical Nutrition*, *72*(3), 690-3.

CHAPTER 6 SOS PROGRAM

Biswas, et al. (January 2005). Curcumin induces glutathione biosynthesis and inhibits NF-kappaB activation and interleukin-8 release in alveolar epithelial cells: mechanism of free radical scavenging activity. *Antioxidants and Redox Signaling*, *7*(1-2), 32-41.

Kidd, P. M. (June 1999). A review of nutrients and botanicals in the integrative management of cognitive dysfunction. *Alternative Medical Review*, *4*(3), 144-61.

Kodam, et al. (2007). Effect of aerobic exercise training on serum levels of high-density lipoprotein cholesterol. *Archives of Internal Medicine, 167,* 999-1008.

Monteleone, P., Maj, M., Beinat, L., et al. (1992). Blunting by chronic phosphatidylserine administration of the stress-induced activation of the hypothalamo-pituitary-adrenal axis in healthy men. *European Journal of Clinical Pharmacology, 42*(4), 385-8.

INDEX

Page numbers followed by an *f* or *t* indicate figures or tables.

ABOUT THE AUTHOR

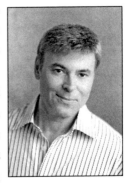

R andy Karp is a leading expert in the field of nutrition and its effects on human behavior and physiology. Born the son of Dr. Edward Karp, a pioneer in prevention and doctor of Naprapathy, the evaluation and treatment of neuro-musculoskeletal conditions, Randy was raised in an environment to observe how foods affected both behavior and health.

As a student of behavioral psychology, he was intrigued by the relationship between maladaptive behavior and a poor diet. Later, he observed a similar correlation while counseling adolescents in substance abuse programs as part of his practicum for his Masters of Science in Human Services. That missing link compelled him to dig deeper into every aspect of our food: how it is grown, processed, prepared and presented. He became a driven and passionate crusader with a finite mission: to understand the impact of food and supplements on one's health and behavior, and to provide options to all those who have been misinformed.

After his mother lost her life to cancer, Randy Karp was dedicated in his single-minded purpose to find the answers that would prevent the onset of disease with exposés that revealed misinformation about food, supplements and nutrition. His extensive research allowed him to discover little-known secrets that would enable us to harness the power of Super-Nutrients.

As Karp continued his research, he successfully demystified the misinformation that has ultimately resulted in the untimely deaths of those we love. According to Dr. Barry Sears of *Zone* book fame, "Randy Karp has performed an extremely valuable service by debunking much of the mythology that surrounds our food supply. If you are truly interested in nutrition, then you should definitely read his book, *Misinformed About Food*."

Randy Karp has served on the Board of Directors and Advisory Board of the Clarinda State Psychiatric Hospital in Clarinda City, Iowa. He also served on the Advisory Board of the Polk County Association of Mental Health in Des Moines, Iowa. He received the Volunteer of the Year award from the President's Council on Voluntary Action, Washington D.C., for improving the lives of those less fortunate in his community. Karp also received the Volunteer of the Year award from the Polk County Association of Mental Health.

After his training in behavioral psychology, he founded a clinic to teach gross motor skills to mentally-challenged and autistic children. In the process, he became a leading advocate for self-care. He would later receive graduate honors for his work on the effects of food on behavior. A former member of the Young Presidents Organization, Randy currently operates Global Solutions LTD, and his newly-formed company, Informed Living LLC, offering life-enhancing products that fill a void, based on the research included in his book, *Misinformed About Food*. This book reveals what most people do not know about food and its effect on one's body, brain and overall well-being.

A uniquely qualified expert on the entire spectrum of food, behavior and anti-aging, Randy is a leading advocate of a new brand of self-health care and continues to advance research in upcoming installments of the *Misinformed* series. Karp is a featured expert on numerous national radio broadcasts and television talk shows. He is also a contributing expert to *New Living* magazine and a noted keynote speaker. Randy and his wife, Kelly, live in northern Arizona.

www.RKInformedLiving.com

Log on for free Tip of the Week

Speaking Engagements

For availability, contact the author at Info@RKInformedLiving.com. Topics address the needs of each respective audience.

Informed Living, LLC ...

The finest products of their kind for the next generation of self-care!

Email Ordering:

www.RKInformedLiving.com
Log on for information that can change your life.

Phone orders:

Please call: 928-778-0070

Global Solutions Press, LLC

Naked truth, real stories—life-altering books—designed to inform. Contact the publisher at GlobalSolutionsPress@gmail.com.

Media Page

www.RKInformedLiving.com/media_page.html

CPSIA information can be obtained at www.ICGtesting.com
Printed in the USA
BVOW082222040113

309817BV00006B/15/P